MEDICAL STATISTICS from A to Z

MEDICAL STATISTICS
from A to Z

A Guide for Clinicians and Medical Students

Third Edition

Brian S. Everitt
King's College London

CAMBRIDGE
UNIVERSITY PRESS

CAMBRIDGE
UNIVERSITY PRESS

University Printing House, Cambridge CB2 8BS, United Kingdom

One Liberty Plaza, 20th Floor, New York, NY 10006, USA

477 Williamstown Road, Port Melbourne, VIC 3207, Australia

314–321, 3rd Floor, Plot 3, Splendor Forum, Jasola District Centre, New Delhi – 110025, India

79 Anson Road, #06–04/06, Singapore 079906

Cambridge University Press is part of the University of Cambridge.

It furthers the University's mission by disseminating knowledge in the pursuit of education, learning, and research at the highest international levels of excellence.

www.cambridge.org
Information on this title: www.cambridge.org/9781108826464
DOI: 10.1017/9781108919739

First published 2003
Second edition 2006
Reprinted 2009
Third edition 2021

Printed in the United Kingdom by TJ Books Limited, Padstow Cornwall

A catalogue record for this publication is available from the British Library.

Library of Congress Cataloging-in-Publication Data
Names: Everitt, Brian, author.
Title: Medical statistics from A to Z : a guide for clinicians and medical students / Brian S. Everitt.
Description: Third edition. | Cambridge, United Kingdom ; New York, NY : Cambridge University Press, 2021. | Includes bibliographical references.
Identifiers: LCCN 2020029461 (print) | LCCN 2020029462 (ebook) | ISBN 9781108826464 (paperback) | ISBN 9781108919739 (epub)
Subjects: MESH: Statistics as Topic | Dictionary, Medical
Classification: LCC R121 (print) | LCC R121 (ebook) | NLM WA 13 | DDC 610.3–dc23
LC record available at https://lccn.loc.gov/2020029461
LC ebook record available at https://lccn.loc.gov/2020029462

ISBN 978-1-108-82646-4 Paperback

To the memory of my dear friend and colleague for almost forty years, Professor Graham Dunn

Figures

Preface to the Third Edition

In the third edition of *Medical Statistics from A to Z,* I have added nearly 150 new definitions, many describing topics that have appeared in the medical statistical literature in the last five years or so. I have also updated many references and improved (I hope) some of the definitions in the first and second editions.

Preface to the Second Edition

In the second edition of *Medical Statistics from A to Z,* I have added many new definitions and taken the opportunity to correct and clarify a number of entries. More references are also provided that point readers to more detailed accounts of topics.

Preface to the First Edition

Clinicians, research workers in the health sciences, and even medical students often encounter terms from medical statistics and related areas in their work, particularly when reading medical journals and other relevant literature. The aim of this guide is to provide such people with nontechnical definitions of many such terms. Consequently, no mathematical nomenclature or formulae are used in the definitions. Those readers interested in such material will be able to find it in one of the many standard statistical texts now available and in *The Cambridge Dictionary of Statistics*. In addition, readers seeking more information about a particular topic will hopefully find the references given with the majority of entries of some help; whenever possible, these involve medical rather than statistical journals, and introductory statistical texts rather than those that are more advanced. (References are not given for terms such as mean, variance and critical region for which further details are easily available in most introductory medical statistics texts.)

Several forms of cross-referencing are used. Terms in Courier New appear as a separate headword elsewhere in the dictionary, although this procedure is used in a relatively limited way with headwords defining frequently occurring terms such as random variable, probability and sample not referred to in this way. Some entries simply refer readers to another entry. This may indicate that the terms are synonymous or that the term is discussed more conveniently under another entry. In the latter case, the term is printed in *italics* in the main entry. Entries are in alphabetical order using the letter-by-letter rather than the word-by-word convention.

Of the many sources of material I have consulted in the preparation of this book, I would like to mention two that have been of particular help, namely the *Encyclopedia of Biostatistics* and the *Dictionary of Epidemiology*.

REFERENCES

Armitage, P. and Colton, T., 1989, *Encyclopedia of Biostatistics*, John Wiley & Sons, Chichester.

Everitt, B. S. and Skrondal, A., 2010, *The Cambridge Dictionary of Statistics*, 4th ed., Cambridge University Press, Cambridge.

Last, J. M., 2001, *Dictionary of Epidemiology*, 4th ed., Oxford University Press, New York.

Abortion rate: The annual number of abortions per 1,000 women of reproductive age (usually defined as age 15–44 years). For example, in the USA in 1970 the rate was 5, in 1980 it was 25 and in 1990 it was 24. [*Family Planning Perspectives*, 1998, 30, 244–7.]

Abortion ratio: The estimated number of abortions per 1,000 live births in a given year. Given by the ratio, 1,000 × (number of abortions divided by the number of live births). For example, in the USA in 1970 the ratio was 52, in 1980 it was 359, and in 1990 it was 344. [*Family Planning Perspectives*, 1998, **30**, 244–7.]

Abscissa: The horizontal (or *x*-axis) on a graph, or a particular point on that axis.

Absolute cause-specific risk: Synonym for **absolute risk**.

Absolute deviation: Synonym for **average deviation**.

Absolute risk: Often used as a synonym for incidence, although also used occasionally for attributable risk, excess risk or risk difference. Defined more properly as the probability that a disease-free individual will develop a given disease over a specified time interval given current age and individual risk factors, and in the presence of competing risks. Absolute risk is a probability and consequently lies between 0 and 1. *See also* **relative risk**. [Kleinbaum, D. G., Kupper, L. L. and Morgenstern, H., 1982, *Epidemiologic Research: Principles and Quantitative Methods*, Lifetime Learning Publications, Belmont.]

Absolute risk reduction: The proportion of untreated people who experience an adverse event minus the proportion of treated people who experience the event. For example, in a clinical trial of mammography, it was found that out of 129 750 women who were invited to begin having mammograms in the late 1970s and early 1980s, 511 died of breast cancer over the next 15 years, a death rate of 0.4 per cent. In the control group of 117 260 women who were not invited to have regular mammograms, there were 584 breast cancer deaths over the same period, a death rate of 0.5 per cent. So, the estimated absolute risk reduction is 0.1 per cent. *See also* **relative risk** and **number needed to treat**. [Strauss, S. E., Glaszziou, P., Scott Richardson, W. and Haynes, R. B., 2018, *Evidence Based Medicine: How to Practice and Teach EBM*, 5th ed., Churchill Livingstone, New York.]

Absorbing barrier: *See* **random walk**.

Accelerated failure time model: A general model for data consisting of `survival times`, in which explanatory variables measured on an individual are assumed to act multiplicatively on the timescale, and so affect the rate at which an individual proceeds along the time axis. Consequently, the model can be interpreted in terms of the speed of progression of a disease. This model, which simply regresses the logarithm of the survival time on the covariates, although used far less often than `Cox's proportional hazards model`, might be a useful alternative in many situations because of this intuitive physical interpretation. [Collett, D., 2015, *Modelling Survival Data in Medical Research*, 3rd ed., Chapman & Hall/CRC, Boca Raton, FL.]

Acceptable quality level: *See* **quality control procedures**.

Acceptable risk: The risk for which the benefits of a particular medical procedure are considered to outweigh the potential hazards. For example, islet transplantation would help to control the many secondary effects of type 1 diabetes, but what is the appropriate level of risk to implement this technology responsibly considering the possible dangers from retroviruses? [*Nature*, 1998, **391**, 326.]

Acceptance region: A term associated with statistical significance tests, which gives the set of values of a `test statistic` for which the null hypothesis is to be accepted. Suppose, for example, that a `z-test` is being used to test the null hypothesis that the mean blood pressure of men and women is equal against the alternative hypothesis that the two means are not equal. If the chosen `significance` of the test is 0.05, then the acceptance region consists of values of the test statistic z between -1.96 and 1.96. [Altman, D. G., 2018, *Practical Statistics for Medical Research*, Chapman & Hall/CRC, Boca Raton, FL.]

Accident proneness: A personal psychological factor that affects an individual's probability of suffering an accident. The concept has been studied statistically under a number of different assumptions for accidents:

- Pure chance, leading to the `Poisson distribution`
- True contagion, that is, the hypothesis that all individuals initially have the same probability of having an accident, but that this probability changes each time an accident happens
- Apparent contagion, that is, the hypothesis that individuals have constant but unequal probabilities of having an accident

The study of accident proneness has been valuable in the development of particular statistical methodologies, although in the last two decades the concept has, in general, been out of favour. Attention now appears to have moved more towards risk evaluation and analysis. [Shaw, L. and Sichel, H. S., 1971, *Accident Proneness*, Pergamon Press, Oxford.]

Accrual rate in clinical trials: The rate at which eligible patients are entered into a `clinical trial`, measured as people per unit time. Often disappointingly low, for reasons that may be both physician and patient related. Low accrual to adult oncology trials is a major barrier to progress in cancer therapy. [*Journal of Clinical Oncology*, 2001, **19**, 3554–61.]

Accuracy: The degree of conformity to some recognized standard value. *See also* **bias**.

Accuracy versus precision: An accurate estimate is close to the quantity being estimated. A precise interval estimate is a narrow one, but it may not be accurate even when quoted to a large number of decimal places.

ACES: Abbreviation for **active control equivalence studies**.

ACF: Abbreviation for **autocorrelation function**.

ACORN: Acronym for 'a classification of residential neighbourhoods'. A system for classifying households according to demographic, employment and housing characteristics of their immediate neighbourhood. Derived by applying cluster analysis to 40 variables, including age, class, tenure, dwelling type and car ownership, used to describe each neighbourhood. [Dorling, D. and Simpson, S., 1999, *Statistics in Society*, Arnold, London.]

Acquiescence bias: The bias produced by respondents in a survey who have the tendency to give positive answers, such as 'true', 'like', 'often' or 'yes' to a question. At its most extreme, the person responds in this way irrespective of the content of the question. Thus, a person may respond 'true' to two statements such as 'I always take my medicine on time' and 'I often forget to take my pills'. *See also* **end-aversion bias**. [*Journal of Intellectual Disability Research*, 1995, **39**, 331–40.]

Active control equivalence studies (ACES): Studies that aim to demonstrate that an experimental treatment is equivalent in efficacy to a standard treatment. The justification for undertaking such studies is that even if the new treatment is no more effective than the existing treatment in alleviating a particular condition, it may still be of use for patients who are resistant to, or who simply cannot tolerate, the standard treatment. So clinical trials are sometimes undertaken when the object is simply to show that the new treatment is at least as good as the existing treatment. [Senn, S., 2008, *Statistical Issues in Drug Development*, 2nd ed., John Wiley & Sons, Chichester.]

Active control trials: Clinical trials in which the new treatment is compared with some other active agent rather than a placebo. For example, a clinical trial investigating treatments for asthma might compare the long-acting beta-agonists salmeterol and formoterol with the shorter-acting beta-agonist salbutomol. [Senn, S., 2008, *Statistical Issues in Drug Development*, 2nd ed., John Wiley & Sons, Chichester.]

Active life expectancy (ALE): Defined for a given age as the expected remaining years free of disability. In life expectancy the end point is death. In active life expectancy the end point is the loss of independence or the need to rely on others for assistance with daily activities. ALE is a useful index of public health and quality of life in a population. Interest in recent years has centred on whether current trends towards longer life expectancy have been accompanied by comparable increases in active life expectancy. *See also* **disability-free life expectancy.** [*New England Journal of Medicine*, 1983, **309**, 1218–24.]

Activities of daily living scale (ADLS): A scale designed to measure physical ability/ disability, which is used in investigations of a variety of chronic disabling conditions such as arthritis. The scale is based on scoring responses to questions about mobility, self-care, grooming, and so on. *See also* **Barthel index** and **health assessment questionnaire**. [*Journal of the American Medical Association*, 1963, **185**, 914–19.]

Actuarial statistics: The statistics used by actuaries to evaluate risks, calculate liabilities and plan the financial course of insurance, pensions, and so on. An example is life expectancy for people of various ages, occupations, etc. *See also* **life table**. [Benjamin, B. and Pollard, J. H., 1993, *The Analysis of Mortality and Other Actuarial Statistics*, 3rd ed., Institute of Faculty of Actuaries, Oxford.]

Adaptation: A heritable component of the phenotype that confers an advantage in survival and reproduction success; the process by which organisms adapt to environmental conditions. [Sham, P. C., 1998, *Statistics in Human Genetics*, Arnold, London.]

Adaptive cluster sampling: A procedure in which an initial set of subjects is selected by some sampling process and, whenever the variable of interest of a selected subject satisfies a given criterion, additional subjects in the neighbourhood of that subject are added to the sample. [*Biometrika*, 1996, **84**, 209–19.]

Adaptive randomization designs: Randomized clinical trials in which treatment allocation probabilities are modified based on accumulating data in the trial to achieve selected experimental objectives while protecting the study from bias and preserving inferential validity of the trial results. Such designs have the potential to outperform traditional parallel group fixed randomization designs by treating trial participants more efficiently, identifying promising treatments more rapidly and minimizing unnecessary expenditures while maintaining validity and integrity of results. *See also* **covariate adaptive randomization** and **Bayesian adaptive randomization**. [*Drug Information Journal*, 2006, **40**, 425–35.]

Adaptive treatment-switching design: A design for clinical trials that allows the investigator to switch a patient's treatment from an initial assignment to an alternative treatment if there is evidence of lack of efficacy or safety of the initial treatment. Such a design is commonly employed in cancer trials.

Adaptive randomization: There are now many methods of adaptive randomization that can be used in clinical trials as an alternative to simple randomization but it might be wise to keep in mind that old piece of advice, 'If it ain't broke, don't fix it'.

Addition rule for probabilities: For two *mutually exclusive events*, that is, events that cannot occur together, the probability of either event occurring is the sum of the two individual probabilities. The rule extends in an obvious way to more than two mutually exclusive events. *See also* **multiplication rule for probabilities**.

Additive effect: A term used when the effect of administering two or more factors together is the sum of the effects that would be produced by each of the factors in the absence of the others.

Additive genetic variance: The variance of a characteristic that can be explained by the additive effects of genes. [Sham, P. C., 1998, *Statistics in Human Genetics*, Arnold, London.]

Add-on trial: A clinical trial that compares treatments, say *A* and *B*, in the presence of a standard treatment, say *S*, the randomized comparisons being *S* + *A* versus *S* + *B*. Under certain conditions, *B* may be a placebo version of *A*. Used routinely in AIDS trials. [*Statistical Methods in Medical Research*, 2002, **11**, 1–22.]

Adequate subset: A term used most often in regression analysis for a subset of the explanatory variables that is thought to be as adequate for predicting the response variable as the complete set of explanatory variables under consideration. *See also* **all-subsets regression** and **selection methods in regression**.

Adherence: Synonym for **compliance**.

Adjectival scales: Scales with adjectival descriptions and discrete or continuous responses. Two examples are:

1. *Discrete response (participants may circle one)*
   How much pain are you suffering today?
   Below average   Average   Above average
2. *Continuous response (participants may mark anywhere on the line)*
   How satisfied are you with your treatment?

Very dissatisfied   Dissatisfied   Neutral   Satisfied   Very satisfied

[Streiner, D. L. and Norman, G. R., 1989, *Health Measurement Scales*, Oxford University Press, Oxford.]

Adjusted R²: The square of the multiple correlation coefficient adjusted for the number of parameters in the model under consideration. [Der, G. and Everitt, B. S., 2008, *A Handbook of Statistical Analysis using SAS*, 3rd ed., Chapman & Hall/CRC, Boca Raton, FL.]

Adjusted treatment means: A term usually applied to the estimates of the treatment means in an analysis of covariance after they have been adjusted for the covariates of interest using the estimated relationship between the covariates and the response variable. [Fisher, L. D. and Van Belle, G., 2004, *Biostatistics: A Methodology for the Health Sciences*, 2nd ed., Wiley-Blackwell, New York.]

Adjusting for baseline: The process of allowing for the effect of `baseline characteristics`, particularly a prerandomization measure of the response variable, on the response variable, usually in the context of a `clinical trial`. A number of methods might be used; for example, the analysis of simple `change scores`, the analysis of percentage change, or, in some cases, the analysis of more complicated variables, such as $100 \times$ change/baseline. In general, it is preferable to use the adjusted variable that has least dependence on the baseline measure. In the context of a `longitudinal study` in which the correlations between the repeated measures over time are moderate to large, then using the baseline values as covariates in an `analysis of covariance` is known to be more efficient than analyzing change scores. *See also* **baseline balance**. [Senn, S., 2008, *Statistical Issues in Drug Development*, 2nd ed., John Wiley & Sons, Chichester.]

Adjusting for baseline: Change scores remain popular despite being less powerful than using analysis of covariance. It is difficult to think why.

ADLS: Abbreviation for **activities of daily living scale**.

Administrative databases: `Databases` derived from information collected routinely and systematically for purposes of managing a healthcare system. Such data can be used to examine admission procedures and lengths of stay and make comparisons across hospitals, communities and regions. [Grady, M. L. and Schwartz, H. A., 1992, *Medical Effectiveness Research Data Methods*, Department of Health and Human Services, Rockville, MD.]

Admixture in human populations: The exchange of `genes` by breeding between members of different linguistic and cultural groups, or the sudden infusion of genes caused by large-scale migration. [*Annals of Human Genetics*, 1971, **35**, 9–17.]

Adoption studies: Studies involving subjects raised by non-biological parents. Such studies have played a prominent role in the assessment of genetic variation in human and animal traits. For example, if the shared environment is influential, then siblings raised in the same family should be more similar than adopted-away siblings (siblings reared apart). [Fuller, J. L. and Thompson, W. R., 1979, *Foundations of Behavior Genetics*, Mosby, St Louis, MO.]

Adverse event: Any undesirable consequences experienced by a patient during a medical investigation or study, particularly a `clinical trial`. These can range from the minor, for example constipation, to the far more serious, for example a heart attack. Such events need to be noted on a case report. [*Quality in Health Care*, 2000, **9**, 47–52.]

Aetiological fraction: Synonym for **attributable risk**.

Age heaping: A term applied occasionally to the collection of data on ages when these are accurate only to the nearest year, half-year or month. *See also* **rounding**. [*Geographical Journal*, 1992, **28**, 427–42.]

Age–incidence curve: A plot of age against the `age-specific incidence rate` for some disease or condition of interest. For example, for cancer of the uterine cervix, the curve rises steeply from puberty to age 40, after which it plateaus. [*Proceedings of the National Academy of Science of the United States of America*, 1977, **74**, 1341–2.]

Ageing models: Models for ageing and biological life span are important to plan for the future of society. The features of lifetime data in ageing research which distinguish such data from typical `survival data` are that (1) all individuals enter the study simultaneously, (2) a cohort is observed until the last member is dead and lifetime normally refers to the entire life span of each individual, (3) censoring is only seldom encountered and (4) the data are usually aggregated in a `life table`. [*Age and Ageing*, 2006, **35**, 607–14.]

Age-of-onset estimation: The estimation of the distribution, as a function of age, of the time a trait or condition first appears. For example, a psychiatrist might be interested in the age-of-onset of schizophrenia. Estimating age-of-onset is important in studies of disease aetiology and crucial to clinical management and in designing disease prevention studies. [*Genetic Epidemiology*, 1989, **6**, 217–20.]

Age–period–cohort analysis: A family of statistical techniques for understanding temporal trends in an outcome measure in terms of three related time variables: the subject's age, the subject's date of birth and the calendar period. Early methods employed informative graphical displays of the data, but recently more formal modelling techniques have been used to try to disentangle the separate contributions of each of the factors. *See also* **Lexis diagram**. [*Annual Reviews of Public Health*, 1991, **12**, 425–57.]

Age-related reference ranges: Range of values of a measurement of interest that identify to upper and lower limits of normality in some population, where the range varies according to the subject's age. An example is shown in Figure 1. [*Statistics in Medicine*, 1993, **12**, 917–24.]

Age–sex pyramid: *See* **population pyramid**. [*British Journal of Medicine*, 1985, **291**, 1391–3.]

Age–sex register: A list of all patients or clients of a medical practice or service classified by age and sex. Such information is often needed for calculating, for example, `age-specific birth rate`, `age-specific death rate` and `sex-specific death rate` for conditions of interest. [*British Medical Journal (Clinical Research Edition)*, 1984, **288**, 1967.]

Age-specific birth rate: The number of live births per 1,000 women in a specific age group. For example, in California in 1990, the rate for women aged 15–19 years was 11.4; in 1998, the corresponding figure was 11.2. [*Child Trends*, 2018.]

Age-specific death rate: Death rate calculated for a specified age group. For example, for 20–30-year-olds:

$$DR(20/30) = \frac{\text{number of deaths among 20–30-year-olds in a year}}{\text{average population size of 20–30-year-olds in the year}}$$

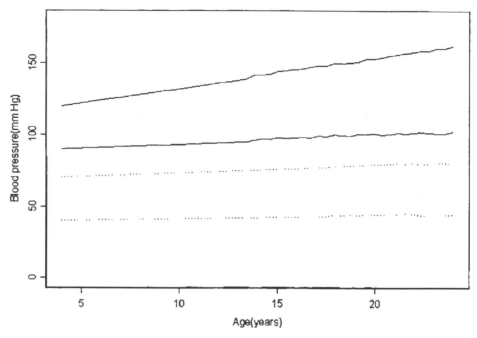

Figure 1 Age-related 95% reference ranges for blood pressure in boys: systolic (solid lines); diastolic (dotted lines).
(Figure after that in age-related reference ranges in *Encyclopaedic Companion to Medical Statistics*, 2nd ed., eds. B. S. Everitt and C. R. Palmer, John Wiley & Sons, Chichester, 2005.)

Calculating death rates in this way is usually necessary since such rates almost invariably differ widely with age, a variation not reflected in the crude death rate. In England and Wales in 1990, the age-specific death rates per 1,000 for men in four age groups were:

- 45–54 years: 4.8
- 55–64 years: 14.8
- 65–74 years: 39.5
- 75–84 years: 94.3

See also **cause-specific death rates** and **standardized mortality rate**. [Fisher, L. D. and Van Belle, G., 2004, *Biostatistics*, 2nd ed., Wiley-Blackwell, New York.]

Age-specific fertility rate: The number of births occurring during a specified period to women of a specified age group, divided by the number of person-years lived during that period by women of that age group. For example, in the period 1990–5, the rate per 1,000 women in the 15–19 years age group in Africa was 136, in Asia 45 and in Europe 27. The corresponding figures for the 40–44-years age group were Africa 82, Asia 22 and Europe 5.

Age-specific incidence rate: Incidence rates calculated within a number of relatively narrow age bands. For example, age is the most important risk factor for prostate cancer, with the incidence rate being very small for men below 45 years but about 1,000 per 100,000 at age 65. [*American Journal of Epidemiology*, 2000, **151**, 1158–71.]

Age standardization: A process of adjusting rates before they are compared in different populations, so as to minimize the effects of possible differences in age composition of the populations. *See also* **standardized mortality rate**.

Agglomerative hierarchical clustering methods: Methods of cluster analysis that begin with each individual defining a separate cluster and proceed by combining individuals and later groups of individuals into larger clusters ending when all the individuals have been combined into a single cluster. At each stage, the individuals or groups of individuals who are closest according to some particular definition of distance are joined. The whole series of steps can be summarized by a dendrogram. Solutions corresponding to a particular number of clusters are found by cutting the dendrogram at some level. *See also* **average linkage clustering, complete linkage cluster analysis, single linkage clustering, Ward's method** and **K-means cluster analysis**. [Everitt, B. S., Landau, S., Leese, M. and Stahl, D., 2011, *Cluster Analysis*, 5th ed., John Wiley & Sons, Chichester.]

Agresti's alpha: A generalization of the odds ratio for two-by-two contingency tables to larger contingency tables arising from data where there are different degrees of severity of a disease and differing amounts of exposure. [Agresti, A., 2010, *Analysis of Ordinal Categorical Data*, 2nd ed., Wiley-Blackwell, New York.]

Aickin's measure of agreement: A chance-corrected measure of agreement that is similar to the kappa coefficient but that uses a different definition of chance agreement. [*Biometrics*, 1990, **46**, 293–302.]

Akaike's information criterion: An index often used as an aid in choosing the most suitable model for a set of observations. The index takes into account both the statistical goodness of fit and the number of parameters that have to be estimated to achieve this degree of fit, by imposing a penalty for increasing the number of parameters. Lower values of the index indicate the preferred model, that is, the one with the fewest parameters that still provides an adequate fit to the data. *See also* **parsimony principle**. [*Psychometrika*, 1987, **52**, 345–70.]

Algorithm: A well-defined set of rules that, when applied routinely, lead to a solution of a particular class of mathematical or computational problem.

Alias: *See* **confounding**.

Allele: One of two or more genes that may occur at a given location in the genes of an individual; essentially alternative forms of a gene occupying the same locus on a chromosome.

Allocation rule: *See* **discriminant analysis**.

Allometric growth: Changes in the shape of an organism associated with different growth rates of its parts. Shape changes in growing organs or whole organisms may be triggered by either biological or physical needs. [Bookstein, F. L., 1978, *The Measurement of Biological Shape and Shape Change*, Springer-Verlag, Berlin.]

All-subsets regression: A form of `regression analysis` in which all possible models are compared and the 'best' selected using some appropriate index of performance of each model. If the number of explanatory variables is q, then there are a total of $2^q - 1$ models to consider, since each explanatory variable can be either 'in' or 'out' of the model and the model with no explanatory variables is excluded. So, for example, with $q = 10$, a total of 1,023 models have to be considered. The `leaps-and-bounds algorithm` is generally used to make the approach computationally feasible when there is a large number of explanatory variables.[Rawlings, J. O., Pantula, S. G. and Dickey, D. A., 2nd ed., 2013, *Applied Regression Analysis: A Research Tool*, Springer, New York.]

Alpha (*a*): The probability of a `type I error`. *See also* **significance level**.

Alpha spending function: An approach to `interim analysis` for `clinical trials` that allows the control of the `type I error` rate while retaining flexibility in the number of interim analyses to be conducted and their timing. [*Statistics in Medicine*, 1996, **15**, 1739–46.]

Alpha-trimmed mean: A statistic for estimating the mean of a population that is less affected by the presence of `outliers` than the arithmetic mean. Involves dropping a proportion (alpha) of the observations from both ends of the sample before calculating the mean of the remainder. [Fisher, L. D. and Van Belle, G., 2013, *Biostatistics*, 2nd ed., John Wiley & Sons, New York.]

Alternate allocation: A method of allocating patients to treatment groups in a `clinical trial` that places alternate patients into the groups. Not to be recommended since it is open to accusations of abuse, with, for example, the treating clinician having the possibility of manipulating that the patient receives each treatment. [Everitt, B. S. and Wessely, S., 2008, *Clinical Trials in Psychiatry*, 2nd ed., Wiley-Blackwell, Chichester.]

> **Alternate allocation:** Never use this method of allocation if you wish your clinical trial to be taken seriously.

Alternative hypothesis: The hypothesis against which the null hypothesis is tested generally in the context of statistical significance tests. [Altman, D. G., 2018, *Practical Statistics for Medical Research*, Chapman & Hall/CRC, Boca Raton, FL.]

Analysis as randomized: Synonym for **intention-to-treat analysis**.

Analysis of covariance: Essentially an application of `multiple linear regression` in which some of the explanatory variables are categorical, often binary, for example treatment group, and others are continuous, for example age. The aim is to increase the sensitivity of the `F-tests` used in assessing treatment differences. [Altman, D. G., 2018, *Practical Statistics for Medical Research*, Chapman & Hall/CRC, Boca Raton, FL.]

Analysis of dispersion: Synonym for **multivariate analysis of variance**.

Analysis of variance: The separation of variation attributable to one factor from that attributed to others. By partitioning the total variance of a set of observations into parts due to particular factors, for example sex, treatment group, etc., differences in the mean values of the dependent variable can be assessed. The simplest analysis of this type involves a *one-way design*: a sample of individuals from a number of different populations is compared with respect to some outcome measure of interest. The total variance in the observations is partitioned into a part due to differences between the group means (*between-groups sum of squares*) and a part due to differences between subjects in the same group (*within-groups sum of squares* or *residual sum of squares*). The results of this division are usually arranged in an *analysis of variance table*. The equality of the means of the populations involved implies that the between-group and within-group variances are both estimating the same quantity, and this can be tested by an appropriate F-test. [Altman, D. G., 2018, *Practical Statistics for Medical Research*, Chapman & Hall/ CRC, Boca Raton, FL.]

Analysis of variance: The model underlying the analysis of variance is essentially the same as that involved in multiple linear regression, with the explanatory variables being dummy variables coding factor levels and interactions between factors.

Analysis of variance table: *See* analysis of variance.

Analytic epidemiology: A term for epidemiological studies, such as case-control studies, that obtain individual-level information on the association between disease status and exposures of interest.

ANCOVA: Acronym for **analysis of covariance**.

Anecdotal evidence: Evidence from case reports or observations on a single patient by a particular clinician rather than from systematically collected data. Although such evidence is not acceptable for drawing conclusions about treatments or therapies, it may be suggestive of procedures worthy of further investigation in an appropriate scientific manner, for example by way of a clinical trial. [Everitt, B. S. and Wessely, S., 2008, *Clinical Trials in Psychiatry*, 2nd ed., Wiley-Blackwell, Chichester.]

Anecdotal evidence: Suitable only for tabloid journalists, not for serious medical researchers.

Angle transformation: Synonym for **arc-sine transformation**.

Angular histogram: A method for displaying circular data, which involves wrapping the usual histogram around a circle. Each bar in the histogram is centred at the midpoint of the group interval with the length of the bar proportional to the frequency of the group. Figure 2 shows such a display for arrival times on a 24-hour

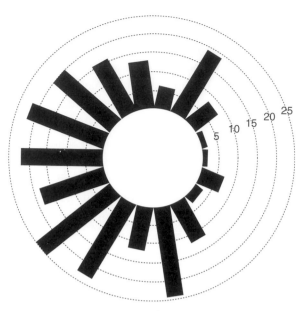

Figure 2 Angular histogram for arrival times at an intensive care unit.
(Reproduced by permission of Cambridge University Press from *Statistical Analysis of Circular Data*, by N. I. Fisher, 1995.)

clock of 254 patients at an intensive care unit, over a period of 12 months. [Fisher, N. I., 1993, *Statistical Analysis of Circular Data*, Cambridge University Press, Cambridge.]

Animal model: A study carried out in a population of laboratory animals that is used to model processes comparable to those that occur in human populations.

ANOVA: Acronym for **analysis of variance**.

Antagonism: *See* **synergism**.

Anthropometry: The subject that deals with the measurement of the size, weight and proportions of the human body. [Tanner, J. M., 1981, *A History of the Study of Human Growth*, Cambridge University Press, Cambridge.]

Antidependence models: Models used in the analysis of `longitudinal data` that assume a particular form for the `variance-covariance matrix` of the repeated measurements, a form that arises from assuming that an observation at a particular time point is dependent on the values of a small number of the immediately preceding observations, but given these values, is conditionally independent of earlier observations. [*Biometrics*, 1986, **42**, 805–20.]

Apgar score: *See* **Likert scale**.

Approximation: A result that is not exact but is sufficiently close to the truth to be of practical value.

A priori comparisons: Synonym for **planned comparisons**.

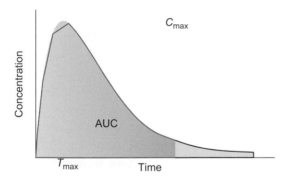

Figure 3 Time course of plasma concentration following a single oral administration of a drug: illustrates area under the curve, C_{max} and T_{max}.
(Taken with permission of the publisher Wiley from *Encyclopedia of Biostatistics*, volume 1, 2nd ed., edited by P. Armitage and T. Colton, 2005.)

Arc-sine transformation: A transformation of a proportion designed to stabilize its variance and produce values more suitable for techniques such as analysis of variance and regression analysis. [Collett, D., 2003, *Modelling Binary Data*, 2nd ed., Chapman & Hall/CRC, Boca Raton, FL.]

Area sampling: A method of sampling in which a geographical region is subdivided into smaller areas (countries, villages, city blocks, etc.), some of which are then selected at random and subsampled or surveyed completely. [*American Journal of Epidemiology*, 2001, **153**, 1119–27.]

Area under curve (AUC): Often a useful way of summarizing the observations made on an individual over time, for example those collected in a longitudinal study or for a dose–response relationship. The measure is illustrated in Figure 3. Usually calculated by adding together the area under the curve between each pair of consecutive observations. The AUC is often a predictor of biological effects, such as toxicity or efficacy, and for measurements taken at regular intervals it is essentially equivalent to using the mean. *See also* **C_{max}**, **T_{max}** and **response feature analysis**. [*International Journal of Clinical Pharmacology, Therapeutics and Toxicology*, 1991, **29**, 394–9.]

Arithmetic mean: *See* mean.

Armitage–Doll model: A model for carcinogenesis in which the central idea is that the important variable determining the change in risk is not age but time. The model proposes that cancers of a particular tissue develop according to the following process:

• A normal cell develops into a cancer cell by means of a small number of transitions through a series of intermediate steps.
• Initially, the number of cells at risk is very large, and for each cell a transition is a rare event.
• The transitions are independent of one another.

[LeCam, L. M. and Neyman, J., 1961, *Proceedings of the Fourth Berkeley Symposium on Mathematic Statistics and Probability*, University of California Press, Berkeley, CA.]

Artefactual associations: *See* association.

Artificial intelligence (AI): A discipline that attempts to understand intelligent behaviour in the broadest sense, by getting computers to reproduce it, and to produce machines that behave intelligently no matter what their underlying mechanism. (Intelligent behaviour is taken to include reasoning, thinking and learning.) *See also* **artificial neural network** and **pattern recognition**. [Russell, S. and Norvig, P., 2002, *Artificial Intelligence: A Modern Approach*, 2nd ed., Prentice Hall, Harlow.]

Artificial neural network: A mathematical structure modelled on the human neural network and designed to attach many statistical problems, particularly in the areas of pattern recognition, multivariate analysis, learning and memory. The essential feature of such a structure is a network of simple processing elements (*artificial neurons*) coupled together (either in the hardware or the software) so that they can cooperate. From a set of inputs and an associated set of parameters, the artificial neurons produce an output that provides a possible solution to the problem under investigation. In many neural networks, the relationship between the input received by a neuron and its output is determined by a generalized linear model. Enthusiasts often assert that neural networks provide a new approach to computing, whereas sceptics point out that they may solve a few 'toy' problems but cannot be taken seriously as a general problem-solving tool. [Garson, G. D., 1998, *Neural Networks: An Introductory Guide for Social Scientists*, Sage, London.]

> **Artificial neural network:** Fashionable, but perhaps not the answer to as many problems as its advocates would have the rest of us believe.

Artifical neurons: *See* **artificial neural network**.

Ascertainment bias: A possible form of bias, particularly in retrospective studies, that arises from a relationship between the exposure to a risk factor and the probability of detecting an event of interest. In a study comparing women with cervical cancer and a control group, for example, an excess of oral contraceptive use amongst the cases might possibly be due to more frequent screening in this group. *See also* **recall bias**. [*American Journal of Epidemiology*, 2002, **155**, 875–80.]

Asher's paradox: According to Richard Asher, a distinguished London physician, if you can believe fervently in the treatment you are suggesting to a patient, even though controlled studies show that it is quite useless, then your results are much better, your patients are much better, and your income is much better too. Asher goes on to suggest that this accounts for the remarkable success of some of the less gifted, but more credulous members of the medical profession, and also for the often violent dislike of statistics and controlled tests, which fashionable and successful doctors are accustomed to display. *See also* **placebo effect**.

ASN: Abbreviation for **average sample number**.

As-randomized analysis: Synonym for **intention-to-treat analysis**.

Assay: An experiment designed to estimate the strength, kind or quality of some physical, chemical, biological, physiological or psychological agent by means of the response induced by that agent in living or nonliving matter. *See also* **bioassay**.

Assay run: A set of consecutive measurements, readings or observations all based on the same batch of reagents.

Assigned treatment: The treatment a patient in a `clinical trial` is designated to receive, as indicated at the time of enrolment. *See also* **compliance**, **intention-to-treat analysis** and **pill count**.

Association: A general term to describe the statistical dependence between two variables; 'positive association' implies that values of one variable increase (decrease) as the other variable increases (decreases), and 'negative' association the reverse. Association can be measured in a variety of ways, for example, `correlation coefficients`, `relative risk`, `odds ratio`, `phi coefficient` and the `Goodman and Kruskal measure of association`. It needs to be remembered that an observed association say between an exposure and a disease, may be artefactual, non-causal or causal. An *artefactual association* may, for example, arise because of `bias` in the study, and a noncasual association can occur if the disease causes the exposure rather than vice versa, or if both disease and exposure are associated with a third variable, known or unknown. *See also* **Berkson's fallacy** and **Simpson's paradox**. [Everitt, B. S., 1992, *The Analysis of Contingency Tables*, 2nd ed., Chapman & Hall/CRC, Boca Raton, FL.]

Association: Remember, an association, if biologically plausible, may suggest a causal link but proof is only obtainable by experiment.

Assortative mating: A process whereby biological parents are more similar for a `phenotype` trait than they would be if the mating occurred at random in the population. Common examples in human populations are height and intelligence. [*Eugenics Quarterly*, 1968, **15**, 128–40.]

Assumptions: The conditions under which statistical techniques give valid results. For example, `analysis of variance` generally assumes normality, homogeneity of variance, and independence of the observations.

Asymmetrical distribution: A `probability distribution` or `frequency distribution` that is not symmetrical about some central value. A `J-shaped distribution` is an example.

Asymptotic method: Synonym for **large sample method**.

Attachment level: A common measure of periodontal disease levels given by the minimum distance between the cement–enamel junction (a reference point on the tooth) and the epithelial attachment. Usually measured in millimetres with a graduated blunt-end probe. [*Journal of Periodontology*, 2002, **73**, 198–205.]

Attack rate: A term often used for the incidence rate of a disease or condition in a particular group, or during a limited period of time, or under special circumstances such as an epidemic. A specific example would be one involving outbreaks of food poisoning, where the attack rates would be calculated for those people who have eaten a particular item and for those who have not. Calculated as the ratio of the number of people ill in the time period over the number of people at risk in the time period. An example involving a well-known brand of soft drink occurred in Belgium in 1999, in which 37 of 280 students were identified as cases and the attack rate was 13.2% overall, 15.6% among girls and 8.9% among boys.

Attenuation: A term applied to the correlation calculated between two variables when both are subject to measurement error to indicate that the value of the correlation between the true values is likely to be underestimated. *See also* **regression dilution**. [Fisher, L. D. and Van Belle, G., 2004, *Biostatistics: A Methodology for the Health Sciences*, 2nd ed., John Wiley & Sons, New York.]

Attributable fraction: A measure that quantifies the proportional reduction in disease prevalence that would be achieved if a risk factor of interest could somehow be eliminated from the population. The measure depends jointly on relative risk and the prevalence on the risk factor within the general population. [*Statistical Methods in Medical Research*, 2001, **10**, 159–93.]

Attributable risk: A measure of the association between exposure to a particular factor and the risk of a particular outcome, calculated as

$$\frac{\text{incidence rate among exposed} - \text{incidence rate among nonexposed}}{\text{incidence rate among exposed}}$$

Measures the amount of the incidence rate that can be attributed to one particular factor. Can be estimated from case-control studies and cross-sectional studies. For example, it has been reported that for lifetime smokers, 31% of all lung cancer is attributable to five nonsmoking risk factors. *See also* **relative risk** and **preventable fraction**. [*American Journal of Epidemiology*, 1995, **142**, 1338–43.]

Attrition: A term used to describe the loss of subjects over the period of a longitudinal study. Such phenomena may cause problems in the analysis of data from such a study. *See also* **missing values**. [Everitt, B. S. and Wessely, S., 2008, *Clinical Trials in Psychiatry*, 2nd ed., Wiley-Blackwell, Chichester.]

AUC: Abbreviation for **area under curve**.

Audit in clinical trials: The process of ensuring that data collected in complex clinical trials are of high quality. [*Controlled Clinical Trials*, 1995, **16**, 104–36.]

Figure 4 Levels of luteinizing hormone in blood samples taken from a healthy woman every 10 minutes (a) and the autocorrelation function with approximately 95% confidence limits for zero correlation (b).
(Taken with permission of the publisher Wiley from *Encyclopedia of Biostatistics*, volume 1, 2nd ed., edited by P. Armitage and T. Colton, 2005.)

Audit trail: A computer program that keeps a record of changes made to a `database`.

Autocorrelation: The internal correlation of the observations in a `time series`, usually expressed as a function of the time lag between observations. A plot of the value of the autocorrelation against the time lag is known as the *autocorrelation function* or *correlogram* and is a basic tool in analysis of time series data. An example of a medical time series and its associated correlogram is shown in Figure 4. [Chatfield, C., 2019, *The Analysis of Time Series: An Introduction*, 7th ed., Chapman & Hall/CRC, Boca Raton, FL.]

Autocorrelation function (ACF): *See* **autocorrelation**.

Auto-encoding: Coding of clinical data by a computer program that matches original text to predetermined dictionary terms.

Autoregressive model: A model used primarily in the analysis of `time series` in which an observation at a particular time is postulated to be a linear function of previous values in the series plus an error term. [Chatfield, C., 2019, *The Analysis of Time Series: An Introduction*, 7th ed., Chapman & Hall/CRC, Boca Raton, FL.]

Available case analysis: An approach to `multivariate data` containing `missing values` on a number of variables, in which means, variances and `covariances`

are calculated from all available subjects with non-missing values on the variable (means and variances) or pair of variables (covariances) involved. Although this approach makes use of as many of the observed data as possible, it does have disadvantages. For example, the summary statistics for each variable may be based on different numbers of observations, and the calculated `variance-covariance matrix` may now not be suitable for methods of `multivariate analysis` such as `principal components analysis` and `factor analysis`. *See also* **missing values** and **imputation**.
[Schafer, J. L., 1997, *Analysis of Incomplete Multivariate Data*, Chapman & Hall/CRC, Boca Raton, FL.]

Available case analysis: Causes problems when the investigator wishes to apply, say, factor analysis to the data. Complete case analysis and imputation of the missing values are possible alternatives.

Average: Used most often for the arithmetic mean of a sample of observations, but can also be used for other measures of location, such as the median.

Average age at death: A flawed statistic for summarizing `life expectancy` and other aspects of mortality. For example, a study comparing average age at death for male symphony orchestra conductors and for the entire US male population showed that, on average, the conductors lived about four years longer. The difference is, however, illusory, because as age at entry was birth, those in the US male population who died in infancy and childhood were included in the calculation of the average life span whereas only men who survived to become conductors could enter the conductor cohort. The apparent difference in longevity disappeared after accounting for `infant mortality rate` and `perinatal mortality rate`.
[Andersen, B., 1990, *Methodological Errors in Medical Research*, Blackwell Scientific, Oxford.]

Average age at death: Beware trying to prove that clinicians (or statisticians) live longer on the basis of this statistic.

Average deviation: A little used measure of the spread of a sample of observations given by the average of the absolute values of deviations of each observation from the sample mean.

Average linkage clustering: An `agglomerative hierarchical clustering method` that uses the average distance from members of one cluster to members of another cluster as its measure of intergroup distance. [Everitt, B. S., Landau, S., Leese, M. and Stahl, D., 2001, *Cluster Analysis*, 5th ed., John Wiley & Sons, Chichester.]

Average sample number (ASN): A quantity often used to describe the performance of a `sequential analysis` and given by the expected value of the sample size required to reach a decision to accept the null hypothesis or the alternative hypothesis and therefore to discontinue sampling.

Axiom: A statement that is considered self-evident and used as a foundation on which arguments can be based.

Back-calculation: A method of estimating past infection rate of an `epidemic` infectious disease by working backwards from observed disease `incidence rate` using knowledge of the `incubation period` between infection and disease. Used mainly for reconstructing plausible HIV incidence curves from AIDS incidence data. Limitations of the approach are that it provides little information about recent infection rates and that projections can be sensitive to recent incidence. [*Statistical Science*, 1993, **8**, 82–119.]

Background level: The usually low concentration of some substance or agent that is characteristic of a particular time or place rather than a specific hazard. This may be naturally occurring, for example, the background level of naturally occurring forms of ionizing radiation to which nearly everybody is exposed or human-made, for example, automobiles of industrial production.

Back-projection: Synonym for **back-calculation**.

Back-to-back stem-and-leaf plots: A method for comparing two distributions by 'hanging' the two sets of leaves in the `stem-and-leaf plots` of the two sets of data, off either side of the same stem. An example appears in Figure 5.

Backward elimination: *See* **selection methods in regression**.

Backward-looking study: An alternative (and unattractive) term for `retrospective study`.

Bagging: Suppose there is some model of interest for a data set, for example, a `linear regression`. If repeated `bootstrap samples` are taken from the original data set and the model fitted, the results will be slightly different in each case and the predictions at each point will vary from model to model. The 'bagged' prediction for each point is an average, over the predictions of all the models for that point. The aim of the process is to reduce the prediction variance. [*Machine Learning*, 1996, **24**, 123–40.]

Balaam's design: A design for testing differences between two treatments, *A* and *B*, in which patients are allocated randomly to one of four sequences, *AA*, *AB*, *BA* or *BB*. *See also* **crossover design**. [*Statistics in Medicine*, 1988, **7**, 471–82.]

Balanced design: A term usually applied to any experimental design in which the same number of observations is taken for each combination of the experimental factors. *See also* **non-orthogonal design**.

```
Before                    After
        : 12 : 9
        : 13 : 1  6
   8  6 : 14 : 5  7  7
      4 : 15 : 1  7
 9  7  0 : 16 : 5  6  8  8
 6  4  3 : 17 : 9
   7  5 : 18 : 0
      8 : 19 :
      0 : 20 : 1
```

Figure 5 Back-to-back stem and leaf plot of systolic blood pressure of 15 subjects before and two hours after taking the drug captopril.
(From Everitt, B. S. and Skrondal, A., 2010, *The Cambridge Dictionary of Statistics*, 4th ed., Cambridge University Press, Cambridge.)

Balanced incomplete block design: An experimental design in which not all treatments are used in all `blocks`. Such designs have the following properties:
- Each block contains the same number of units.
- Each treatment occurs the same number of times in all blocks.
- Each pair of treatment combinations occurs together in a block the same number of times as any other pair of treatments.

In medicine, this type of design might be used to avoid asking subjects to attend for treatment an unrealistic number of times, and thus perhaps to avoid creating problems arising from the occurrence of `missing values`. [Herzog, M. H., Francis, G. and Clarke, A., 2019, *Understanding Statistics and Experimental Design: How Not to Lie with Statistics*, Springer, New York.]

Balanced longitudinal data: `Longitudinal data` for which observations at the same number of time points are available on each subject, and time intervals between pairs of corresponding observations are the same for all subjects. The observations need not be spaced equally. [*Biometrics*, 1992, **48**, 743–50.]

Bar chart: A form of graphical representation for displaying data classified into a number of (usually unordered) categories. Equal-width rectangular bars are constructed over each category, with height equal to the observed frequency of the category. An example of such a chart is shown in Figure 6. *See also* **histogram** and **component bar chart**.

Barefoot statistician: A user (and sometimes producer) of information, whose expertise lies in a balance of basic statistical skills and communication links with their community. [*Statistical Science*, 1990, **5**, 372–402.]

Barrett and Marshall model for conception: A biologically plausible model for the probability of conception in a particular menstrual cycle that assumes that batches of sperm introduced on different days behave independently. Day-specific pregnancy probabilities can be calculated from the model. *See also* **EU model**. [*Population Studies*, 1969, **23**, 455–61.]

Barthel index: A `quality-of-life` variable used to assess the ability of a patient to perform daily activities such as feeding, bathing, dressing, etc. Can be used to

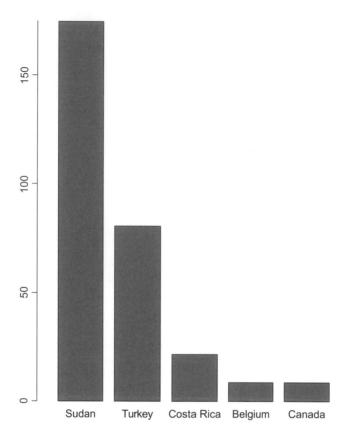

Figure 6 Bar chart of mortality rates per 1,000 live births for children under 5 years of age in five different countries.

determine a baseline level of functioning and to monitor improvements in activities of daily living over time. A score of 0 corresponds to complete dependence on others, and a score of 10 implies that the patient can perform all usual daily activities without assistance. *See also* **activities of daily living scale** and **U-shaped distribution**. [*International Disability Study*, 1988, **10**, 61–3.]

Bartlett's test: A test for the equality of the variances of more than two populations. Very sensitive to non-normality, so that a significant result might be interpreted as an indication of the nonequality of the population variances when in reality it is due to the nonnormality of the observations. *See also* **Box's test** and **Hartley's test**.

Bartlett's test: Do not take the results of this test too seriously.

Baseline balance: A term used to describe, in some sense, the equality of the observed baseline characteristics among the groups in, say, a clinical trial. Conventional practice dictates that before proceeding to assess the treatment effects from the clinical outcomes, the groups must be shown to be comparable in terms of these baseline measurements and observations, usually by carrying out appropriate significant tests. Such tests are criticized frequently by statisticians, who usually prefer important prognostic variables to be identified before the trial and then used in an `analysis of covariance`. [Senn, S., 2008, *Statistical Issues in Drug Development*, 2nd ed., John Wiley & Sons, Chichester.]

Baseline balance: Avoid the foolish but common use of baseline measurements to check that the groups in a randomized clinical trial are 'balanced'.

Baseline characteristics: Observations and measurements collected on subjects or patients at the time of entry into a study before undergoing any treatment, for example, sex, age and weight. [*Statistician*, 1985, **1**, 125–36.]

Basic reproduction number: A term used in the theory of infectious diseases for the number of secondary cases that one case would produce in a completely susceptible population. The number depends on the duration of the infectious period, the probability of infecting a susceptible individual during one contact, and the number of new susceptible individuals contacted per unit time, with the consequences that it may vary considerably for different infectious diseases and also for the same disease in different populations. When the basic reproduction number is less than one, the infection will die out, but if it is greater than one then the disease will spread exponentially causing a large `epidemic`. If the basic reproduction number equals one, then the infection will become endemic in the population. The larger the value of the basic reproduction number, the larger the fraction of the population that must be immunized to prevent an epidemic. For AIDS, for example, the basic reproduction number is between 2 and 5, and for measles between 16 and 18. [*Journal of Biological Dynamics*, 2009, **3**, 116–29.]

Bathtub hazard: The shape taken by the `hazard function` for the event of death in human beings; it is relatively high during the first year of life, decreases fairly soon to a minimum, and begins to climb again sometime around ages 45–50. Such a curve is shown in Figure 7.

Battery reduction: A general term for reducing the number of variables of interest in a study for the purposes of analysis and perhaps later data collection. For example, an overly long questionnaire may not yield accurate answers to all questions, and its size may need to be reduced. Techniques such as `factor analysis` and `principal component analysis` are generally used to achieve the required reduction.

Bayesian adaptive randomization: A method of randomization used in `clinical trials` in which treatment randomization probability is based on the value of a `posterior probability` that one treatment is better than the other. *See also* **adaptive randomization designs** and **covariate-adaptive randomization**. [*European Journal of Cancer*, 2007, **43**, 860–7.]

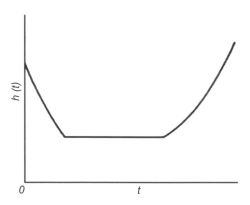

Figure 7 Bathtub hazard for death in human beings.

Bayesian confidence interval: An interval of a `posterior distribution` that is such that the density at any point inside the interval is greater than the density at any point outside and that the area under the curve for that interval is equal to a pre-specified probability level. For any probability level, there is generally only one such interval, which is also known as the *highest posterior density region*. Unlike the usual `confidence interval` associated with `frequentist inference`, here the intervals specify the range within which the parameters lie with a certain probability. [Berry, D. A. and Stangl, D. K., 2019, *Bayesian Biostatistics*, CRC, Boca Raton, FL.]

Bayesian meta-analysis: This approach to `meta-analysis` provides a flexible modelling strategy that accounts for uncertainty in all the parameter estimates. The method can be easily extended to non-normal distribution of random effects. This approach also allows additional information from other trials or studies to be incorporated in the form of a `prior distribution`. The Bayesian approach is computationally intensive because of the need to compute the `posterior distributions` of parameters, but this can now be handled routinely using the `Markov chain Monte Carlo` (MCMC) method. [Gibbons, R. D. and Amatya, A. K., 2016, *Statistical Methods for Drug Safety*, Chapman & Hall/CRC, Boca Raton, FL.]

Bayesian methods: An approach to inference based on `Bayes's theorem`, in which prior knowledge in the form of a specified `probability distribution` for the unknown parameters (the `prior distribution`) is updated in the light of the observed data to give a revised probability distribution for the parameters (the `posterior distribution`). This form of inference differs from the classical form of `frequentist inference` in several respects, particularly in the use of a prior probability distribution for the parameters; this is absent from classical inference. The prior distribution represents the investigator's knowledge before collecting the data. [Spiegelhalter, D. J., Abrams, K. R. and Myles, J. P., 2004, *Bayesian Approaches to Clinical Trials and Health-Care Evaluation*, John Wiley & Sons, Chichester.]

Bayesian persuasion probabilities: A term for particular posterior distributions used to judge whether a new therapy is superior to the standard as derived from the prior distributions of two hypothetical experts, one of whom believes that the new therapy is highly effective and another who believes that it is no more effective than other treatments. The *persuade-the-pessimist probability* is the posterior probability that the new therapy is an improvement on the standard assuming the sceptical expert's prior, and the *persuade-the-optimist probability* is the posterior probability that the new therapy gives no advantage over the standard assuming the enthusiast's prior. Large values of these probabilities should persuade the a priori most opinionated parties to change their views. [*Statistics in Medicine*, 1997, **16**, 1792–802.]

Bayes's theorem: A procedure for revising and updating the probability of some event in the light of new evidence. For example, an estimate of the probability that a woman has breast cancer will change if she is tested positive on a mammograph. The theorem originates in an essay by the Reverend Thomas Bayes. *See also* **conditional probability, positive predictive value** and **negative predictive value**. [Everitt, B. S., 2008, *Chance Rules*, 2nd ed., Springer, New York.]

Begg's test: A test for funnel plot asymmetry based on the size of the rank correlation coefficient between the effect size estimates and their sampling variances. *See also* **Egger's test**. [*Nephrology, Dialysis and Transplantation*, 2004, **19**, 2747–53.]

Behrens–Fisher problem: The problem of testing for the equality of the means of two normal distributions that do not have the same variance. Various test statistics have been proposed but none is completely satisfactory. *See also* **Student's *t*-test**. [*Computer Methods and Programs in Biomedicine*, 2003, **70**, 259–63.]

Believe the negative rule: *See* **believe the positive rule**.

Believe the positive rule: A rule for combining two diagnostic tests, *A* and *B*, in which 'disease present' is the diagnosis given if either *A* or *B* or both are positive. An alternative, *believe the negative rule*, assigns a patient to the disease class only if both *A* and *B* are positive. These rules do not necessarily have better positive predictive values than a single test; whether they do depends on the association between test outcomes. [*Biometrics*, 1989, **45**, 1213–22.]

Bellman–Harris process: A branching process evolving from an initial individual in which each individual lives for a random length of time and at the end of its life produces a random number of offspring of the same type.
[Jagers, P., 1975, *Branching Processes with Biological Applications*, John Wiley & Sons, Chichester.]

Bell-shaped distribution: A probability distribution having the overall shape of a vertical cross section of a bell. The normal distribution is the most well-known example, but Student's *t*-distribution is also this shape.

Benchmark dose: A term used in risk assessment studies where human, animal or ecological data are used to set safe low dose levels of a toxic agent, for the dose that is associated with a particular level of risk. [*Applied Statistics*, 2005, **54**, 245–58.]

Benchmarking: A procedure for adjusting a less reliable series of observations to make it consistent with more reliable measurements or *benchmarks*. For example, data on hospital bed occupation collected monthly will not necessarily agree with figures collected annually, and the monthly figures (which are likely to be less reliable) may be adjusted at some point to agree with the more reliable annual figures. [*International Statistical Review*, 1994, **62**, 365–77.]

Benchmarks: *See* benchmarking.

Bench-to-bedside research: Synonymous to **translational medicine**.

Benefit–cost ratio: The ratio of net present value of measurable benefits to cost. Used to determine the economic feasibility of success of a health intervention programme.

Berkson's bias: Synonym for **Berkson's fallacy**.

Berkson's fallacy: The existence of artefactual associations between two medical conditions, or between a disease and a risk factor, arising from the interplay of differential admission rates with respect to the suspected causal factor. First described in 1946 by Joseph Berkson, a physician in the Division of Biometry and Medical Statistics at the Mayo Clinic. A classic example is a study of autopsies in which fewer autopsies than expected find both tuberculosis and cancer to occur together apparently implying that the frequency of cancer is lower among tuberculosis victims. But any conclusion that we may infer from this (that tuberculosis is protective against cancer) is erroneous, simply because not every death is autopsied. Here perhaps people who die with both diseases are less likely to have been autopsied, leading to an artificially low number of autopsies with both diseases. *See also* **Simpson's paradox**. [Everitt, B. S. and Palmer, C. (eds.), 2011, *Encyclopedic Companion to Medical Statistics*, John Wiley & Sons, Chichester.]

Berkson's fallacy: Be on the lookout for associations generated by differential admission rates; it is not possible to correct for these during analysis.

Berkson's paradox: Synonym for **Berkson's fallacy**.

Bernoulli sequence: A set of n independent `binary variables` with the probability of, 'success' being the same for all trials.

Berry–Esseen theorem: A theorem relating to how rapidly the distribution of the mean approaches normality. *See also* **central limit theorem**. [*Theory of Probability and Its Applications*, 2007, **51**, 549–53.]

Best linear unbiased estimator (BLUE): A `linear estimator` of a parameter that has smaller variance than any similar estimator of the parameter.

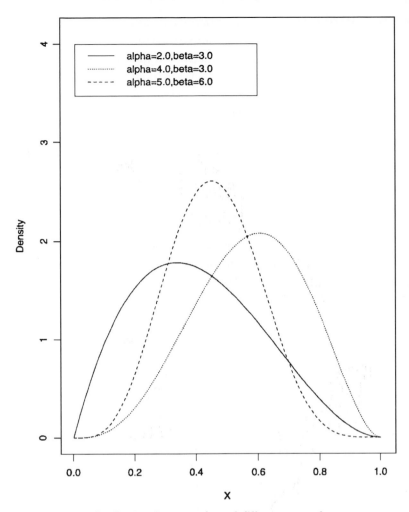

Figure 8 Beta distribution for a number of different sets of parameters.

Beta coefficient: A regression coefficient that is standardized so as to allow for a direct comparison between explanatory variables as to their relative power for predicting the response variable. Calculated from the raw regression coefficients by multiplying them by the standard deviation of the corresponding explanatory variable. [Lewis-Beck, M. S., 1993, *Regression Analysis*, volume 2, Sage Publications, London.]

Beta distribution: A probability distribution, the shape of which depends on the values of two parameters. Can vary from a U-shaped distribution to a J-shaped distribution. Some examples are shown in Figure 8. [Evans, M., Hastings, N. and Peacock, B., 2000, *Statistical Distributions*, 3rd ed., John Wiley & Sons, New York.]

Beta error: Synonym for **type II error**.

Beta-geometric distribution: A probability distribution arising from assuming that the parameter of a geometric distribution has a beta distribution. The distribution has been used to model the number of menstrual cycles required to achieve pregnancy. [*Statistics in Medicine*, 1993, **12**, 867–80.]

Beta regression: An increasingly popular method for analyzing bounded data in medical research. In most cases, the method is applied to model outcomes such as proportions or patient reported outcomes lying in the interval zero to one. This form of regression is useful for two main reasons, because it can accommodate a broad range of probability distributions for the data and its ability to model-bounded data. [*Statistics in Medicine*, 2018, **27**, 1024–44.]

Between-groups sum of squares: *See* **analysis of variance**.

Bias: Deviation of results or inferences from the truth, or processes leading to such deviation. More specifically, the extent to which the statistical method used in a study does not estimate the quantity thought to be estimated or does not test the hypothesis to be tested. Bias can occur at any stage of the research process from the literature review through to the publication of results. Essentially a systematic error that skews all data. *See also* **ascertainment bias**, **recall bias**, **selection bias** and **biased estimator**. [*British Medical Journal*, 2002, **325**, 1437–8.]

Biased coin method: A method of random allocation sometimes used in a clinical trial in an attempt to avoid major inequalities in numbers of subjects allocated to the different treatments. At each point in the trial, the treatment with the fewest number of subjects thus far is assigned a probability greater than a half of being allocated the next subject. If the treatments have an equal number of subjects at any stage, then simple randomization is used to allocate the next subject. [*Statistics in Medicine*, 1986, **5**, 211–30.]

Biased estimator: An estimator of a parameter whose expected or average value is not equal to the true value of the parameter. The reason for sometimes using such estimators rather than those that are unbiased rests in their potential for leading to a value that is closer, on average, to the parameter being estimated than would be obtained from the latter. This is so because it is possible for the variance of such an estimator to be sufficiently smaller than the variance of one that is unbiased to more than compensate for the bias introduced. [Rawlings, J. O., Pantula, S. G. and Dickey, D. A., 2013, *Applied Regression Analysis: A Research Tool*, 2nd ed., Springer, New York.]

Biased estimator: Not always a disaster.

Bias/variance trade-off: A term that summarizes the fact that if you want less bias in an estimate of a model parameter, it usually costs you more variance.

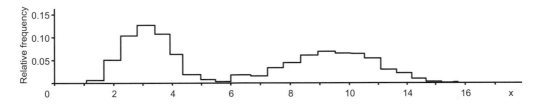

Figure 9 Bimodal probability and frequency distributions.

Big Mac index: An index that attempts to measure different aspects of the economy by comparing the cost of hamburgers between countries. [Hand, D. J., 2004, *Measurement Theory and Practice*, Arnold, London.]

Bilateral dichotomous data: Data generated when patients receive treatments on two organs or body parts, for example eyes, hips and joints. Ignoring the obvious dependence feature of such data can lead to very misleading estimates of treatment differences. [*Statistics in Medicine*, 2006, **25**, 2271–83.]

Bimodal distribution: A probability distribution, or a frequency distribution, with two modes. Figure 9 shows an example of each.

Bimodal distribution: Such distributions can be modelled using finite mixtures.

Binary sequence: A sequence whose elements take one of only two possible values, usually denoted 0 or 1. *See also* **Bernoulli sequence** and **binomial distribution**.

Binary variable: Observations that occur in one of two possible states, these often being labelled 0 and 1. Such data are encountered frequently in medical investigations; commonly occurring examples include dead/alive, improved/not improved and depressed/not depressed. Data involving this type of variable often require specialized techniques such as logistic regression for their analysis. *See also* **Bernoulli sequence**.

Binomial distribution: The probability distribution of the number of occurrences of a binary event in a series of n independent trials in which the

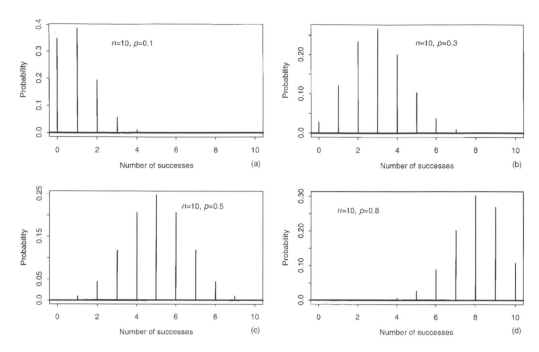

Figure 10 A number of binomial distributions.

probability of the occurrence of the event remains fixed at some value p. The mean of the distribution is np and the variance is $np(1 - p)$. A number of binomial distributions are displayed in Figure 10. [Evans, M., Hastings, N. and Peacock, B., 2000, *Statistical Distributions*, 3rd ed., John Wiley & Sons, New York.]

Bioassay: The process of evaluating the potency of a stimulus by analyzing the response it produces in biological organisms. Examples of a stimulus in this context are a drug, a hormone, radiation and an environmental effect. *See also* **probit** analysis. [Finney, D. J., 1978, *Statistical Methods in Biological Assay*, 3rd ed., Arnold, London.]

Bioavailability: The study of variables that influence and determine the amount of active drug that gets from the administered dose to the site of pharmacological action, as well as the rate at which it gets there. The extent and rate of absorption determine the bioavailability of a drug. [Chow, S. C. and Liu, J. P., 2008, *Design and Analysis of Bioavailability and Bioequivalence Studies*, 3rd ed., Chapman & Hall, Boca Raton, FL.]

Bioequivalence: Two drug products are bioequivalent if they will reach the same therapeutic effect or they are therapeutically equivalent and hence can be used interchangeably. [Chow, S. C. and Liu, J. P., 2008, *Design and Analysis of Bioavailability and Bioequivalence Studies*, 3rd ed., Chapman & Hall, Boca Raton, FL.]

Bioequivalence trials: Clinical trials carried out to compare two or more formulations of a drug containing the same active ingredient in order to determine whether the different formulations give rise to comparable blood levels.

[Chow, S. C. and Liu, J. P., 2008, *Design and Analysis of Bioavailability and Bioequivalence Studies*, 3rd ed., Chapman & Hall, Boca Raton, FL.]

Bioinformatics: A discipline of computational biology that encompasses mathematics, statistics, physics and chemistry and has as its aims exploring models for biological systems and creating tools that biologists can use to analyze data, for example, to assess the similarity between two or more DNA sequences. [*Nature Genetic Supplement*, 2003, **33**, 305–10.]

Biological assay: Synonym for **bioassay**.

Biological efficacy: The effect of treatment for all people who receive the therapeutic agent to which they were assigned. Measures the biological action of treatment among compliant people. [*European Respiratory Journal*, 2003, **22**, 575–675.]

Biological marker (biomarker): A characteristic that is objectively measured and evaluated as an indicator of normal biological processes, pathogenic processes or pharmacologic responses to a therapeutic intervention. Use of biomarkers may help to predict and monitor the clinical response to an intervention and they are often used as surrogate endpoints when measuring the clinical endpoint of interest is difficult. [*Pharmacoepidemiology and Drug Safety*, 2001, **10**, 497–508.]

Biometry: The application of statistical methods to the study of numerical data based on observation of biological phenomena.

Biostatistics: Strictly the branch of science that applies statistical methods to biological problems, although now used more often to include statistics applied to medicine and health sciences. [Rosner, B., 2015, *Fundamentals of Biostatistics*, 8th ed., Duxbury Press, MA.]

Bipolar factor: *See* **factor rotation**.

Birth-cohort study: A prospective study of people born in a defined period. For example, a study following up, perhaps for many years, all children born in a particular week, in a particular year, in respect of the possible effect of breastfeeding on adult intelligence. [*Paediatric and Perinatal Epidemiology*, 1992, **6**, 81–110.]

Birth–death ratio: The ratio of number of births to number of deaths within a given time in a population. According to the World Bank, for every 1,000 people in the world, an average of 7.75 people will die each year and 19.35 will be born, a ratio of 2.5 births for every death.

Birth defect registries: Organized databases containing information on individuals born with specified congenital disorders. Important in providing information that may help to prevent birth defects. [*International Journal of Epidemiology*, 1981, **10**, 247–52.]

Birth interval: The time interval between the completion of one pregnancy and the completion of the next. A study of families in part of Finland, for example, found that the average birth interval where the previous child survived until the birth of the next sibling was 33.2 months. [*Injury Prevention*, 2000, **6**, 219–22.]

Birth order: The ranking of siblings according to age, starting with the eldest in the family.

Birth rate: The number of births occurring in a region in a given time period divided by the size of the population of the region at the middle of the time period, usually expressed per 1,000 members of the population. For example, the birth rates for a number of countries in 1990 were as follows:

Country	Birth rate/1,000
Cambodia	40.6
China	20.2
Malaysia	28.9
Thailand	19.9

Birthweight: Infant's weight recorded at the time of birth. Low birthweight is defined as a value below 2,500 g; very low birthweight is defined as a value below 1,500 g.

Birthweight is an important predictor of an infant's future well-being; the mortality of babies varies considerably according to birthweight, with very high mortality rates among very small babies. The weight of a newborn infant depends on its growth rate and its gestational age when born. Any factor that shortens gestational age will reduce mean birthweight, but does not necessarily cause an intrauterine growth retardation. [*Lancet*, 1996, **348**, 1478–80.]

Biserial correlation coefficient: A coefficient measuring the association between a continuous variable and a binary variable. *See also* **point-biserial correlation**. [*Psychometrika*, 1963, **28**, 81–5.]

Bit: A unit of information consisting of one binary digit.

Bivariate distribution: A probability distribution describing the joint statistical behaviour of a pair of random variables, for example systolic blood pressure and the number of cigarettes smoked per day. A well-known example is the *bivariate normal distribution*, a distribution that involves five parameters, the mean of each variable, the variance of each variable, and the correlation between the variables. Figure 11 shows a number of examples of bivariate normal distributions. [Hutchinson, T. P. and Lai, C. D., 1990, *Continuous Bivariate Distributions, Emphasizing Applications*, Rumsby Scientific Press, Adelaide.]

Bivariate normal distribution: *See* **bivariate distribution**.

Bivariate survival data: Data in which two related survival times are of interest. For example, in familial studies of disease incidence rates, data may be available on the ages and causes of death of fathers and their sons. [*Statistics in Medicine*, 1993, **12**, 241–8.]

Blinding: A procedure used in clinical trials to avoid the possible bias that might be introduced if the patient and/or doctor knows which treatment the patient is receiving. If neither the patient nor the doctor is aware of which

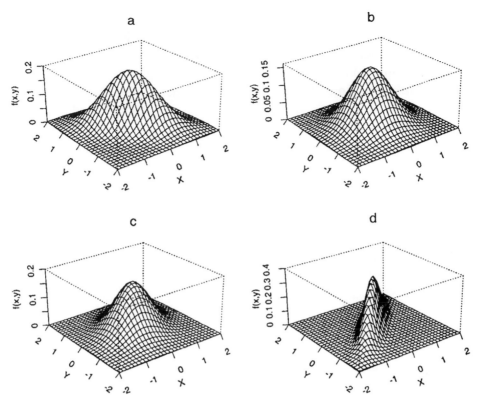

Figure 11 Perspective plots of four bivariate normal distributions each with zero means and unit standard deviations: (a) correlation is 0.6; (b) correlation is 0.0; (c) correlation is 0.3; (d) correlation is 0.9.

treatment has been given, then the trial is termed *double-blind*. If only one of the patient or doctor is unaware, then the trial is called *single-blind*. Clinical trials should use the maximum degree of blindness that is possible, although in some areas, for example surgery, it is often impossible for an investigation to be double-blind. Trials that are not double-blinded are more likely than blinded studies to demonstrate (falsely) a treatment effect in favour of the active intervention group. Although double-blinding is the gold standard for clinical trials, there is evidence that it is often not particularly effective, since both patients and their treating clinicians can frequently detect which treatment the patient is receiving. *See also* **sham procedures in medicine**. [Everitt, B. S. and Wessely, S., 2008, *Clinical Trials in Psychiatry*, 2nd ed., Wiley-Blackwell, Chichester.]

Blinding: Beware of overstated claims for blinding: the practice does not always match the intent. For example, in a double-blind trial of propranolol against placebo in patients who had recently had a heart attack, nearly 70% of physicians and over 80% of patients guessed correctly which substance had been administered.

Block: A term used in experimental design to refer to a homogeneous grouping of experimental units (often subjects) designed to enable the experimenter to isolate and, if necessary, eliminate, variability due to extraneous causes. *See also* **randomized block design**.

Block randomization: A random allocation procedure used to keep the number of subjects in the different groups of a `clinical trial` balanced closely at all times. For example, if subjects are considered in sets of four at a time, then there are six ways in which two treatments, *A* and *B*, can be allocated so that two subjects receive *A* and two receive *B*, namely:

1. *AABB*
2. *ABAB*
3. *ABBA*
4. *BBAA*
5. *BABA*
6. *BAAB*

If only these six combinations are used for allocating treatments to each block of four subjects, then the numbers in the two treatment groups can never differ by more than two. *See also* **biased coin method** and **minimization**. [*Controlled Clinical Trials*, 1988, **9**, 375–82.]

BLUE: Abbreviation for **best linear unbiased estimator**.

Blunder index: A measure of the number of gross errors made in a laboratory and detected by an external quality assessment exercise.

BMI: Abbreviation for **body mass index**.

Body mass index (BMI): An index that uses your height and weight to indicate whether your weight is 'healthy'. The index is given by weight in kilograms divided by the square of height in metres. Values below 18.5 indicate an underweight individual, values between 18.5 and 24.9 indicate an individual in the healthy weight range, between 25 and 29.9 suggests an individual is overweight and over 30 indicates an individual is obese. The index correlates with body fat content, a relationship that differs with age and gender. [*Statistical Methods in Medical Research*, 2018, **27**, 798–811.]

Bonferroni correction: A procedure for guarding against an increase in the `type I error` when performing multiple significance tests. To maintain the type I error at some selected value *a*, each of the *m* tests to be performed is judged against a significance level, *a/m*. For a small number (up to 5) of simultaneous tests, this method provides a simple and acceptable answer to the problem of multiple testing. It is, however, highly conservative and is not recommended if a large number of tests are to be applied, when one of the many other `multiple comparison tests` available is generally preferable. *See also* **least significant difference test**, **Scheffé's test** and **Newman–Keuls test**. [*British Medical Journal*, 1998, **316**, 1236–8.]

Bootstrap method: A method for estimating the possible `bias` and the precision of parameter estimates by repeatedly drawing random samples with replacement from the observations available. These *bootstrap samples* each provide an estimate of the parameter of interest, with a large number of them providing the required empirical distribution from which bias, precision and `confidence intervals` can be extracted. Such methods are applied in circumstances in which the form of the population from which the observed data have been drawn is unknown; they are particularly useful when very limited sample data are available and traditional parametric modelling and analysis are difficult to apply. *See also* **jackknife**. [*Statistical Science*, 1986, **1**, 54–77.]

Bootstrap samples: *See* **bootstrap method**.

Borrowing effect: A term used when abnormally low `standardized mortality rates` for one or more causes of death may be a reflection of an increase in the `proportional mortality ratios` for other causes of death. For example, in a study of vinyl chloride workers, the overall proportional mortality rate for cancer indicated approximately a 50% excess compared with cancer death rates in the male US population. (One interpretation of this is a possible deficit of non-cancer deaths due to the `healthy worker effect`.) Because the overall proportional mortality rate must by definition be equal to unity, a deficit in one type of mortality must entail a 'borrowing' from other causes.

Bowker's test for symmetry: A test that can be applied to square `contingency tables` to assess the hypothesis that the chance of being in cell *i,j* of the table is equal to the chance of being in cell *j,i*. In the case of a `two-by-two contingency table`, the test becomes `McNemar's test`. *See also* **marginal homogeneity**. [Everitt, B. S., 1992, *The Analysis of Contingency Tables*, 2nd ed., Chapman & Hall/ CRC, Boca Raton, FL.]

Box-and-whisker plot: A graphical method of displaying the important characteristics of a set of observations. The display is based on the `five-number summary` of the data, with the 'box' part covering the `interquartile range` and the 'whiskers' extending to include all but `outside observations`, these being indicated separately. Such diagrams are often particularly useful for comparing the characteristics of samples from different populations, as shown in Figure 12.

Box-counting method: A method for estimating `fractal dimension` of self-similar patterns in space that consists of plotting the number of `pixels` that intersect the pattern under consideration versus the length of the pixel unit. [Falconer, K., 2014, *Fractal Geometry*, 3rd ed., Wiley-Blackwell, Oxford.]

Box–Cox transformations: A family of data transformations designed to achieve normality. [Rawlings, J. O., Pantula, S. G. and Dickey, D. A., 2013, *Applied Regression Analysis: A Research Tool*, 2nd ed., Springer, New York.]

Box plot: Synonym for **box-and-whisker plot**.

Box's test: A test for assessing the equality of the variances in a number of populations that is less sensitive to departures from normality than `Bartlett's test`. *See also* **Hartley's test**.

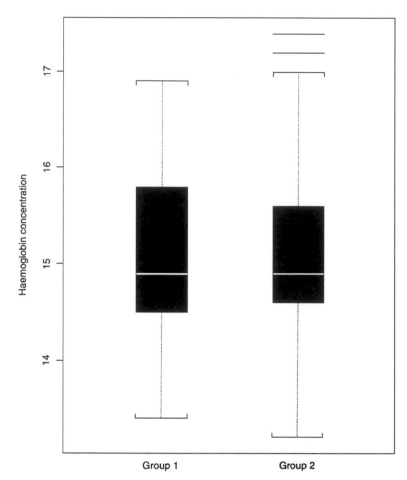

Figure 12 Box-and-whisker plot of haemoglobin concentration for two groups of men.

Branching process: A stochastic process in which individuals give rise to offspring, the distribution of descendants being likened to branches of a family tree. [Jagers, P., 1975, *Branching Processes with Biological Applications*, John Wiley & Sons, Chichester.]

Breadline index: An index of poverty that incorporates measures of unemployment, long-term illness and social class. [Gordon, D. and Pantazis, C. (eds.), 1997, *Breadline Britain in the 1990s*, Ashgate, Aldershot.]

Breakdown point: A measure of insensitivity of an estimator to multiple outliers in the data. Roughly, it is given by the smallest fraction of data contamination needed to cause an arbitrarily large change in the estimate. [*Computational Statistics*, 1996, **11**, 137–46.]

Breslow–Day test: A test of the null hypothesis of homogeneity of the odds ratio across a series of two-by-two contingency tables. [Breslow, N. E. and Day, N. E., 1957, *Statistical Methods in Cancer Research*, volume I: The Analysis of Case Control Studies, IARC, Lyon.]

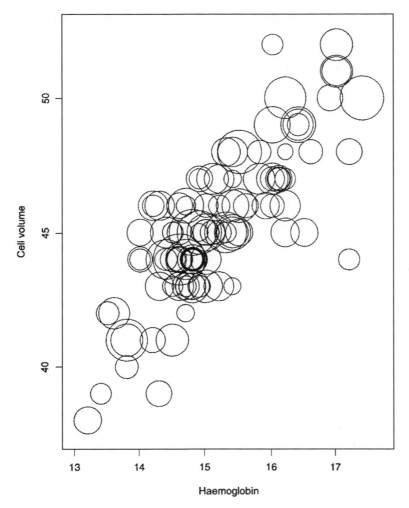

Figure 13 Bubble plot of haemoglobin concentration versus cell volume with radii of circles proportional to white blood count.

Bridging clinical trials: `Clinical trials` designed to evaluate whether a proposed dose of a particular drug for use in one population, for example, children, gives similar pharmacokinetic levels, or has similar effects on a surrogate marker as an established dose of the same drug used in another population, for example adults. [*Biometrics*, 2008, **64**, 1117–25.]

Brownian motion: A phenomenon first reported by an English botanist, Robert Brown, in 1827, when he observed that pollen particles in an aqueous suspension performed a continuous haphazard zigzag movement. It was only in 1905 that the motion could be explained by assuming that the particles are subject to continual bombardment of the molecules in the surrounding medium. [Bailey, N. T. J., 1990, *The Elements of Stochastic Processes with Applications to the Natural Sciences*, John Wiley & Sons, New York.]

Bubble plot: A method for displaying observations that involve three variable values. Two of the variables are used to form a `scatter diagram` and values of the third variable are represented by circles with differing radii centred at the appropriate position. An example is shown in Figure 13. [Everitt, B. S. and Rabe-Hesketh, S., 2001, *The Analysis of Medical Data using S-PLUS*, Springer, New York.]

Burdens of diseases: A name given to a concept dealing with a range of medical statistics that aim to give a comprehensive picture of how different diseases impact on society. The main burdens covered are mortality, morbidity and costs of care and treatment. The main interest is how the burdens of different diseases compare; for example, is heart disease a bigger killer than cancer. [*British Journal of Social and Preventative Medicine*, 1975, **29**, 222–7.]

Byte: A unit of information, as used in digital computers, equal to eight `bits`.

Calendarization: A generic term for **benchmarking**.

Calendar plot: A method of describing `compliance` for individual patients in a `clinical trial`, where the number of tablets taken per day are set in a calendar-like form (see Figure 14). *See also* **chronology plot.** [*Statistics in Medicine*, 1997, 16, 1653–64.]

Calibration: A procedure that enables a series of easily obtainable but possibly less precise measurements to be used in place of more expensive or more-difficult-to-obtain measurements of some quantity of interest. Suppose, for example, that there is a well-established, accurate method of measuring the concentration of a given chemical compound, but that it is too expensive and/or cumbersome for routine use. A cheap and easy-to-apply alternative is developed which is, however, known to be imprecise and possibly subject to `bias`. By using both methods over a range of concentrations of the compound, and applying `regression analysis` to the values from the cheap method and the corresponding values from the accurate method, a *calibration curve* can be constructed that may, in future applications, be used to read off estimates of the required concentration from the values given by the less involved, inaccurate method. [*International Statistical Institute*, 1991, **59**, 309–36.]

Calibration curve: *See* **calibration.**

California score: A score used in studies of sudden infant death syndrome that gives the number from eight adverse conditions present for a given infant. The events include fewer than 11 antenatal visits, male sex, birthweight under 3,000 g and mother under 25 years old.

Caliper matching: *See* **matching.**

Campbell collaboration: An international group of scientists whose mission is to promote access to systematic evidence of the effects of interventions in areas such as crime, social welfare, education and other social and behavioural sectors. [**www.campbellcollaboration.org**]

	Mon	Tue	Wed	Thu	Fri	Sat	Sun
						0	1
3	1	1	2	1	0	1	1
10	1	1	1	1	1	0	0
17	0	1	1	2	0	2	0
24	1	1	1	0	1	0	0
31	1						

Figure 14 Calendar plot of the number of tablets taken per day.
(Reproduced from *Statistics in Medicine* with permission of the publisher Wiley.)

Canonical correlation analysis: A method of analysis for investigating the relationship between two groups of variables by finding linear functions of one of the sets of variables which maximally correlate with linear functions of the variables in the other set. In many respects, the method can be viewed as an extension of `multiple linear regression` to situations involving more than a single response variable. Alternatively, it can be considered as analogous to `principal components analysis`, except that a correlation rather than a variance is maximized. A simple example of where this type of technique might be of interest is when the results of tests for, say, reading speed (x_1), reading power (x_2), arithmetical speed (y_1) and arithmetical power (y_2) are available from a sample of schoolchildren, and the question of interest is whether reading ability (measured by x_1 and x_2) is related to arithmetical ability (as measured by y_1 and y_2). [*Pain*, 1992, **51**, 67–73.]

Canonical correlation analysis: Results are often difficult to interpret, even by statisticians.

Capture–recapture sampling: A sampling scheme used in situations where the aim is to estimate the total number of individuals in a population. An initial sample is obtained and the individuals in that sample are marked or otherwise identified. A second sample is subsequently obtained independently, and it is noted how many individuals in that sample are marked. If the second sample is representative of the population as a whole, then the sample proportion of marked individuals should be about the same as the corresponding population proportion. From this relationship, the total number of individuals in the population can be estimated. Used originally to estimate the size of animal populations, the method is now also used to assess the size of many populations of great interest in medicine, for example the number of drug users in a particular area or the completeness of cancer registry data. [*Epidemiological Reviews*, 1995, **17**, 243–64.]

Care pathways: Longer `life expectancies` and medical advances have led to a steady increase in the number of individuals living with a chronic disease. The necessary coordination of the multidisciplinary care required for such patients had led to the

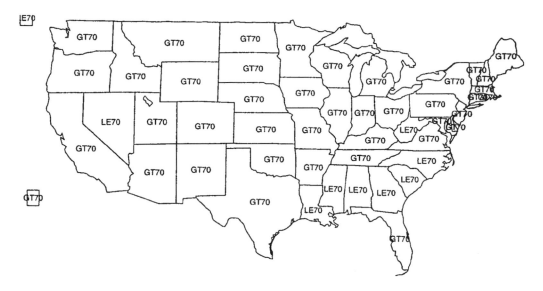

Figure 15 Cartogram of life expectancy in the USA by state. LE70 = 70 years or less, GT70 = more than 70 years.

concept of a care pathway, the aim of which is to enhance the quality of care by improving patient outcomes, promoting patient safety, increasing patient satisfaction and optimizing the use of resources. [*International Journal of Integrated Care*, 2012, **12**, e192.]

Carrier: A person that harbours a specific infectious agent in the absence of discernible clinical disease and serves as a potential source of infection. [*Acta Pathologica Microbiologica Scandinavica*, 1956, **39**, 107–8.]

Carry-over effects: *See* **crossover design**.

Cartogram: A diagram in which descriptive statistical information is displayed on a geographical map by means of shading, by using a variety of different symbols or by some more involved procedure. Figure 15 shows a simple example and Figure 16 shows a more complex example. *See also* **disease mapping**.

Case: A term used most often in `epidemiology` for a person in the population or study group identified as having the disease or condition of interest.

Case–cohort study: A study that has the same aims as a `cohort study` but tries to achieve them at less expense by following all cohort members for disease outcomes but following only a sample of members for all other information of interest. For example, only 20% of the cohort members in an investigation of breast cancer may have the full range of covariates of interest measured. [*American Journal of Epidemiology*, 1990, **131**, 169–76.]

Case-control study: *See* **retrospective study**.

Case-crossover design: A procedure for the analysis of transient effects on the risk of acute illness events that uses cases as their own controls. The idea behind the method is to ask a patient whether he or she was engaged in some activity or

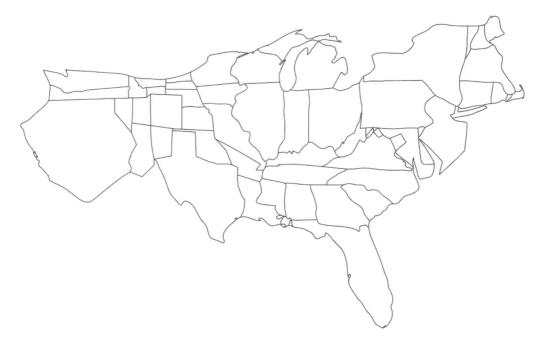

Figure 16 A 1996 US population cartogram (all states are resized relative to their population).

exposed to a suspected cause immediately before the event, and to compare the response to the usual frequency with which he or she engages in the activity or is exposed. In this way, each case is its own control. The hypothesis that vigorous exercise predisposes to heart attacks, for example, might be investigated by such a design, with cases being asked about their usual frequency of taking vigorous exercise and about whether they were engaged in such activity immediately before their heart attack. [*American Journal of Epidemiology*, 1991, **133**, 144–53.]

Case-fatality rate: The probability of death amongst diagnosed cases of a disease. Specifically defined as number of deaths due to the disease in a specified time period divided by the number of cases of the disease at the beginning of the period. Typically used in acute infectious diseases such as AIDS, although the use of a survivorship table is often preferable. Not so useful for chronic diseases because the period from onset to death is typically long and variable. [Morton, R. F., Hebel, J. R. and McCarter, R. J., 2011, *A Study Guide to Epidemiology and Biostatistics*, 7th ed., Jones & Bartlett, Burlington, MA.]

Case-heterogeneity study: A procedure for the estimation of relative risks not against a set of non-diseased population referents but against a set of subjects with other diseases, some of which may also have an association with the same exposure factors or their correlates. [*Statistics in Medicine*, 1986, **5**, 49–60.]

Case mix: The characteristics of the patients and/or the medical problems treated by an individual clinician, hospital or clinic.

Case–parent–triad design: A design useful for studying genetic risk factors in reproductive `epidemiology`. The central idea of the design is to use parents of affected children to serve as genetic controls. [*International Journal of Epidemiology*, 2002, **31**, 669–78.]

Case series: A method that is typically used to evaluate the association between a transient exposure and an acute event, using only cases. The method is self-controlled because time-invariant confounders, such as sex, location, genetics and underlying state of health are controlled for implicitly. [*Biometrics*, 1995, **51**, 228–35.]

Catalytic epidemic models: Models concerned with the age distribution at attack of infectious disease. The simplest such model assumes that a constant force of infection acts upon members of a susceptible population. More generally, the force of infection is allowed to be a function of the age of a susceptible individual. [*Applied Statistics*, 1974, **23**, 330–9.]

Catchment area: A region from which the clients of a particular clinic or hospital are drawn.

Categorical variable: A variable that gives the appropriate label of an observation after allocation to one of several possible categories, for example gender: male or female; marital status: married, single or divorced; blood group: A, B, AB or O. Categorical variables separate observations into groups. The categories are often given numerical labels, but for this type of data these have no numerical significance. *See also* **binary variable**, **continuous variable** and **measurement scale**. [Altman, D. G., 2018, *Practical Statistics for Medical Research*, Chapman & Hall/CRC, Boca Raton, FL.]

Categorizing continuous variables: A procedure common in medical research in which continuous variables are converted into categorical variables by grouping values into two or more categories, for example age might become 'young' (<40) and 'old' (≥ 40). The use of such grouping for descriptive purposes is probably unobjectionable, but when carried forward to data analysis it can cause serious problems and should be avoided since, in essence, the procedure introduces an extreme form of measurement error. [Altman, D. G., 2018, *Practical Statistics for Medical Research*, Chapman & Hall/CRC, Boca Raton, FL.]

Categorizing continuous variables: Although seemingly very popular with clinical researchers, a procedure that is best avoided.

Causality: The relating of causes to the effects they produce. Many investigations in medicine seek to establish causal links between events, for example that receiving treatment *A* causes patients to live longer when compared with taking treatment *B*. In general, the strongest claims to have established causality come from data collected in experimental studies. Relationships established in `observational studies` may be very suggestive of a causal link, but they are almost always open to alternative explanations. *See also* **Hill's criteria of causality**. [*American Journal of Epidemiology*, 1991, **133**, 635–45.]

Causal mediation analysis: A method that seeks to decompose the effect of a treatment or exposure among multiple possible paths and provide casually interpretable path-specific effect estimates. The goal of such an analysis is to illuminate the mechanisms through which the exposure affects the outcome. The simplest example of such an analysis is when the exposure effect is apportioned between the direct effect and the indirect effect of a single mediator. *See also* **path analysis**. [*Statistical Science*, 2010, **25**, 51–71.]

Causal risk difference: The difference between the rate of disease that would have been observed if the entire study population had been exposed and the rate of disease that would have been observed if the entire study population had been unexposed.

Cause-specific death rate: A death rate calculated for people dying from a particular disease. For example, the following are the rates per 1,000 people for three disease classes for developed and developing countries in 1985:

	C1	C2	C3
Developed	0.5	4.5	2.0
Developing	4.5	1.5	0.6

C1 = Infectious and parasitic diseases; C2 = Circulatory diseases; C3 = Cancer.

See also **crude death rate** and **age-specific death rate**. [Parkin, M., Whelan, S., Ferlay, J., Teppo, L. and Thomas, D. B., 2003, *Cancer Incidence in Five Continents*, volume VIII, IARC Scientific Publications, Lyon.]

Ceiling effect: A term used to describe what happens when many subjects in a study have scores on a variable that are at or near the possible upper limit (ceiling). Such an effect may cause problems for some types of analysis because it reduces the possible amount of variation in the variable. A medical example is the use of morphine where increasing the dose leads to smaller and smaller gains in pain relief. The converse, or *floor effect*, causes similar problems. [*Annals of Thoracic Surgery*, 2002, **73**, 1222–8.]

Cell-cycle models: Mathematical models for the study of the variation in the cell-cycle time and phase durations. [*Acta Biotheoretica*, 1995, **43**, 3–25.]

Censored regression models: A general class of models for analyzing truncated and censored data where the range of the dependent variable is constrained, for example, below or above a certain threshold value. [*Statistics in Medicine*, 2018, **3**, 143–52.]

Censoring: The loss of subject from a study before the event of interest has occurred. Arises most often in studies of survival times when, at the end of the study, some patients remain alive. The survival time of these patients is known only to be longer than the time they have been observed (right-censored). Data containing censored observations need appropriate techniques for their analysis, for example

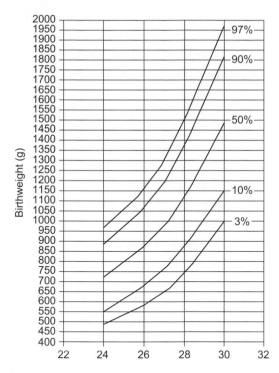

Figure 17 Centile reference chart for birthweight for gestational age.

Cox's proportional hazards model. [Collett, D., 2015, *Modelling Survival Data in Medical Research*, 3rd ed., Chapman & Hall/CRC, London.]

Census: A study that involves making observations of every member of a population of interest. Intended originally for the purposes of taxation and military service, censuses are now used to provide the facts essential to governmental policymaking, planning and administration. Age, birth date, occupation, national origin and marital status are some of the variables generally recorded. [Garoogian, D. (ed.), 2003, *The American Tally*, Grey House Publishing, Amenia, NY.]

Centile: Synonym for **percentile**.

Centile reference charts: Charts used in medicine to observe clinical measurements on individual patients in the context of population values. If the population `centile` corresponding to the subject's value is atypical, then this may indicate an underlying pathological condition. The chart can also provide a background with which to compare the measurement as it changes over time. An example is given in Figure 17. [*Statistics in Medicine*, 1996, **15**, 2657–68.]

Centralized database: A `database` held and maintained in a central location, particularly in a `multicentre study`.

Central limit theorem: A theorem that asserts that the sum of a large number of random variables is distributed approximately normally, no matter what the probability distribution of the original variables. Important to statistical theory because it provides the general conditions under which the distribution of an arithmetic mean is approximated by the `normal distribution`. The theorem allows the use of the `normal distribution` in creating `confidence intervals` and hypothesis testing. [Altman, D. G., 2018, *Practical Statistics for Medical Research*, Chapman & Hall/CRC, Boca Raton, FL.]

Central range: The range within which the central 90% of values of a set of observations lie.

Central tendency: A property of the frequency distribution of a variable, usually measured by statistics such as the mean, median and mode.

CFA: Abbreviation for **confirmatory factor analysis**.

Chain-binomial models: Models arising in the mathematical theory of infectious diseases that postulate that at any stage in an `epidemic` there are a certain number of infected individuals and susceptible individuals, and that it is reasonable to suppose that the latter will yield a fresh crop of cases at the next stage, the number of new cases having a `binomial distribution`. This results in a chain of binomial distributions, the actual probability of a new infection at any stage depending on the numbers of infected individuals and susceptible individuals at the previous stage. [Bailey, N. T. J., 1975, *The Mathematical Theory of Infectious Diseases*, Arnold, London.]

Chain-of-events data: Data on a succession of events that can only occur in a prescribed order. One goal in the analysis of this type of data is to determine the distribution of times between successive events. [*Biometrics*, 1999, **55**, 178–87.]

Chain referral sampling: Synonymous with **snowball sampling**.

Chains of infection: A description of the course of an infection among a set of individuals. The susceptible individuals infected by direct contact with the introductory cases are said to make up the first generation of cases; the susceptible individuals infected by direct contact with the first generation are said to make up the second generation, and so on. The enumeration of the number of cases in each generation is called an *epidemic chain*. Thus, the sequence 1–2–1–0 denotes a chain consisting of one introductory case, two first-generation cases, one second-generation case and no cases in later generations. A concrete example is provided by the transmission of HIV by unprotected sexual intercourse between, say, men from one area of the world and women in another region. [*Proceedings of the National Academy of Science of the United States of America*, 2003, **100**, 11143–7.]

Change point studies: Studies involving chronologically ordered data collected over a period of time during which it is known (or suspected) that there has been a change in the underlying data-generation mechanism. Interest then lies in making inferences about the time in the sequence that the change occurred. [*International Statistical Institute*, 1980, **48**, 83–93.]

Change scores: Scores obtained by subtracting a post-treatment value on some response variable from the value pre-treatment. Often used as the basis of analysis for a pre–post study but known to be less powerful than using `analysis of` covariance of post-treatment scores with pre-treatment as a covariate. *See also* **adjusting for baseline**. [Senn, S., 2008, *Statistical Issues in Drug Development*, 2nd ed., John Wiley & Sons, Chichester.]

Chance events: According to Cicero, these are events that occurred or will occur in ways that are uncertain; events that may happen, may not happen, or may happen in some other way. Cicero's characterization of such events is close to one dictionary definition of chance, namely 'the incalculable element in existence that renders events unpredictable'. But for Leucippus (circa 450 BC) the operation of chance was associated with some hidden cause and such a view was held widely in the Middle Ages where chance had no place in the universe, rather than that all events were thought of as predetermined by God or by extrinsic causes determined by God. But in the twentieth century, the deterministic view of the Universe was overthrown by the successful development of quantum mechanics with its central tenet being that it is impossible to predict exactly the outcome of an atomic system and where this uncertainty is not due to measurement error or experimental clumsiness but is a fundamental aspect of the basic physical laws themselves. [Everitt, B. S., 2008, *Chance Rules*, 2nd ed., Springer, New York.]

Chaos: Apparently random behaviour exhibited by a deterministic system. The concept has been used in medicine in investigations of measles `epidemics`. [Gleik, J., 1987, *Chaos*, Sphere Books, London.]

Chaos: Said to have been discovered in the 1970s, although Clerk Maxwell was well aware of its consequences nearly 150 years earlier.

Child death rate: The number of deaths of children aged 1–14 years in a given year per 1,000 or per 100,000 children in this age group. For example, in Massachusetts, USA in 1997, the rate per 100,000 was 15, and in Alaska in the same period it was 42.

Chi-squared distribution: The distribution of the sum of squares of a number (n) of normal variables each with zero mean and standard deviation one. The shape of the distribution depends on n, as shown in Figure 18. Important as the distribution (in large samples) of the `chi-squared test`. [Evans, M., Hastings, N. and Peacock, B., 2000, *Statistical Distributions*, 3rd ed., John Wiley & Sons, New York.]

Chi-squared goodness-of-fit test: *See* **chi-squared test**.

Chi-squared test: Most commonly used to refer to the test of the independence of the two categorical variables forming a `contingency table`, although the test is used in several other ways, for example to assess the fit of a theoretical `probability distribution` to observed data, when it is generally referred to as the *chi-squared goodness-of-fit test*. The test is based on squared differences between the observed and `expected frequencies`. [Greenwood, P. E. and Nikulin, M. S., 1996, *A Guide to Chi-Squared Testing*, John Wiley & Sons, New York.]

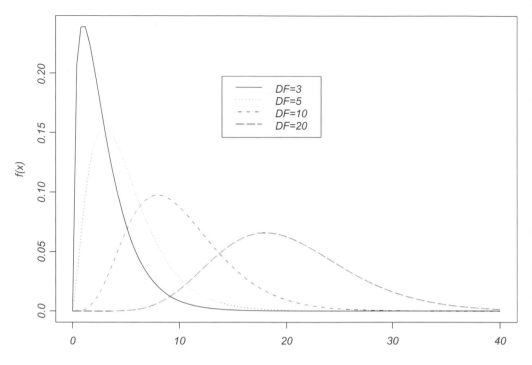

Figure 18 Chi-squared distributions for different parameter values. DF, degrees of freedom.

Chi-squared test for trend: A test applied to a two-dimensional `contingency table` in which one variable has two categories and the other has k ordered categories to assess whether there is a difference in the trend of the proportions in the two groups. The result of using the ordering in this way is a test that has more `power` for detecting departures from the null hypothesis than using the `chi-squared test` for independence. [Everitt, B. S., 1992, *The Analysis of Contingency Tables*, 2nd ed., Chapman & Hall/CRC, Boca Raton, FL.]

Chloropleth mapping: Synonymous with **disease mapping**.

Chow test: A test of the equality of two independent set of regression coefficients under the assumption of normally distributed error. [*Biometrical Journal*, 1996, **38**, 819–28.]

Chronic disease models: Chronic diseases are diseases of long duration and generally slow progression. Because of the long natural history of such diseases there is more potential to interact with other diseases, risk factor exposures and age-related declines in physiology. The possibility of multiple age-dependent interactions with the chronic disease process leads to models for such processes having a number of statistical problems. [*Global Journal of Heath Science*, 2015, **7**, 210–27.]

Chronology plot: A method of describing `compliance` in individual patients taking part in a `clinical trial` by plotting times when they take their tablets over the course of the study. See Figure 19 for an example. *See also* **calendar plot**. [*Statistics in Medicine*, 1997, **16**, 1653–64.]

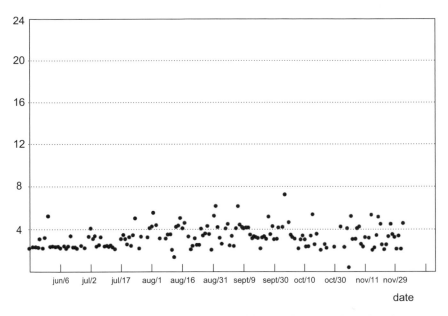

Figure 19 Chronology plot of times that a tablet is taken in a clinical trial.
(Reproduced from *Statistics in Medicine* with permission of the publisher Wiley.)

Chronomedicine: The study of the effects of circadian and other natural time structures on health, disease risk, etc. [*Annual Review of Physiology*, 1969, **31**, 675–725.]

C-Index: Synonym for **concordance index**.

Circadian variation: The variation that takes place in variables such as blood pressure and body temperature over a 24-hour period. Such variations may arise directly from the effects of the varying levels of electromagnetic radiation from the sun at different times of the day. In addition, many living organisms have evolved internally generated rhythms that do not depend entirely on external stimuli. *See also* **seasonal variation**. [*Cell*, 1994, **78**, 261–4.]

Class frequency: The number of observations in a class interval of the observed frequency distribution of a variable.

Classification and regression trees (CART): An alternative to procedures such as `multiple linear regression` and `logistic regression` for investigating the relationship between a response variable and a set of explanatory variables. The essential feature of this approach is the repeated division of the observations into smaller and smaller groups within which the response variable becomes more and more homogeneous. In this way, a tree structure is generated. An example is shown in Figure 20. Various procedures are available to help decide when further division is unnecessary. Binary response variables lead to what are known as *classification trees*, and continuous response variables lead to *regression trees*. [Everitt, B. S., 2003, *Modern Medical Statistics*, Arnold, London.]

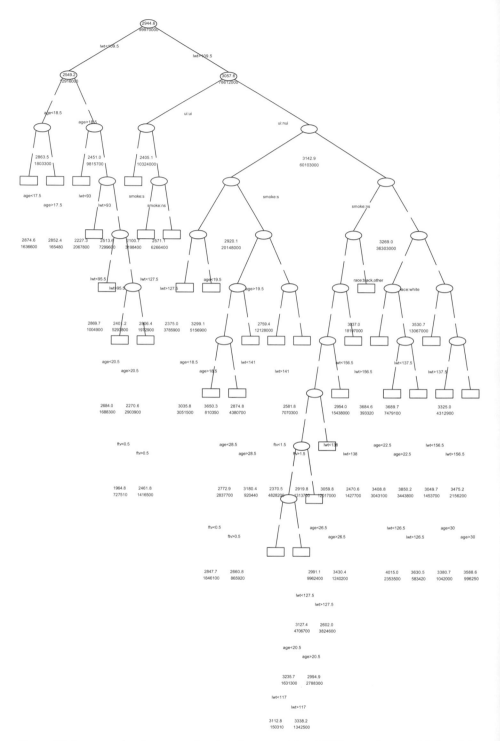

Figure 20 An example of a regression tree from applying CART procedures to birthweight of babies.

Classification and regression trees: The seductive diagrams that result from this approach should not cloud the fact that it remains largely exploratory.

Classification of medical and surgical procedures: Classification designed to facilitate statistical analysis, with the structure and composition of categories reflecting their frequency of occurrence and surgical importance. [World Health Organization, 1978, *International Classification of Procedures in Medicine*, World Health Organization, Geneva.]

Classification rule: *See* discriminant analysis.

Classification tree: *See* classification and regression trees.

Class intervals: The intervals of the frequency distribution of a set of observations.

Clemmesen's hook: A phenomenon sometimes observed when interpreting parameter estimates from age-period-cohort analysis, where rates increase to some maximum but then fall back slightly before continuing their upward trend. [*Anticancer Research*, 1995, **15**, 511–15.]

Clinical endpoint: A characteristic or variable that reflects how a patient feels, functions or survives. True clinical endpoints may be difficult to measure or may be affected by concomitant medications or competing risks from comorbidity, in which case a surrogate endpoint may be preferred.

Clinical epidemiology: The application of methods derived from epidemiology and other fields to the study of clinical phenomena, particularly diagnosis, treatment decisions and outcomes. [Fletcher, R. H., Fletcher, S. W. and Wagner, E. H., 2013, *Clinical Epidemiology: The Essentials*, 5th ed., Williams & Wilkins, Baltimore, MD.]

Clinical prediction models: Models for predicting the natural course of diseases or the response of patients to healthcare interventions, with regard to specific endpoints and observable characteristics. For example, clinicians and others may be interested in assessing the risk of dying within a particular time of undergoing a heart bypass operation. [Steyerberg, E. W., 2008, *Clinical Prediction Models: A Practical Approach to Development, Validation, and Updating*, Springer, New York.]

Clinical prior: *See* prior distributions.

Clinical signals: Signals obtained when human subjects are monitored by measuring electrical activity in a particular part of the body; examples are electrical activity from the brain (EEG) and from the heart (ECG). Time series are usually used to analyze clinical signals in hospitals and often provide life-saving information. [*Statistical Methods in Medical Research*, 1996, **5**, 51–66.]

Clinical trial: A prospective study involving human subjects designed to determine the effectiveness of a treatment, a surgical procedure, or a therapeutic regimen administered to patients with a specific disease. There is a well-established categorization of such studies into the following types:

- *Phase I study:* Initial clinical trial on a new compound, usually conducted among healthy volunteers with a view to assessing safety.

- *Phase II study:* Once a drug has been established as safe in a phase I study, the next stage is to conduct a clinical trial in patients to determine the optimum dose and to assess the efficacy of the compound.
- *Phase III study:* Large multicentre comparative clinical trials to demonstrate the safety and efficacy of the new treatment with respect to the standard treatments available. These are the studies that are needed to support product licence applications.
- *Phase IV study:* Studies conducted after a drug is marketed to provide additional details about its safety, efficacy and usage profile. *See also* **high-risk trials** and **vulnerable-population trials.** [Everitt, B. S. and Wessely, S., 2008, *Clinical Trials in Psychiatry*, 2nd ed., Oxford University Press, Oxford.]

Clinical trial: About 8,000 trials are carried out each year. The randomized clinical trial is probably the greatest contribution by statisticians to medical research.

Clinical trial protocol: A guideline for the conduct of a `clinical trial` that describes in a clear and detailed manner how the trial is to be performed so that all the investigators are aware of the procedures to be used. Particularly important in `multicentre studies`. [Everitt, B. S. and Wessely, S., 2008, *Clinical Trials in Psychiatry*, 2nd ed., Oxford University Press, Oxford.]

Clinical trial simulator: A computer program which can be used to model real-world `clinical trials`, and which is capable of rendering the implications of different designs and analysis decisions more tangible to individuals whose background and primary interests lie in medicine rather than statistics. See **www.certara.com/trial-simulator**

Clinical trials quality control: Procedures for monitoring the data collected in possibly complex `clinical trials` to prevent the possibility of errors arising in the data from honest mistakes, sloppiness or even, in rare cases, deliberate fraud. *See also* **audit in clinical trials**. [*Controlled Clinical Trials*, 1981, **1**, 327–32.]

Clinical versus statistical significance: The distinction between the possible clinical importance of results obtained in a medical investigation as opposed to the statistical significance obtained by applying some statistical test. With large samples, for example, very small differences that have little or no clinical importance may turn out to be statistically significant. The practical implications of any finding in a medical investigation must be judged on clinical as well as statistical grounds. [Ward, H. et al., 2019, *Oxford Handbook of Epidemiology for Clinicians,* Oxford University Press, Oxford.]

Clinical versus statistical significance: Beware the researcher who tries to convince you that a difference of 4 mm Hg in blood pressure between two groups with $P < 0.05$ is of any clinical relevance. With large samples, even tiny differences will be statistically significant.

Clinimetrics: The study of indices and rating scales used to describe or measure symptoms, physical signs and other clinical phenomena in clinical medicine. [*Psychotherapy and Psychosomatics*, 2004, **73**, Special Issue.]

Clinstat Guidelines: Advice on interim data monitoring in `clinical trials` for `data monitoring committees`. The advice is as follows. The process of examining and analyzing data accumulating in a clinical trial, either formally or informally, can introduce bias. Therefore, all interim analyses, formal or informal, by any study participant, sponsor staff member, or data monitoring group should be described in full, even if the treatment groups were not identified. The need for statistical adjustment because of such analyses should be addressed. Minutes of meetings of a data monitoring group may be useful (and may be requested by the review division). [Ellenberg, S. S., Fleming, T. R. and DeMets, D. L., 2002, *Data Monitoring Committees in Clinical Trials*, Wiley, New York.]

Clonogenic assay: An `assay` designed to predict the chemosensitivity of a patient's tumour. A portion of the tumour is disaggregated and then planted in single-cell suspension. A proportion of the tumour cells divide and multiply into colonies that can be counted after a fixed time of growth. The inhibition of formation of these colonies by a chemotherapeutic agent suggests that this agent may also be of use in the treatment of the patient. [*Proceedings of the Fifth NCI-EORTC Symposium on New Drugs in Cancer Therapy*, 1986, Amsterdam, the Netherlands.]

Closed and open birth interval data: The lengths of the 'closed' intervals from the ith to the $(i + 1)$th birth and of the 'open' intervals since the most recent birth for women who have had the same number of children. Considered useful indicators of current changes in natality patterns. *See also* **birth interval**. [*Journal of the American Statistical Society*, 1970, **65**, 678–93.]

Closed and open populations: A closed population adds no new members over time, and loses members only to death, whereas an open population may gain numbers over time, through immigration or birth, and lose members who are still alive through emigration.

Closed population: *See* **closed and open populations**.

Cluster analysis: A set of methods for constructing a (hopefully) sensible and informative classification of an initially unclassified set of data, using the variable values observed on each individual. *See also* **agglomerative hierarchical clustering methods, K-means cluster analysis** and **finite-mixture distribution**. [Everitt, B. S., Landau, S., Leese, M. and Stahl, D., 2011, *Cluster Analysis*, 5th ed., John Wiley & Sons, Chichester]

Clustered data: A term applied both to data in which the sampling units (usually people) are grouped into clusters sharing some common feature, for example animal litters, families or geographical regions, and to `longitudinal data`, in which a cluster is defined by a set of repeated measurements made on the same individual. A distinguishing feature of such data is that they tend to exhibit intracluster correlation, which needs to be accounted for in any analysis. Methods of analysis that ignore this aspect of the data are inadequate and will usually give standard error estimates for model parameters that are too low. *See also* **multilevel models**, **mixed-effects models**, **marginal models** and **generalized estimating equations**. [*Statistics in Medicine*, 1992, **11**, 67–100.]

Clustering: Most commonly used for the irregular grouping of events in either space or time or simultaneously in both space and time, which may demand investigation to identify a possible causal agent. *See also* **disease clusters** and **scan statistics**. [*Journal of Chronic Diseases*, 1980, **33**, 703–12.]

Cluster randomization: The random allocation of groups or clusters of individuals, for example families, hospital wards, classrooms, rather than individuals, in the formation of treatment groups. Although not as statistically efficient as individual randomization, the procedure frequently offers important economic, feasibility or ethical advantages. [Donner, A. and Klar, N., 2010, *Cluster Randomization Trials in Health Research*, John Wiley & Sons, New York.]

Cluster sampling: A method of sampling in which the members of a population are arranged in groups (the clusters). A number of clusters are selected at random and those chosen are then subsampled. The clusters generally consist of natural groupings, for example families, hospitals, schools, etc. *See also* **random sample**, **area sampling** and **quota sample**. [Levy, P. S. and Lemeshow, S., 2008, *Sampling of Populations: Methods and Applications*, 4th ed., John Wiley & Sons, New York.]

C_{max}: A measure traditionally used to compare treatments in `bioequivalence trials`. The measure is simply the highest recorded response value for a subject. *See also* **area under curve**, **response feature analysis** and T_{max}.

Coale and Trussell model: A model for describing the variation in the age pattern of human fertility that states that marital fertility is the product of natural fertility and fertility control. [*Journal of Mathematical Biology*, 1983, **18**, 201–11.]

Coarse data: A term sometimes used when the exact values in a data set are not observed. Examples include data containing `missing values` and data containing censored observations.

Cochran-Armitage test: Commonly used in both `epidemiology` and genetics to test for linear trend in two-way tables with a binary outcome, for example, testing the association between dose and treatment effect in `clinical trials` and the associations between exposure and a binary outcome in `observational studies`. [*Biometrics*, 1955, **11**, 375–86.]

Cochrane central register of controlled trials: Part of the `Cochrane Collaboration`, this register contains a comprehensive source of records relating to controlled trials of healthcare interventions. As of January 2004, the register contains over 400,000 citations of reports of randomized trials and other studies potentially relevant for inclusion in systematic reviews of healthcare interventions. [*Evaluation and Health Professions*, 2002, **25**, 38–64.]

Cochrane Collaboration: An international network of individuals committed to preparing, maintaining and disseminating `systematic reviews` of the effects of healthcare. The collaboration is guided by six principles: collaboration, building on people's existing enthusiasm and interests, minimizing unnecessary duplication, avoiding bias, keeping evidence up to date, and ensuring access to the evidence. Most concerned with evidence from randomized clinical trials. *See also* **evidence-based medicine**. [Higgins, J. P. T. et al. (eds.), 2019, *Cochrane Handbook for Systematic Reviews of Interventions*, 2nd ed., John Wiley & Sons, Chichester.]

> **Cochrane Collaboration:** An extremely important contribution to improving the standards of clinical trials and systematic reviews.

Cochran's C-test: A test to see whether the variances of a number of populations are equal. *See also* **Bartlett's test**, **Box's test** and **Hartley's test**. [Fleiss, J. L., Levin, B. and Cho Paik, M., 2003, *Statistical Methods for Rates and Proportions*, 2nd ed., Wiley, New York.]

Cochran's Q-test: A procedure for assessing the hypothesis of no interobserver bias in situations where a number of raters judge the presence or absence of some characteristic on a number of subjects. Essentially a generalized McNemar's test. [*Biometrika*, 1950, **37**, 256–66.]

Coefficient of alienation: A name sometimes used for one minus the square of the correlation coefficient of two variables. *See also* **coefficient of determination**.

Coefficient of concordance: A coefficient used to assess the degree of agreement among raters ranking *n* individuals according to some specific considerations. [Sprent, P., 1981, *Quick Statistics*, Penguin Books, London.]

Coefficient of determination: The square of the correlation coefficient between two variables. Gives the proportion of the variation in one variable that is accounted for by the other. [Rawlings, J. O., Pantula, S. G. and Dickey, D. A., 2013, *Applied Regression Analysis: A Research Tool*, 2nd ed., Springer, New York.]

Coefficient of inbreeding: *See* **Wright's inbreeding coefficient**.

Coefficient of kinship: The probability that two homologous genes drawn at random, one from each of the two parents, will be identical and therefore homozygous in an offspring. [*Circulation*, 2004, **110**, 3143–8.]

Coefficient of variation: A measure of spread for a set of data, defined as

$100 \times$ standard deviation/mean

Proposed originally as a way of comparing the variability in different distributions, but found to be sensitive to errors in the mean.

Cohen's d: A standardized mean difference estimate calculated as the difference between two group means divided by a standard deviation pooled across both groups (or where homogeneity of variance can be assumed the standard deviation of one of the groups). The statistic is often used as a measure of effect size for

Figure 21 Time series for daily mortality and sulphur dioxide (SO₂) concentration in London during the winter months of 1958.

continuous response variables in a `meta-analysis`. [Rosenthal, R., 1991, *Meta-Analytic Procedures for Social Research*, Sage Publications, Thousand Oaks, CA.]

Coherence: A term used most often for the strength of the association between two `time series`. Figure 21, for example, shows daily mortality and sulphur dioxide concentration time series for London during the winter months of 1958; the obvious question is whether the pollution was in any way affecting mortality, and answering this would involve calculating some measure of the coherence of the two series. The relationship is generally measured by the time series analogue of the `correlation coefficient`, although the result is no longer a single number but a function. [Chatfield, C., 2019, *The Analysis of Time Series: An Introduction*, 7th ed., Chapman & Hall/CRC, Boca Raton, FL.]

Cohort: *See* **cohort study.**

Cohort component method: A widely used method for forecasting the age- and sex-specific population in future years in which the initial population is stratified by age and by sex and projections are generated by application of survival ratios and birth rates, followed by an additive adjustment for net migration. [*Journal of the American Planning Association*, 1959, **1,** 45–64.]

Cohort study: An investigation in which a group of individuals (the *cohort*) is identified and followed prospectively, perhaps for many years, and their subsequent medical history recorded. An example is the 1970 British Cohort Study in which data were collected about the births and the families of babies born in the United Kingdom between 5 and 11 April 1970. The aim was to look at the sociological and biological characteristics of the mother in relation to neonatal `mortality rates`. The cohort may be subdivided at the onset into groups with different characteristics, for example exposed and not exposed to some risk factor, and at some later stage a comparison made of the `incidence rate` of a particular disease in each group. As described, this type of study is perhaps more properly termed a *concurrent cohort study*, in contrast to a *historical cohort study* (or *nonconcurrent cohort study*) where data on exposure and occurrence of disease are collected after the events have taken place. For example, in an investigation of the possible link between exposure to a certain chemical and lung cancer, the investigator might use employee records dating back many years to identify comparable employees who did and did not handle that chemical. The price for this convenience is both a greater chance of `bias` (including in some instances, uncertainty that exposure preceded disease), and potential knowledge of disease status when selecting for exposure. *See also* **prospective study**. [Morton, R. F., Hebel, J. R. and McCarter, R. J., 1990, *A Study Guide to Epidemiology and Biostatistics*, 3rd ed., Aspen, Gaithersburg, MD.]

Coincidences: Surprising co-occurrence of events perceived as meaningfully related with no apparent causal connection. Such events abound in everyday life and are often the source of some amazement. As pointed out by Sir Ronald Fisher, however, 'the one chance in a million will undoubtedly occur, with no less and no more than its appropriate frequency, however surprised we may be that it should occur to us'. [Everitt, B. S., 2008, *Chance Rules*, 2nd ed., Springer, New York.]

Collapsing categories: A procedure often applied to `contingency tables` in which two or more row or column categories are combined, often so as to yield a smaller table in which there are a larger number of observations in particular cells. Not to be recommended in general since it can give rise to misleading conclusions. *See also* **categorizing continuous variables** and **Simpson's paradox**. [Feinstein, A. R., 1996, *Multivariable Analysis*, New York University Press, New York.]

Collinearity: *See* **multicollinearity**.

Commensurate variables: Variables that are on the same scale or expressed in the same units, for example systolic and diastolic blood pressure.

Common factor: *See* **factor analysis**.

Common vehicle spread: The spread of a disease agent from a source that is common to those who acquire the disease, that is, the 'vehicle' of the spread. Common vehicles include air, water and food. Communicable diseases that are spread in this way do not characteristically manifest themselves in an `epidemic` with large numbers of cases all occurring at once.

Communicable diseases: Diseases due to a specific infectious agent.

Community controls: *See* **control group**.

Community intervention study: An `intervention study` in which the experimental unit to be randomized to different treatments is not an individual patient or subject but a group of people, for example a school or a factory. *See also* **cluster randomization**. [*American Journal of Epidemiology*, 1994, **140**, 279–89.]

Community medicine: A broad medical speciality developed during the latter part of the twentieth century to cover various aspects of medicine and healthcare in relation to communities rather than individuals. [*British Medical Journal*, 1974, **2**, 186–7.]

Comorbidity: A term applied to two disorders to indicate their potential co-occurrence in the same patient or family, etc. The illnesses can be medical or psychiatric conditions, as well as drug-use disorders, including alcoholism. Comorbid illnesses may occur simultaneously or sequentially. The fact that two illnesses are comorbid does not, however, necessarily imply that one is the cause of the other. [*Statistics in Medicine*, 1995, **14**, 721–33.]

Comparative bioavailability trial: A clinical trial in which different formulations of a drug are administered to a number of subjects and blood samples obtained at various times following administration. Assay of the drug in the blood sample gives, for each administration of a formulation to a given subject, a sequence of concentrations of drug in the blood. The purpose of such trials is to assess the in vivo performances of the different formulations. [*European Journal of Drug Metabolism and Pharmacokinetics*, 2001, **26**, 257–62.]

Comparative calibration: A term applied to the problem of comparing several distinct models of measuring a given quantity.

Comparative exposure rate: A measure of association for use in a matched case-control study, defined as the ratio of the number of case–control pairs, where the case has greater exposure to the risk factor under investigation, to the number where the control has greater exposure. In simple cases, the measure is equivalent to the odds ratio or a weighted combination of odds ratios. In more general cases, the measure can be used to assess association when an odds ratio computation is not feasible. [*Statistics in Medicine*, 1994, **13**, 245–60.]

Comparative risk assessment: A process in which scientific methods are used to gather data, classify the type and severity of risks, and identify and verify relationships between outcomes and risk factors. *See also* **quantitative health risk assessment**. [*The Lancet*, 2005, **366**, 1784–93.]

Comparative trial: Synonym for **controlled trial**.

Comparison group: Synonym for **control group**.

Comparison-wise error rate: Synonym for **per-comparison error rate**.

Compartmental models: Models used widely in tracer kinetic studies to investigate the time course of a drug through some or all of the stages of absorption, distribution, metabolism and elimination. [Jacquez, J. A., 1972, *Compartmental Analysis in Biology and in Medicine*, Elsevier, New York.]

Compensatory equalization: A process applied in some clinical trials and intervention studies, in which comparison groups not given the perceived preferred treatment are provided with compensations that make these comparison groups more equal than originally planned. [Conrad, K. J. (ed.), 1994, *Critically Evaluating the Role of Experiments in Program Evaluation*, Jossey-Bass, San Francisco, CA.]

Competing risks: A term used in the study of mortality patterns in a population of individuals all subject to a number of risk factors. For example, in a study of smoking as a risk factor for lung cancer, coronary heart disease is a competing risk. Interest generally lies in isolating the effects of individual risks, although in many situations it may not be clear which of the possible competing causes resulted in death. [Crowder, M., 2001, *Classical Competing Risks*, Chapman & Hall/CRC, New York.]

Complier average causal effect (CACE): The treatment effect among true compliers in a clinical trial. For a suitable response variable, the CACE is given as the mean difference in outcome between compliers in the treatment group and those controls who would have complied with the treatment had they been randomized to the treatment group. The CAE may be viewed as a measure of 'efficacy' as opposed to 'effectiveness'. [*Journal of School Psychology*, 2017, **60**, 7–24.]

Complete case analysis: An analysis that uses only the individuals in a data set who have no missing values on any variable. This approach can reduce the effective sample size and introduce bias into many types of analysis. *See also* **available case analysis**. [*Journal of the American Statistical Association*, 1992, **87**, 1227–37.]

> **Complete case analysis:** In the past, a procedure often used for dealing with data from longitudinal studies in which some participants drop out. No longer needed since approaches such as the fitting of mixed-effects models can now use all the available data effectively.

Complete linkage cluster analysis: An agglomerative hierarchical clustering method in which the distance between two clusters is defined as the greatest distance between a member of one cluster and a member of the other. [Everitt, B. S., Landau, S., Leese, M. and Stahl, D., 2011, *Cluster Analysis*, 5th ed., John Wiley & Sons, Chichester.]

Compliance: The extent to which patients in a clinical trial follow the trial protocol. Because poor patient compliance can adversely affect the outcome of a trial, it is important to use methods to both improve and monitor the level of compliance. The most frequently used measure of compliance is the pill count, although it is likely that this overestimates compliance. [*Controlled Clinical Trials*, 1996, **17**, 805–15.]

> **Compliance:** Clinical researchers should remember that there are no worse experimental animals on earth than human beings, and sometimes they do not take their medicine.

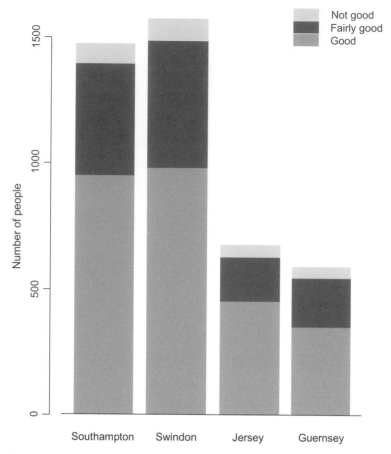

Figure 22 Component bar chart showing subjective health assessment in four regions of the United Kingdom.

Complementary log-log model: An alternative to logistic regression for investigating the relationship between a binary response variable and a set of explanatory variables of interest. Often used in toxicology studies. [Collett, D., 2003, *Modelling Binary Data*, 2nd ed., Chapman & Hall/CRC, London.]

Component bar chart: A bar chart that shows the component parts of the aggregate represented by the total length of the bar. The component parts are shown as sectors of the bar with lengths in proportion to their relative size. Shading or colour can be used to enhance the display. An example is shown in Figure 22.

Compositional data: A set of observations each of which is a proportion and for which the sum is constrained to be one. For example, a number of blood samples might be analyzed and the proportion, in each, of a number of chemical elements recorded. [Aitchison, J., 2003, *The Statistical Analysis of Compositional Data*, Chapman & Hall, London.]

Composite hypothesis: A hypothesis that specifies more than a single value for a parameter. For example, the hypothesis that the mean of a population is greater than some value.

Compound symmetry: A particular pattern for the entries in the `variance-covariance` matrix of a set of `multivariate data`, namely that variances of each variable are equal to one another and the covariances of each pair of variables are the same. Occurs most commonly in discussions of methods of analysis for `longitudinal data`. [Everitt, B. S., 2001, *Statistics for Psychologists*, LEA, Mahwah, FL.]

Comprehensive cohort design: A type of `clinical trial` in which all participants are followed up regardless of their randomization status. In such trials, people agreeing to participate are randomized to one of the study interventions. People who do not agree to be randomized because of a preference for one of the interventions are given their preference and followed up as part of a cohort study. At the end, the outcomes of people who participated in the randomized clinical trial can be compared with those who participated in the cohort study to assess their similarities and differences. [*Methods Inform Medicine*, 1985, **24**, 131–4.]

Computer-aided diagnosis: Computer programs designed to support clinical decision-making. In general, such systems are based on the repeated application of `Bayes's theorem`. In some cases, a reasoning strategy is implemented that enables the programs to conduct clinically pertinent dialogue and explain their decisions. Such programs have been developed in a number of areas of medicine, for example the investigation of dyspepsia and of acute abdominal pain.

See also **expert systems**. [*New England Journal of Medicine*, 1994, **330**, 1792–6.]

Computer-assisted interviews: A method of interviewing subjects in which the interviewer reads the question from a computer screen instead of a printed page and uses the keyboard to enter the answer. Skip patterns (i.e., 'if so-and-so, go to question such-and-such') are built into the program so that the screen automatically displays the appropriate question. Checks can be built in and an immediate warning given if a reply lies outside an acceptable range or is inconsistent with previous replies; revision of previous replies is permitted, with automatic return to the current question. The responses are entered directly on to the computer record, avoiding the need for subsequent coding and data entry. The program can make automatic selection of subjects who require additional procedures, such as special tests, supplementary questionnaires or follow-up visits. [*Journal of Official Statistics*, 1994, **10**, 181–95.]

Computer-intensive methods: Statistical procedures that make use of a large amount of computer time. Examples include the `bootstrap method` and the `jackknife`. [Everitt, B. S., 2001, *Statistics for Psychologists*, LEA, Mahwah, FL.]

Computer languages: Artificial languages that give instructions to computer systems. Sets of instructions combine into *computer programs*. Examples include Fortran, C and the current *lingua-franca* of statisticians, R.

Computer programs: *See* **computer languages**.

Computer virus: A computer program designed to sabotage by carrying out unwanted and often damaging operations. Viruses can be transmitted via discs or over networks. A number of procedures are available that provide protection against the problem.

Conception rates: Estimating conception rates is not straightforward. Counting the number of pregnancies conceived in a population and then using these figures to drive conception rates will be incomplete because pregnancies that end very early before the woman realizes she is pregnant will be missing. An alternative approach is to estimate the numbers of conceptions indirectly through data collection systems designed to count the outcomes of pregnancy in terms of miscarriage, legal abortion and registrable birth. But early miscarriages can still cause problems because they are less likely to appear in national systems. [*Birth Statistics*, 2001, Office of National Statistics.]

Concomitant variables: Synonym for **covariates**.

Concordance: Pairs of groups of individuals of identical phenotype. In twin studies, a condition in which birth twins exhibit or fail to exhibit a trait of interest.

Concordance index: A statistic that gives the probability that a randomly selected patient who experienced an event (e.g. specific disease of interest) had a higher risk score calculated from logistic regression than a patient who had not experienced the event. [*Statistical Methods in Medical Research*, 2018, **27**, 2359–73.]

Concurrent cohort study: *See* **cohort study**.

Conditional distribution: The probability distribution of a random variable (or the joint distribution of several variables) when the values of one or more other variables are held fixed.

Conditional mortality rate: Synonym for **hazard function**.

Conditional power: *See* **stochastic curtailment**.

Conditional probability: The probability that an event, A, occurs given the outcome of some other event, B. Usually written $P(A|B)$. For example, the probability of a person being colour-blind given that the person is male is about 0.1, and the corresponding probability given that the person is female is approximately 0.0001. It is not, of course, necessary that $P(A|B) = P(B|A)$. The probability of having spots given that a patient has measles, for example, is very high; the probability of having measles given that a patient has spots is, however, much less. The two conditional probabilities are actually related by a form of Bayes's theorem, namely $P(A|B) = P(B|A) \times P(A)/P(B)$. If $P(A|B) = P(A)$, then the events A and B are said to be independent. *See also* **specificity** and **sensitivity**. [Everitt, B. S., 2008, *Chance Rules*, 2nd ed., Springer, New York.]

Conditional regression models: Models used particularly for the analysis of longitudinal data in which the conditional expectation of each response is modelled, given either the values of previous responses (*transition model*) or a set of random effects that reflect natural heterogeneity among individuals due to unmeasured factors. For normally distributed responses, the results of fitting such models are essentially equivalent to the results from using marginal models with the same correlational structure. For non-normal responses, however, this is not the case, and the estimated regression coefficients from a conditional regression model and a marginal model have different interpretations. For the latter, the coefficient represents the effect for a given individual; for the former, it represents the average effect in the population. *See also* **mixed-effects models**. [Everitt, B. S., 2002, *Modern Medical Statistics*, Arnold, London.]

Confidence interval: A range of values calculated from the sample observations, which is believed, with a particular probability, to contain the true parameter value. A 95% confidence interval, for example, implies that if the estimation process was repeated again and again, then 95% of the calculated intervals would be expected to contain the true parameter value. Note that the stated probability level refers to properties of the interval and not to the parameter itself, which is not considered a random variable (but *see* **Bayesian methods**). [Everitt, B. S. and Palmer, C. (eds.), 2011, *Encyclopedic Companion to Medical Statistics*, 2nd ed., John Wiley & Sons, Chichester.]

Confidence limits: The upper and lower values of a confidence interval.

Confirmatory factor analysis: *See* **factor analysis**.

Confounders: Variables, which whilst not of direct interest themselves, are thought to be related to the outcome of interest and to other variables which are of direct interest to the investigator.

Confounding: A phenomenon that occurs when it is not possible to disentangle the effects of two or more processes. In epidemiology, for example, a factor that is associated with both disease risk and exposure status. The two effects are usually referred to as *aliases*.

Conservative and non-conservative tests: Terms usually encountered in discussions of multiple comparison tests. Non-conservative tests provide poor control over the per-experiment error rate. Conservative tests, on the other hand, may limit the per-comparison error rate to unnecessarily low values, and tend to have low power unless the sample size is large.

Consistency: A term used for a particular property of an estimator, namely that its bias tends to zero as sample size increases.

Consistency checks: Checks built into the collection of a set of observations to assess their internal consistency. For example, data on age might be collected directly and also by asking about date of birth.

Consolidated standards for reporting trials (CONSORT) statement: A protocol for reporting the results from clinical trials. The core contribution of the protocol consists of a flow diagram (see Figure 23) and a checklist. The flow diagram enables reviewers and readers to grasp quickly how many eligible participants were assigned randomly to each arm of the trial, etc. [*Journal of the American Medical Association*, 1996, **276**, 637–9.]

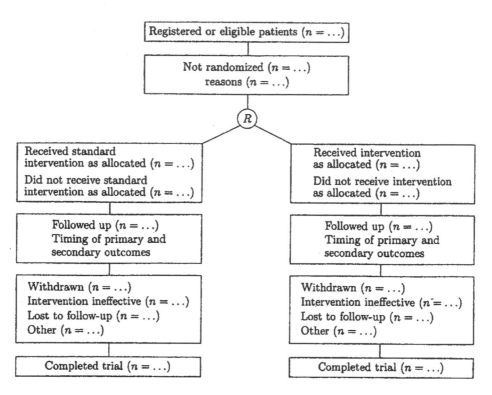

Figure 23 Consolidated standards (CONSORT) for reporting clinical trials.

Consolidated standards for reporting trials (CONSORT) statement: A valuable attempt to improve the reporting of clinical trials, although having a tendency to be over-prescriptive.

CONSORT statement: Abbreviation for **consolidated standards for reporting trials statement**.

Construct: Generally used for a concept that exists theoretically but is not directly observable. Essentially a `latent variable`.

Construct validity: The extent to which a set of `manifest variables` adequately measure `constructs` of interest.

Content analysis: The coding of statements or answers to open-ended questions made in relatively unstructured interviews that allows the systematic analysis of written and spoken material. [*Journal of Health Communication*, 2002, **7**, 123–37.]

Contingency coefficient: A measure of the strength of an association between two categorical variables. [Fleiss, J. L., 1981, *Statistical Methods for Rates and Proportions*, John Wiley & Sons, New York.]

Contingency tables: The tables arising when observations on a number of categorical variables are cross-classified. Entries in each cell are the number of individuals with the corresponding combination of variable values. Most common are tables

involving two categorical variables known as two-dimensional `contingency`
`tables`, an example of which is shown in the following table:

Retarded activity amongst psychiatric patients

	Affectives	Schizo	Neurotics	Total
Retarded activity	12	13	5	30
No retarded activity	18	17	25	60
Total	30	30	30	30

The analysis of such two-dimensional tables generally involves testing for the
independence of the two variables using the familiar `chi-squared test`. Three-
and higher-dimensional tables are now analyzed routinely using `log-linear`
`models`. [Everitt, B. S., 1992, *The Analysis of Contingency Tables*, 2nd ed.,
Chapman & Hall/CRC, Boca Raton, FL.]

Continuity correction: *See* **Yates's contingency correction**.

Continuous variable: A measurement not restricted to particular values except in so far
as this is restricted by the accuracy of the measuring instrument. Common
examples include weight, height, temperature and blood pressure. For such a
variable, equal-sized differences on different parts of the scale are equivalent. *See
also* **categorical variable** and **measurement scale**.

Contour plot: A topographical map drawn from data involving observations of three
variables. One variable is represented on the horizontal axis and a second variable is
represented on the vertical axis. The third variable is represented by isolines
(lines of constant value). Used most often for displaying graphically `bivariate`
`distributions`, in which case the z-axis usually represents the probability
density function (or an estimate of it) corresponding to the values of the other two
variables. An example is given in Figure 24. An alternative method of display is the
perspective plot, in which the values of the third variable are represented by a series
of lines constructed to give a three-dimensional view of the data. This type of
display is illustrated in Figure 25.

Contrast: A comparison of population characteristics for a number of populations. For
example, in a `clinical trial` it may be of interest to compare the mean
response of a control group with the average of two treatment groups. *See also*
Helmert contrast. [Rosenthal, R. and Rosnow, R. L., 1985, *Contrast Analysis*,
Cambridge University Press, Cambridge.]

Control chart: *See* **quality control procedures**.

Control group: In experimental studies, a collection of individuals to which the
experimental procedure of interest is not applied. In `observational`
`studies`, used most often for a collection of individuals not subjected to the risk

Figure 24 Contour plot of the natural log of the lung cancer incidence rates for Connecticut women by age and period.
(Taken with permission of the publisher Wiley from *Encyclopedia of Biostatistics*, volume 1, edited by P. Armitage and T. Colton, 2005.)

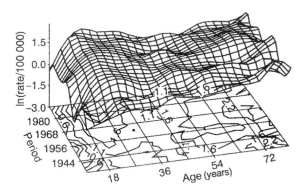

Figure 25 Perspective and contour plot for the natural log of Hodgkin's disease incidence rates for Connecticut women by age and period.
(Taken with permission of the publisher Wiley from *Encyclopedia of Biostatistics*, volume 1, edited by P. Armitage and T. Colton, 2005.)

factor under investigation. In many studies, the controls are drawn from the same clinical source as the cases to ensure that they represent the same catchment population and are subject to the same selective factors. These would be termed *hospital controls*. An alternative is to use controls taken from the population from which the cases are drawn (*community controls*). The latter is suitable only if the source population is well defined and the cases are representative of the cases in this population. [Everitt, B. S. and Wessely, S., 2008, *Clinical Trials in Psychiatry*, 2nd ed., Oxford University Press, Oxford.]

Control group: Remember, the best way to improve the results on any treatment is to leave out the controls!

Controlled trial: A phase III study in which an experimental treatment is compared with a control treatment, the latter being either the current standard treatment or a placebo.

Control statistic: *See* **quality control procedures**.

Convenience sample: A non-random sample chosen because it is easy to collect, for example, people who walk by in the street. Such a sample is unlikely to be representative of the population of interest, but it might be useful for pilot testing.

Conway-Maxwell-Poisson distribution: A probability distribution that accommodates and generalizes several other discrete distributions according to the value of a parameter labelled as the dispersion parameter. Very useful for modelling cure rate models. [*Journal of the Royal Statistical Society, Series C*, 2005, **54**, 127–42.]

Cooperative study: A term sometimes used for multicentre study.

Coplot: A powerful visualization tool for studying how a response depends on an explanatory variable given the values of other explanatory variables. The plot consists of a number of panels, one of which (the 'given' panel) shows the values of a particular explanatory variable divided into a number of intervals, while the others (the 'dependence' panels) show the scatter diagrams of the response variable and another explanatory variable corresponding to each interval in the given panel. The plot is examined by moving from left to right through the intervals in the given panel, while simultaneously moving from left to right and then from bottom to top through the dependence panels. The example shown in Figure 26 involves the relationship between packed cell volume and white blood cell count for a given haemoglobin concentration. [Everitt, B. S. and Rabe-Hesketh, S., 2001, *Analysing Medical Data Using S-PLUS*, Springer, New York.]

Copas model: A model for assessing publication bias in a meta-analysis. [*Statistical Methods in Medical Research*, 2001, **10**, 251–65.]

Correlated samples *t*-test: Synonym for **matched pairs *t*-test**.

Correlation: A general term for interdependence between pairs of variables. *See also* **association** and **correlation coefficient**.

Correlation coefficient: An index that quantifies the linear relationship between a pair of variables. Various correlation coefficients are available, all taking values between -1 and 1, with the extreme values indicating a perfect linear relationship and the sign indicating the direction of the relationship. A value of zero indicates that there is not a linear relationship between the two variables, although there may be a more esoteric nonlinear relationship. The most common such coefficient is *Pearson's product moment correlation coefficient*, which acts as an estimator of the

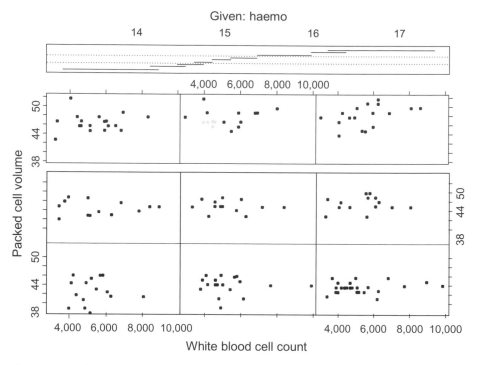

Figure 26 Coplot of haemoglobin concentration, packed cell volume and white blood cell count.

population correlation in a bivariate normal distribution. Some examples of data sets with different degrees of correlation are shown in Figure 27. *See also* **Kendall's tau statistic** and **Spearman's rank correlation**.

Correlation matrix: A square table or array of correlation coefficients between pairs of variables in some set of variables of interest. For example, in investigating muscle and body fat, an investigator may take measurements on the following four variables:

- Tricep (thickness, mm)
- Thigh (circumference, mm)
- Midarm (circumference, mm)
- Bodyfat (%)

Pearson's product moment correlation coefficients might then be calculated for each pair of variables and arranged conveniently as the following correlation matrix, usually denoted by **R**:

$$\mathbf{R} = \begin{array}{c} \\ V1 \\ V2 \\ V3 \\ V4 \end{array} \begin{array}{cccc} V1 & V2 & V3 & V4 \\ \left[\begin{array}{cccc} 1.00 & 0.92 & 0.46 & 0.84 \\ 0.92 & 1.00 & 0.08 & 0.88 \\ 0.46 & 0.08 & 1.00 & 0.14 \\ 0.84 & 0.88 & 0.14 & 1.00 \end{array} \right] \end{array}$$

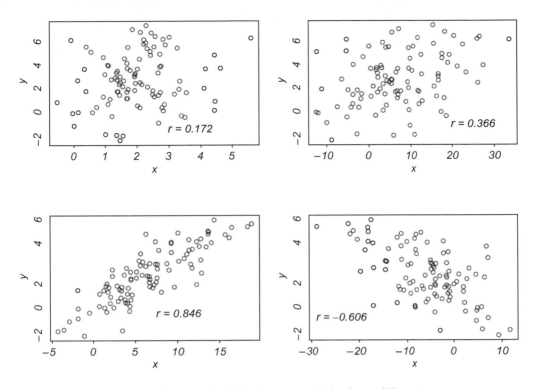

Figure 27 Scatter diagrams in which the two variables have different correlation coefficients.

The arrangement is symmetrical: the values in the ith row and jth column are the same as those in row j and column i, and the NW to SE diagonal contains ones, the 'correlation' of a variable with itself. Correlation matrices are the basis of many methods of multivariate analysis, for example principal components analysis. [Everitt, B. S. and Dunn, G., 2001, *Applied Multivariate Analysis*, 2nd ed., John Wiley & Sons, Chichester.]

Correlogram: *See* **autocorrelation**.

Correspondence analysis: A method for displaying the information in a contingency table graphically. In most applications, a set of xy coordinates is derived to represent the row categories of the table and another set is derived to represent the column categories. The relative positions of points representing row categories and column categories, relative to the origin, reflect the degree of association between them. Figure 28 illustrates the results of applying the method to the following contingency table of eye colour and hair colour: The points representing blue eyes and fair hair, for example, are close to one another in Figure 28 and relatively distant from the origin, implying a positive association. There are more observations in the corresponding cell of the table than

Eye colour	Hair colour				
	Fair	Red	Medium	Dark	Black
Light	688	116	584	188	4
Blue	326	38	241	110	3
Medium	343	84	909	412	26
Dark	98	48	403	681	81

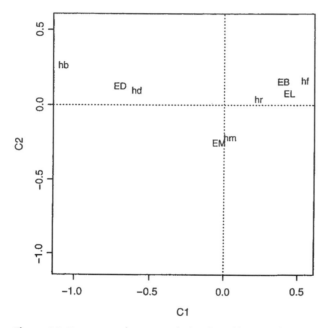

Figure 28 Correspondence analysis plot of hair and eye colour data.

would be expected if eye colour and hair colour were independent variables. [Le Rouk, B., 2010, *Multiple Correspondence Analysis*, Sage, New York.]

Correspondence analysis: Often a useful procedure to be used alongside the chi-squared test of independence of the two variables in a contingency table.

Cosinor analysis: The analysis of biological rhythm data, that is data with `circadian variation`, generally by fitting a single sinusoidal regression function having a known period of 24 hours together with independent and identically distributed error terms. [*Chronobiologia*, 1982, **9**, 397–439.]

Cost–benefit analysis: An economic analysis in which the costs of medical care and the loss of net earnings due to death or disability are considered by translating all costs and benefits into monetary units. [Brent, R. J., 2017, *Advanced Introduction to Cost-Benefit Analysis*, Edward Elgar Publishing, Cheltenham.]

Cost-effectiveness analysis: An economic analysis that compares the incremental medical costs and health outcomes of alternative healthcare programmes. In contrast to `cost-benefit analysis`, health effects are expressed in units such as life-years gained, days free of symptoms, cases avoided, etc. rather than in monetary units. Under most conditions, however, results from both cost–benefit analysis and cost–effectiveness analysis lead to similar conclusions. [Drummond, M. and McGuire, A., 2001, *Economic Evaluation in Health Care: Merging Theory with Practice*, Oxford University Press, Oxford.]

Cost-effectiveness ratio: The ratio of the difference in cost between a test and a standard health programme to the difference in benefits. Generally used as a summary statistic to compare competing healthcare programmes relative to their cost and benefit. [*Statistics in Medicine*, 2001, **20**, 1469–77.]

Cost-minimization analysis: An analysis in which health effects which are known to be equal, are assessed only in terms of costs, and the least costly alternative chosen. [*British Medical Journal*, 1993, **307**, 726.]

Cost of living extremely well index: An index that tries to track the price fluctuations of items which are affordable only to those of very substantial means. The index is used to provide a barometer of economic forces at the top end of the market. The index is made up of prices for 42 goods and services, including a kilogram of beluga malossal caviar and a face lift. [Hand, D. J., 2004, *Measurement Theory and Practice*, Arnold, London.]

Count data: Data obtained by counting the number of occurrences of some event of interest, rather than by making measurements on some scale. An example is the number of decayed teeth in each of a sample of individuals. Often analyzed using the `Poisson distribution` and `Poisson regression`.

Counter-matching: An approach to selecting controls in `nested case-control studies`, in which a covariate is known on all cohort members, and controls are sampled to yield covariate-stratified case-control sets. This approach has been shown to be generally efficient relative to matched case-control designs for studying interaction in the case of a rare risk factor X and an uncorrelated risk factor Y. [*Journal of Epidemiology*, 2003, **13**, 193–202.]

Covariable: Synonym for **covariate**.

Covariance: A measure of the association of two variables given by the average of the product of deviations of each variable from their respective mean values. Unlike `correlation coefficients`, covariances are not constrained to lie between -1 and 1.

Covariance matrix: *See* **variance–covariance matrix**.

Covariance structure modelling: Synonym for **structural equation modelling**.

Covariate-Adaptive Randomization: A class of randomization procedures used for `clinical trials` that attempt to prospectively balance treatment assignments

Figure 29 Critical region.

across selected baseline prognostic factors (covariates) such as age, gender and disease severity known to be correlated with the outcome of a patient while maintaining allocation randomness. In this way, interpretable results are achieved. *See also* **adaptive randomization designs** and **Bayesian adaptive randomization**. [*Drug Information Journal*, 2003, **15**, 293–308.]

Covariates: Often used simply as an alternative term for explanatory variable in regression analysis, but used primarily for variables that must be controlled for in an analysis but are not of specific interest. *See also* **analysis of covariance**.

Coxian phase-type distribution: A special type of Markov model which can be used in two ways; to uncover underlying stages of a survival process and to make inferences about the rates of flow of individuals through these latent stages before an event of interest occurs. Can be used to identify individuals who are likely to deteriorate faster through a series of disease states and so require more aggressive treatment. [*Statistical Methods in Medical Research*, 2018, **27**, 3577–94.]

Cox–Mantel test: A distribution-free method for assessing the equality of two survival curves. [*Cancer Chemotherapy Reports*, 1966, **50**, 163–70.]

Cox's proportional hazards model: A method used to evaluate the effects of a set of explanatory variables on survival times. Essentially a linear regression model for the logarithm of the hazard function, in which the ratio of the hazards for two individuals is assumed constant over time. Explanatory variables are considered to act multiplicatively on the hazard function. Estimated regression coefficients in the model can be exponentiated to give estimated relative risks. [Collett, D., 2015, *Modelling Survival Data in Medical Research*, 3rd ed., Chapman & Hall/CRC, London.]

Cox's regression model: Synonym for **Cox's proportional hazards model**.

Critical region: The values of a test statistic that lead to rejection of a null hypothesis. The size of the critical region is the probability of obtaining an outcome belonging to this region when the null hypothesis is true, that is, the probability of a type I error. Some typical critical regions are shown in Figure 29. *See also* **acceptance region**.

Critical value: The value with which a statistic calculated from sample data is compared in order to decide whether a null hypothesis should be rejected. The value is related to the particular significance level chosen. [Altman, D. G., 2018, *Practical Statistics for Medical Research*, Chapman & Hall/CRC, Boca Raton, FL.]

Cronbach's alpha: An index of the internal consistency of a psychological test consisting of a series of binary items. [*Psychometrika*, 1951, **16**, 297–334.]

Cross-cultural study: A study in which data from different cultural groups are compared. [*Journal of Dental Research*, 1999, **78**, 643–9.]

Crossover design: Clinical trials in which patients are allocated to sequences of treatments with the purpose of studying differences between individual treatments. Random allocation is used to determine the order in which the treatments are received. The simplest such design involves two groups of subjects: patients in one group receive each of two treatments, *A* and *B*, in the order *A* followed by *B*; the patients in the other group receive the treatments in the order *B* followed by *A*. This is known as a *two-by-two crossover design*. Since the treatment comparison is 'within subject' rather than 'between subject', it is likely to require fewer patients to achieve a given statistical power. The analysis of such designs is complicated by the possible presence of *carry-over effects*; when we come to study results from a given period for a given patient, the results may reflect not only the effect of the current treatment but also the effect of the previous treatment. This may make the disentangling of one effect from another extremely difficult. An attempt is often made to minimize the potential problem by including a washout period between receiving each treatment, but some authorities have suggested that this type of design should be used only if such carry-over effects can be ruled out a priori. Crossover designs are applicable only to chronic conditions for which short-term relief of symptoms rather than a cure is the goal. The main advantages of crossover designs are efficiency and the ability to study individual reaction to treatment. [Senn, S., 2002, *Crossover Trials in Clinical Research*, 2nd ed., John Wiley & Sons, Chichester.]

Crossover rate: The proportion of patients in a clinical trial transferring from the treatment decided by an initial random allocation to an alternative one. Also used in genetics for genetic recombination by sexual reproduction.

Cross-sectional study: A study that looks at the relationship between a response variable and some explanatory variables in a particular population at a specific point in time. Many surveys are of this type. An association between outcome and explanatory variables may suggest causality, although a causal link cannot be established because such studies give no information on the temporal ordering of possibly causal events. *See also* **retrospective study** and **prospective study**. [Everitt, B. S. and Palmer, C. (eds.), 2011, *Encyclopedic Companion to Medical Statistics*, 2nd ed., John Wiley & Sons, Chichester.]

Cross-validation: A procedure for assessing the fit of a particular model for a data set. The data are divided at random into two approximately equally sized parts, one of which is then used to estimate the parameters of the model of interest. The fit of this model is then assessed on the second subset of observations. The procedure is needed since estimating the model and testing its fit on the same observations is known to give optimistic conclusions about the model's suitability. *See also* **bootstrap method** and **jackknife**. [*American Statistician*, 1990, **44**, 140–7.]

Crowding index: The mean number of people per room in a housing unit. [*Journal of Epidemiology and Community Health*, 2004, **58**, 476–80.]

Crude birth rate: Synonym for **birth rate**.

Crude death rate: The total deaths during a year divided by the total midyear population. To avoid many decimal places, it is customary to multiply death rates by 100,000 and express the results as deaths per 100,000 population. For example, in 1999 the death rates in the following countries per 100,000 were:

- Zambia: 2384
- Burma: 1239
- UK: 1064
- Mexico: 483

The crude death rate expresses the actual observed mortality rate in a population under study and is the starting point for further development of adjusted rates. *See also* **age-specific death rates** and **cause-specific death rates**. [Morton, R. F., Hebel, J. R. and McCarter, R. J., 1990, *A Study Guide to Epidemiology and Biostatistics*, 3rd ed., Aspen, Gaithersburg, MD.]

Crude risk: The probability that an individual will develop a particular disease in a given time interval in the presence of other competing risks of death. An example is the probability that a 30-year-old woman will develop breast cancer by the time she is 60. Synonymous with **absolute risk**.

C-statistic: A commonly used measure of how well a model can differentiate between individuals who have the outcome of interest and those that do not, calculated as the proportion of all possible pairs (of individuals in which one had the outcome of interest and the other did not) that are concordant, that is, the predicted probability is higher for the individual that had the outcome compared to the predicted probability for the individual that did not. The closer the C-statistic is to the value one, the better the model discriminates between individuals that did and did not have the outcome. A value of 0.5 suggests that the model predicts no better than chance alone. [Harrel, F. E., 2001, *Regression Modelling Strategies with Applications to Linear Models, Logistic Regression and Survival Analysis*, Springer, New York.]

Cumulative frequency distribution: A listing of the sample values of a variable together with the proportion of the observations less than or equal to each value. The

Hormone assay values (nmol/l)

Class limits	Cumulative frequency
75–79	1
80–84	3
85–89	8
90–94	17
95–99	27
100–104	34
105–109	38
110–114	40
≥115	41

empirical equivalent of the `cumulative probability distribution`. An example of such a tabulation is shown below. *See also* **frequency distribution**.

Cumulative hazard: The cumulative probability of death.

Cumulative incidence: The proportion of individuals in a cohort initially free of a given disease who develop that disease in a defined age or time interval. Synonymous with **absolute risk**.

Cumulative incidence ratio: Synonymous with **relative risk**.

Cumulative meta-analysis: The repeated performance of `meta-analysis` with at each step an extra study being included. Studies are often ordered chronologically, allowing an examination of how the pooled `effect size` changes with time. [*Journal of Clinical Epidemiology*, 1995, **48**, 45–57.]

Cumulative probability distribution: A distribution showing how many values of a random variable are less than or more than given values. For grouped data, the given values correspond to the class boundaries.

Cure rate models: Models for `survival times` where there is a significant proportion of people who are cured. In general, some type of `finite-mixture distribution` is involved. [*Statistics in Medicine*, 1987, **6**, 483–9.]

Current status data: Data arising frequently in many experimental or `cohort studies` in which the exact time to an event of interest cannot be observed directly but is only known to have occurred before or after a random monitoring time. The right- or left-censored observation occurs if the `survival time` exceeds or does not exceed the monitoring time, respectively. [*Statistical Methods in Medical Research*, 2020, **29**, 3–14.]

Cusum chart: Acronym for cumulative sum of a series of measurements. Often useful for investigating the influence of time even when it is not part of the design of the study. If there is no time trend, then the cusum is basically flat. A change in level

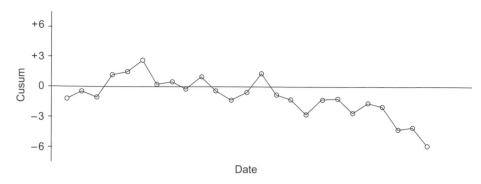

Figure 30 Cusum chart.

over time appears as a change in the slope of the cusum. An example is given in Figure 30. [*Journal of Quality Techniques*, 1975, **7**, 183–92.]

Cyclical variation: The systematic and repeatable variation of some variable over time. Most people's blood pressure, for example, shows such variation over a 24-hour period, being lowest at night and highest during the morning. Such circadian variation is also seen in many hormone levels. *See also* **seasonal variation**. [Chatfield, C., 2019, *The Analysis of Time Series: An Introduction*, 7th ed., Chapman & Hall/CRC, Boca Raton, FL.]

Data and safety monitoring board: A committee set up to monitor a `clinical trial` for patient safety and for evidence of benefit. Needed to ensure minimal acceptable risks to trial participants and to continually reassess the risks versus benefits of trial interventions. [Ellenberg, S., Fleming, T. R. and DeMets, D. L., 2002, *Data Monitoring Committees*, Chapman & Hall/CRC, Boca Raton, FL.]

Data archives: Generally large sets of data that can be accessed and utilized by researchers intending to perform secondary data analysis. Such archives preserve important data against disposal or deterioration. [*British Medical Journal*, 1994, **308**, 1519–20.]

Database: A structured collection of data that is organized in such a way that it may be accessed easily by a wide variety of applications programs. Large clinical databases are becoming increasingly available to clinical and policy researchers and are generally used for two purposes: to facilitate healthcare delivery and for research. An example of such a database is that provided by the US Health Care Financing Administration, which contains information about all Medicare patients' hospitalizations, surgical procedures and surgery visits. *See also* **administrative databases**. [Elmasri, R. and Navathe, S. B., 2016, *Fundamentals of Database Systems*, 7nd ed., Addison-Wesley, Reading, MA.]

Database management system: A computer system organized for the systematic management of a large, structured collection of information that can be used for storage, modification and retrieval of data. [*Controlled Clinical Trials*, 1995, **16**, 30S–65S.]

Data dredging: A term used for comparisons made within a data set not specifically listed before the start of the study. An attempt to find patterns in a data set that are statistically significant but which in fact are largely false positives. *See also* **post hoc comparisons**. [Altman, D. G., 2018, *Practical Statistics for Medical Research*, CRC/Chapman & Hall, London.]

Data editing: The action of removing format errors and keying errors from data.

Data matrix: *See* **multivariate data**.

Data mining: The nontrivial extraction of implicit, previously unknown, potentially useful information from data. The approach uses `expert systems` and statistical and graphical techniques to discover and present knowledge in a form that is easily comprehensible to humans. A wide variety of data mining approaches have proven useful to detect safety signals in report databases. [Witten, I. H., 2016, *Practical Machine Learning Tools*, Morgan Kaufmann, Burlington, MA.]

Data mining: Increasingly used in medical contexts to detect unexpected associations or patterns in large clinical databases.

Data Quality: Analyses can only be as good as the data that underlie them, a statement that can be registered more succinctly in terms of the aphorism, 'Garbage in, garbage out'.

Data reduction: The process of summarizing large amounts of data by forming, for example, frequency distributions and calculating summary statistics such as means, variances, etc., and by representing the data graphically in the form of histograms, scatterplots, etc. Also used for reducing the dimensionality of multivariate data by using principal components analysis or factor analysis. *See also* **battery reduction** and **initial data analysis**. [Dunn, G. and Everitt, B. S., 2010, *Applied Multivariate Data Analysis*, 2nd ed., John Wiley & Sons, Chichester.]

Data screening: The initial assessment of a set of observations to determine whether they appear to satisfy the assumptions of the methods to be used in their analysis. *See also* **initial data analysis**.

Data set: A general term for observations and measurements collected during any type of scientific investigation.

Data Squashing: An approach to reducing the size of very large data sets in which the data are first 'binned' and then statistics such as the mean and variance/covariance are computed on each bin. These statistics are then used to generate a new sample in each bin to construct a reduced data set with similar statistical properties to those of the original. [DuMouchel, W., 2002, *Handbook of Massive Data Sets*. Massive Computing, volume 4, chapter 16. Springer, Boston, MA.]

Death certification: The registration of the facts (cause of death, decedent's name, sex, age, place of residence, etc.) about each death occurring in a region. Legal registration of death before a body may be buried or cremated has been required since 1837 in England and Wales. Doctors in England have been required to certify the cause of death for patients under their care since 1841. [*BMA*, November, 2019.]

Death rate: *See* **crude death rate**.

Debugging: The process of locating and correcting errors in a computer routine or of isolating and eliminating malfunctions of a computer itself.

Deciles: The values of a variable that divide its probability distribution or its frequency distribution into ten equal parts. *See also* **percentiles**.

Decimal reduction time: A parameter used to measure the efficacy of the thermal disinfection of microbial populations, given by the time required to reduce the population by 90%. [*Journal of Food Protection*, 2002, **65**, 419–22.]

Decision analysis: A quantitative method for identifying the optimal course of action among a well-defined set of alternatives under conditions of uncertainty. Of considerable importance in medicine because of the uncertainty that is inherent in diagnosis and treatment choice. The optimal course of action is one that maximizes the average value of the outcome of interest, for example `life expectancy` or `quality-adjusted life-years`. A `decision tree` is the basic structure underlying most applications of decision analysis in medicine. [*Annals of Internal Medicine*, 1987, **106**, 275–91.]

Decision function: *See* **decision theory**.

Decision theory: A unified approach to all problems of estimation, prediction and hypothesis testing. It is based on the concept of a *decision function*, which tells the experimenter how to conduct the statistical aspects of an experiment and what action to take for each possible outcome. Choosing a decision function requires a *loss function* to be defined, which assigns numerical values to making good or poor decisions. [Peterman, M., 2017, *An Introduction to Decision Theory*, Cambridge University Press, Cambridge.]

Decision tree: A graphic representation of the alternatives in a decision-making problem that summarizes all the possibilities foreseen by the decision-maker. For example, suppose we are given the following problem: A physician must choose between two treatments. The patient is known to have one of two diseases, but the diagnosis is not certain. A thorough examination of the patient was not able to resolve the diagnostic uncertainty. The best that can be said is that the probability that the patient has disease A is p. A simple decision tree for the problem is given in Figure 31. [Smith, C., 2019, *Decision Trees and Random Forests: A Visual Introduction for Beginners*, Independently Published.]

Deep models: A term used for those models applied in `screening studies` that incorporate hypotheses about the disease process that generates the observed events. The aim of such models is to attempt an understanding of the underlying disease dynamics. *See also* **surface models**. [Cornel, R. G., 1984, *Statistical Methods for Cancer Studies*, Marcel Dekker, New York.]

Degrees of freedom (df): An elusive concept that occurs throughout statistics. Essentially, the term means the number of independent units of information in a sample relevant to the estimation of a parameter or calculation of a statistic. For example, in a `two-by-two contingency table` with a given set of marginal totals, only one of the four cell frequencies is free, and therefore the table has a single degree of freedom. In many cases, the term corresponds to the number of parameters in a model. Also used to refer to a parameter of various families of distributions, for example `Student's t-distribution` and the

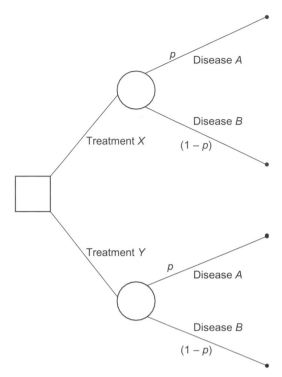

Figure 31 Simple decision tree.

F-distribution. [Altman, D. G., 2018, *Practical Statistics for Medical Research*, Chapman & Hall/CRC, Boca Raton, FL.]

Delay distribution: The probability distribution of the delay in reporting an event. Particularly important in AIDS research, since AIDS surveillance data need to be corrected appropriately for reporting delay before they can be used to reflect current AIDS incidence. *See also* **back-projection**. [*Philosophical Transactions of the Royal Society of London, Series B*, 1989, **325**, 135–45.]

Delayed entry: In survival analysis this refers to situations where units do not come under observation when they become at risk of an event of interest but only after a delay. [Klein, J. P., 2010, *Survival Analysis: State of the Art*, Springer, New York.]

Delta technique: A procedure for finding means and variances of functions of random variables. [Dunn, G., 2004, *Statistical Evaluation of Measurement Errors*, Arnold, London.]

Demand curve data: Data obtained from a self-administration experiment used in substance abuse research which describes how a patient's demand for a drug or non-drug reinforcer varies as a function of price. Self-administration studies have been widely used to evaluate the reinforcing strength of various substances such as hallucinogens, food, nicotine and alcohol. [*Proceedings of the National Academy of Science*, 2014, **111**, 11822–7.]

Demography: The study of human populations with respect to their size, structure and dynamics. The aim of formal demographic analysis is to isolate the components of

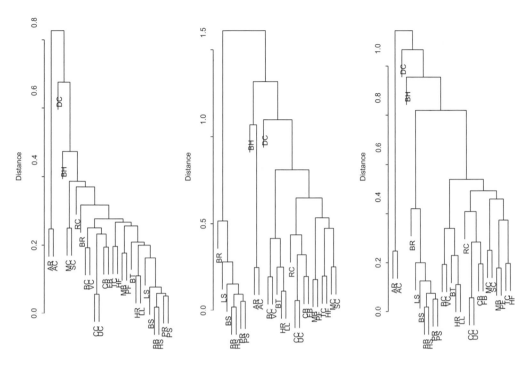

Figure 32 Example of a dendrogram.

demographic patterns by dividing a population into relatively homogeneous subgroups, with analysis by age and sex generally being of greatest importance. [Bangarats, J., Burch, T. and Warchter, K., 1987, *Family Demography: Methods and Their Applications*, Clarendon Press, Oxford.]

Dendrogram: A term encountered in the application of agglomerative hierarchical clustering methods. Refers to a tree-like diagram that describes the stages in the clustering process as individuals and then groups are joined together to form fewer, larger clusters. Examples of such a structure are shown in Figure 32. *See also* **group average clustering**, **single linkage clustering** and **Ward's method**. [Everitt, B. S., Leese, M., Landau, S. and Stahl, D., 2011, *Cluster Analysis*, 5th ed., John Wiley & Sons, Chichester.]

Density sampling: A method of sampling controls in a case–control study that can reduce bias due to possibly changing patterns in exposure. Controls are sampled from the population at risk over the period of accrual of the cases rather than simply at one point in time, such as the end of the period. [*American Journal of Epidemiology*, 1982, **116**, 547–53.]

Dependent variable: *See* **response variable**.

Descriptive statistics: A general term for methods of summarizing and tabulating data that make their main features more transparent, for example calculating means and variances and plotting histograms. *See also* **exploratory data analysis** and **initial data analysis**. [Altman, D. G., 2018, *Practical Statistics for Medical Research*, Chapman & Hall/CRC, Boca Raton, FL.]

Detectable preclinical period: Synonym for **sojourn time**.

Detection bias: *See* **ascertainment bias**.

Detection limits: Limits established within a chemical laboratory to designate low-level data that cannot be distinguished from a zero concentration. Measurements below the limit are considered not significantly different from zero and reported as a non-detect. [*Analytical Chemistry*, 1968, **48**, 586–93.]

Deterministic model: A `mathematical model` that contains no random or probabilistic elements. *See also* **random model**.

Deviance: A measure of the fit of a `generalized linear model`. Essentially a `likelihood ratio test`. [Everitt, B. S., 2003, *Modern Medical Statistics*, Arnold, London.]

Deviate: The value of a variable measured from some standard point of location, usually the mean.

Df (or df): Abbreviation for **degrees of freedom**.

***Diagnostic and Statistical Manual* (DSM):** An attempt to standardize the definitions of mental disorders developed by the American Psychiatric Association by giving all the clinical and other criteria needed to establish a particular diagnosis. [American Psychiatric Association, 2013, *Diagnostic and Statistical Manual of Mental Disorders*, 5th ed., APA, Washington, DC.]

Diagnostics: A generic term for procedures useful for identifying and understanding differences between a model and the data to which it is fitted. The best-known example is the use of `residuals` in `multiple linear regression`. [Cook, R. D. and Weisberg, S., 1994, *An Introduction to Regression Graphics*, John Wiley & Sons, New York.]

Diagnostic tests: Procedures used in clinical medicine and also in `epidemiology` to screen for the presence or absence of a disease. In the simplest case, the test will result in a positive (disease likely) or negative (disease unlikely) finding. Ideally, all those with the disease should be classified by the test as positive and all those without the disease as negative. Two indices of the performance of a test that measure how often such correct classifications occur are its `sensitivity` and `specificity`. Examples include amniocentesis in pregnant women and mammography in screening for breast cancer. *See also* **believe the positive rule** and **receiver operating characteristic curves**. [Nicoll, D., McPhee, S. J., Pigone, M., Detmer, W. M. and Chou, T. M., 2008, *Pocket Guide to Diagnostic Tests*, 5th ed., Lange/McGraw-Hill, New York.]

Dichotomous variable: Synonym for **binary variable**.

Differences versus totals plot: A graphical procedure used most often in the analysis of data from a two-by-two `crossover design`. For each subject, the difference between the response variable values on each treatment is plotted against the total of the two treatment values. The two groups, corresponding to the order in which

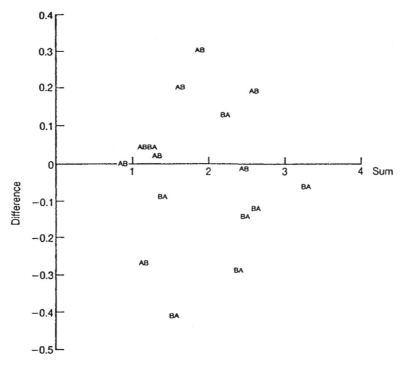

Figure 33 Example of a difference versus total plot.

the treatments were given, are differentiated on the plot by different plotting symbols (in the example given in Figure 33, 'AB' and 'BA' are used). A large shift between the groups in the horizontal direction implies a differential carry-over effect. If this shift is small, then the shift between the groups in a vertical direction is a measure of the treatment effect. Hand, D. J. and Everitt, B. S., 1986, *The Statistical Consultant in Action*, Cambridge University Press, Cambridge.]

Diggle–Kenward model for dropouts: A model for longitudinal data that contains a part that models the probability of dropping out using logistic regression. By using a latent variable to represent the value of the response variable at time of dropout, it is possible to determine the type of missing value in the data and, in particular, accommodate informative missing values. [Diggle, P. J., Liang, K. Y. and Zeger, S. L., 2013, *Analysis of Longitudinal Data*, 2nd ed., Oxford Science Publications, Oxford.]

Diggle–Kenward model for dropouts: A welcome addition to the methodology available for analyzing longitudinal data in which dropouts occur, although how many researchers would feel happy about relying on technical virtuosity if 60% or more of their data were missing?

Digit preference: The personal and often subconscious bias that frequently occurs in the recording of observations. Usually most obvious in the final recorded digit of a

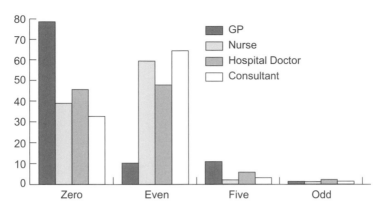

Figure 34 Digit preference among different groups of observers for zero, even, odd and five numerals.

measurement. Figure 34 illustrates this phenomenon. An example of digit preference was observed in the recording of birthweight, where preference for the terminal digit 0 increased progressively with increasing birthweight over the whole range of birthweights. Correction for digit preference led to an increase of nearly 2% in the number of low birthweight babies. [*Journal of Human Hypertension*, 2001, **15**, 365.]

Direct standardization: The process of adjusting a crude mortality or morbidity rate estimate for one or more variables by using a known reference population. It might, for example, be required to compare cancer mortality rates of single and married women with adjustment being made for the age distribution of the two groups, which is very likely to differ with the married women being older. Age-specific death rates derived from each of the two groups would be applied to the population age distribution to yield mortality rates that could be compared directly. *See also* **indirect standardization**. [*Statistics in Medicine*, 1993, **12**, 3–12.]

Disability adjusted life years (DALYs): An attempt to measure the suffering caused by an illness, which takes into account both the years of potential life lost due to premature mortality as well as the years lost due to disease or health condition. One DALY represents the equivalent of the loss of one year of full health. Useful in comparisons across diseases and in setting national and international health priorities. *See also* **health-adjusted life expectancy (HALE)**. [*Journal of Health Economics*, 1997, **16**, 685–702.]

Disability-free life expectancy: The average number of years an individual is expected to live free of disability if current patterns of mortality and disability continue to apply. This measure combines data on both mortality and disabling morbidity, and tends to be highly sensitive to social inequality; for example, it shows that the greater life expectancy of women is, on the whole, made up of time spent in a state of disability. [*European Journal of Public Health*, 1996, **6**, 21–8.]

Discontinuation rate: A term specific to studies of contraceptives given by the total number of discontinuations of a device divided by the number of people continuing to use the device. For example, around half of the women who start using hormonal pills and injectables stop using them within a year. *See also* **Pearl rate**. [*Contraception*, 1996, **53**, 357–61.]

Discordant: A term used in `twin analysis` to describe a twin pair in which one twin exhibits a particular trait and the other does not.

Discrete choice data: Data obtained from presenting patients with sets of health states described by various attributes and asking them to make choices from among them. For example, a patient might be asked to choose between a health state with long life expectancy and poor quality of life and a health state with shorter life expectancy and high quality of life. Such data give information about preferences for different aspects of health-related quality-of-life. [*Health Economics*, 2012, **21**, 141–72.]

Discrete variables: Variables having only integer values, for example number of births, number of pregnancies and number of teeth extracted.

Discriminant analysis: A generic term for a variety of techniques designed to generate rules for classifying individuals to a priori defined groups on the basis of a set of measurements on the individual. In medicine, for example, such methods are generally applied to the problem of using optimally the results from a number of tests or the observations of a number of symptoms to make a diagnosis that can perhaps be confirmed only by post-mortem examination. In the two-group case, the most commonly used method is *Fisher's linear discriminant function*, in which a linear function of the variables giving maximal separation between the groups is determined. This results in a *classification rule* (also known as an *allocation rule*) that may be used to assign a new patient to one of the two groups. The derivation of this linear function assumes that the `variance–covariance matrices` of the two groups are the same. The sample of observations from which the discriminant function is derived is often known as the *training set*. [Huberty, C. J., 1994, *Applied Discriminant Analysis*, John Wiley & Sons, New York.]

Disease cluster: An unusual aggregation of health events, real or perceived. The events may be grouped in a particular area or in some short period of time, or they may occur among a certain group of people, for example those having a particular occupation. The significance of studying such clusters as a means of determining the origins of public health problems has long been recognized. In 1850, for example, the Broad Street pump in London was identified as a major source of cholera by plotting cases on a map and noting the cluster around the well. More recently, recognition of clusters of relatively rare kinds of pneumonia and tumours among young homosexual men led to the identification of AIDS and eventually to the discovery of HIV. *See also* **clustering** and **scan statistic**. [*Statistics in Medicine*, 1995, **14**, 799–810.]

Rate (per 100 000)

▨	0 to 10
⬚	10 to 20
▦	20 to 30
■	More than 30

Figure 35 Standardized mortality rates from breast cancer in the departments and regions of Argentina.

Disease cluster: It has to be recognized that reports of disease clusters lead only rarely to new aetiological insights, and in many cases the political and scientific dimensions that are often involved in their investigation quickly become confused.

Disease mapping: The process of displaying the geographical variability of disease on maps using different colours, shading, etc. An example is shown in Figure 35. The idea is not new, but the advent of computers and computer graphics has made it simpler to apply and it is now used widely in descriptive epidemiology to display, for example, morbidity or mortality information for a region or country. However, it has to be recognized that traditional maps do not always provide the most appropriate projection to look for patterns of disease. *See also* **cartogram**. [Lawson, A. B., 2006, *Statistical Methods in Spatial Epidemiology*, 2nd ed., John Wiley & Sons, New York.]

Disease prevalence: Determined by classifying patients according to whether a disease has been contracted. Classification can be based on high-cost gold standard tests or low-cost screening tests, the latter being subject to misclassification of patients. As a compromise between the two, many studies use partially validated data sets in which all patients are classified by fallible tests and then some patients' classification is validated by the completely accurate gold-standard test. [*Biometrika*, 1992, **79**, 355–65.]

Disease registers: An important tool for clinicians, epidemiologists and health service planners which relate to individuals with, or at high risk of, a specified chronic disease. One of the most common conditions for which disease registers are used is diabetes mellitus. [*Archives of Disease in Childhood*, 1995, **72**, 474–7.]

Disease-specific quality indicators (Qis): Indicators that measure structural, process or outcome elements related to the care of a particular condition. [*Journal of the American Medical Association*, 1988, **260**, 1743–8.]

Disease surveillance: A process that aims to use health and health-related data that precede diagnosis and/or confirmation to identify possible outbreaks of a disease, mobilize a rapid response and therefore reduce morbidity and mortality. Such a process provides essential information for control and response planning, helping to identify changes in incidence and affected group, thereby providing valuable time for public health interventions. [*The Lancet*, 1997, **349**, 794–5.]

Dispersion: The amount by which a set of observations deviate from their mean. When the values of a set of observations are close to their mean, the dispersion is less than when they are spread out widely from their mean. *See also* **variance**.

Distributed database: A `database` that consists of a number of component parts that are situated at geographically separate locations. [Ozsu, M. T. and Valduriez, P., 2020, *Principles of Distributed Database Systems*, 4th ed., Springer, New York.]

Distribution-free methods: Statistical techniques of estimation and inference that are based on a function of the sample observations, the `probability distribution` of which does not depend on a complete specification of the probability distribution of the population from which the sample was drawn. Consequently, the techniques are valid under relatively general assumptions about the underlying population. Often, such methods involve only the ranks of the observations rather than the observations themselves. Examples are `Wilcoxon's signed rank test` and `Friedman's two-way analysis of variance`. In many cases, these tests are only marginally less powerful than their analogues, which assume a particular population distribution (usually a `normal distribution`) even when that assumption is true. Also known as *nonparametric methods*. [Hollander, M. and Wolfe, D. A., 2014, *Nonparametric Statistical Methods*, 3rd ed., Wiley-Blackwell, Oxford.]

DMF index: A measure often used in dentistry that is calculated by adding the number of permanent teeth that are decayed (D), the number that are missing (M) and the number that have been filled (F).

Dorfman scheme: An approach to investigations designed to identify a particular medical condition in a large population, usually by means of a blood test, which may result in a considerable saving in the number of tests carried out. Instead of testing each person separately, blood samples from, say, *k* people are pooled and analyzed together. If the test is negative, then this one test clears *k* people. If the test is positive, then each of the k individual blood samples must be tested separately, and $k + 1$ tests are required for these k people. If the probability of a positive test (p) is small, then the scheme is likely to result in far fewer tests being necessary. For example, if $p = 0.01$, then it can be shown that the value of k that minimizes the expected number of tests per person is 11, and the expected number of tests is 0.2, resulting in 80% saving in the number of tests compared with testing each individual separately. [*Statistics in Medicine*, 2001, **20**, 1957–69.]

Dose-ranging trial: A clinical trial undertaken to identify the range of doses of a new compound that are safe and effective. Effective in this context means that the expected pharmacological effects are observed. Clinical efficacy is not generally at stake at this stage. Most common is the *parallel-dose design*, in which one group of subjects is given a placebo and the other groups are given different doses of the active treatment. [*Controlled Clinical Trials*, 1995, **16**, 319–30.]

Dose–response relationship: The relationship between the dose of a drug received or the level of an exposure and the degree or probability of an outcome in an individual or population. Increasing disease risk with increasing exposure is often taken as an indicator of a causal relationship between exposure and risk. For example, the observation that the risk of lung cancer increases with the number of cigarettes smoked daily and with the duration of smoking was of considerable importance in identifying cigarette smoking as the cause of lung cancer (see Figure 36). [Finney, D. J., 1978, *Statistical Methods in Biological Assay*, 3rd ed., Arnold, London.]

Dot plot: A graphical display for representing labelled quantitative data. An example is given in Figure 37.

Double-blinding: *See* blinding.

Double-dummy technique: A technique sometimes used in clinical trials when it is possible to make an acceptable placebo for an active treatment but not to make two active treatments identical. In this instance, patients can be asked to take two sets of tablets throughout the trial, one representing treatment A (active or placebo) and one representing treatment B (active or placebo). Often particularly useful in a crossover design. [*Journal of the American Medical Association*, 1995, **274**, 545–9.]

Double-masked: Synonym for **double-blind**.

Double sampling: A procedure in which initially a sample of subjects is selected for obtaining only auxiliary information, and then a second sample is selected in which the variable of interest is observed in addition to the auxiliary information. The second sample is often selected as a subsample of the first. The purpose of this type of sampling is to obtain better estimators by using the relationship between the auxiliary variables and the variable of interest. *See also* **two-phase sampling**. [*Survey Methodology*, 1990, **16**, 105–16.]

Doubling time: A term used in describing epidemics for the time taken for the number of infectives to double. Also used in cell biology for the time it takes for a cell to fully divide.

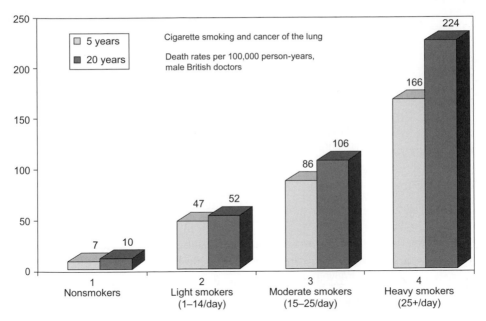

Figure 36 Dose–response relationships for lung cancer and other causes of death in relation to smoking.
(Taken with permission from the *British Medical Journal*.)

Doubly multivariate data: A term sometimes used for the data collected in those `longitudinal studies` in which more than a single response variable is recorded for each subject on each occasion. For example, in a `clinical trial`, weight and blood pressure might be recorded for each subject on each of several planned visits.

Draughtsman plot: Synonym for **scatterplot matrix**.

Drop-in: A subject in a `clinical trial` who takes another treatment during the trial instead of the one to which he or she was allocated and remains available for follow-up. *See also* **intention-to-treat**.

Dropout: A patient who withdraws from a study for whatever reason, which may or may not be known. The fate of patients who drop out of an investigation must be determined whenever possible, and it is important to try to minimize the number of dropouts in a study. *See also* **attrition**, **missing values** and **Diggle–Kenward model for dropouts**. [Everitt, B. S. and Wessely, S., 2008, *Clinical Trials in Psychiatry*, 2nd ed., John Wiley & Sons, Chichester.]

Drug benefit–risk assessment: An assessment and comparison of the favourable therapeutic effects of a drug versus adverse reactions that the drug may induce. The benefit–risk balance is a strong predictor of the drug's long-term viability and a key element for decision-making during the drug's development. In the past, qualitative methods have been used to establish a drug's profile but recently

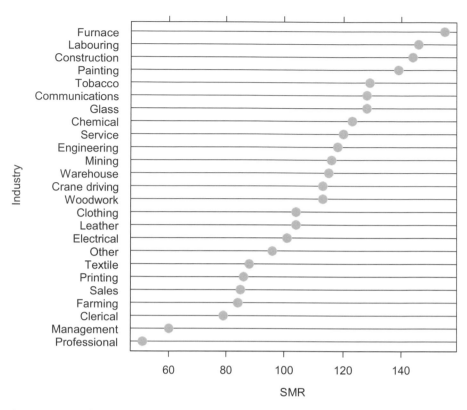

Figure 37 Dot plot of standardized mortality rates (SMR).

structured frameworks and quantitative methodologies have been proposed to make a benefits–risk assessment more comprehensive and consistent. [*Pharmaceutical Statistics*, 2015, **15**, 324–32.]

Drug combinations trials: Trials that are motivated by the fact that individual drugs may target the same disease but via different routes. A combination of such drugs may then have an overall improved effect that the individual treatments, an improvement that needs to be verified by a `clinical trial`. The primary questions that arise in a drug combination therapy trial are: (1) Does there exist a drug combination that shows better effect than placebo control?; (2) Does there exist a drug combination that is superior to the individual treatments?; (3) What are the specific combinations the are both effective and superior to the monotherapies? [*Statistical Methods in Medical Research*, 2020, **29**, 1799–817.]

Drug interaction: The alteration of the effect of one drug owing to the presence of a second drug. Such `interactions` arise from a variety of complex physiological conditions.

Drug stability studies: Studies conducted in the pharmaceutical industry to measure the degradation of a new drug product or an old drug formulated or packaged in a new way. The main study objective is to estimate a drug's shelf life, defined as the time point where the 95% lower confidence limit for the regression line crosses the lowest acceptable limit for drug content according to the *Guidelines for Stability Testing*. [European Medicines Agency, March 2014.]

Drug utilization studies: In most such studies, the purpose is to determine whether a class of drugs or a specific drug is associated with a greater risk of adverse outcomes than either other drugs or no drug. A number of methodological challenges are present in these types of observational studies, irrespective of the source of information. [*Annals of Internal Medicine*, 1997, **127**, 764–8.]

DSM: Abbreviation for *Diagnostic and Statistical Manual*.

Dummy variables: The variables resulting from recoding categorical variables with more than two categories into a series of binary variables. Marital status, for example, if labelled originally as 1 for married, 2 for single and 3 for divorced, widowed or separated, could be redefined in terms of two variables, as follows:
Variable 1: 1 if single, 0 otherwise
Variable 2: 1 if divorced, widowed or separated, 0 if otherwise
For a married person, both new variables could be 0. In general, a categorical variable with k categories would be recoded in terms of $k - 1$ dummy variables. Such recoding is used before polychotomous variables are used as explanatory variables in a regression analysis to avoid the unreasonable assumption that the original numerical codes for the categories, that is, the values 1, 2, ... , k, correspond to an interval scale. *See also* **categorical variables**. [Everitt, B. S. and Palmer, C. (eds.), 2011, *Encyclopedic Companion to Medical Statistics*, 2nd ed., John Wiley & Sons, Chichester.]

Dunnett's test: A multiple comparison test intended for comparing each of a number of treatment groups with a control group. [Fisher, L. D. and Van Belle, G., 2004, *Biostatistics*, 2nd ed., Wiley-Blackwell, Oxford.]

Duplicate data entry: Entering data into a database more than once and comparing results in an effort to record observations as accurately as possible. *See also* **data editing**.

Duration time: A time that elapses before an epidemic ceases. [*Infectious Disease Modelling*, 2018, **3**, 60–73.]

Dynamic population: A population that gains and loses members.
Membership is defined by current status, so membership is not permanent.
A person is a member of the population as long as they meet the definition of the population, and they cease to be a member of the population when they no longer meet the definition.

Dynamic treatment regimes: A set of decision rules for determining which treatment should be chosen at each decision time point for an individual patient, depending on the patient's medical history. Each rule takes as input information on the patient, such as demographics, prior medical history, genetic and genomic characteristics and clinical variables. The result is a personalized medical response tailored to the time-varying states of the patient. [(1) *Annual Review of Statistics and Its Applications*, 2014, **1**, 447–64, (2) *Statistical Methods in Medical Research*, 2017, **26**, 1605–10.]

E

Early detection programme: Synonymous with **screening studies**.

Early warning system: A term used in disease surveillance for any procedure designed to detect as early as possible any departure from usual or normally observed frequency of phenomena. For example, in developing countries, a change in children's average weights is an early warning signal of nutritional deficiency. [*Canadian Medical Association*, 2002, **166**, 1–2.]

EBM: Abbreviation for **evidence-based medicine**.

Ecological fallacy: A term used when spatially aggregated data are analyzed and the results assumed to apply to relationships at the individual level. In most cases, analyses based on area-level means give conclusions very different from those that would be obtained from an analysis of unit-level data. An example from the literature is a correlation coefficient of 0.11 between illiteracy and being foreign-born calculated from person-level data in the USA, compared with a value of -0.53 between percentage illiteracy and percentage foreign-born calculated from summary state summary statistics. [*Journal of Epidemiology and Community Health*, 2000, **54**, 326–7.]

Ecological risk assessment (ERA): A generic term used to describe any formal process whereby ecological threats are identified, their likelihood of occurrence estimated and their consequences described. [*Human and Ecological Risk Assessment*, 2006, **12**, 120–9.]

Ecological statistics: Procedures for studying the dynamics of natural communities and their relation to environmental variables. [Gotelli, N. J. and Ellison, A. M., 2004, *A Primer of Ecological Statistics*, Oxford University Press, Oxford.]

Ecological study: A study in which the units of analysis are populations or groups of individuals rather than individuals. Used widely in epidemiology, despite their methodological limitations (*see* **ecological fallacy**), because of their low cost and convenience. [*American Journal of Public Health*, 1982, **72**, 1336–44.]

Ecological study: The value of ecological studies remains a subject of controversy among epidemiologists. Biases can arise from a variety of sources, and these give some cause for doubting the worth of such studies.

EDA: Abbreviation for **exploratory data analysis**.

ED50: Abbreviation for **median effective dose**.

Effect: Generally used for the change in a response variable produced by a change in one or more explanatory variables.

Effective sample size: Could be defined as the sample size after dropouts, deaths and other specified exclusions from the original sample, but most often is an estimate of the sample size that a survey conducted using random sampling would have required to achieve the same sampling error as computed in the study that did not employ simple random sampling. [*The American Statistician*, 2001, **55**, 187–93.]

Effect size measures: Measures of the effect magnitude of, most often, some form of intervention, for example, in a clinical trial. A variety of statistics are used to measure effect magnitude. Depending on the type of response variable, the effect size might be a difference between means (usually standardized in some way), an odds ratio or a relative risk. [Davis, S. F. (ed.), 2003, *Handbook of Research Methods in Experimental Psychology*, Blackwell Science, Oxford.]

Efficacy: The effect of treatment relative to a control in the ideal situation where all people comply fully with the treatment regimen to which they were assigned by random allocation. [*Archives of General Psychiatry*, 1981, **38**, 1203–8.]

Efficiency: A term applied in the context of comparing different methods of estimating the same parameter with the estimate having the lowest variance being regarded as the most efficient. Also used when comparing competing experimental designs, with one design being more efficient than another if it can achieve the same precision with fewer resources.

Egger's test: A test for funnel plot asymmetry based on a linear regression of effect size divided by its standard error, against precision (the reciprocal of the standard error). *See also* **Begg's test**. [*American Journal of Epidemiology*, 2005, **162**, 925–42.]

Ehrenberg's equation: An equation linking the height and weight of children between the ages of 5 and 13, given by

$$\log \bar{w} = 0.8\bar{h} + 0.4$$

where $\bar{w}$ is the mean weight in kilograms and $\bar{h}$ is the mean height in metres. The relationship has been found to hold in England, Canada and France. [*Indian Journal of Medical Research*, 1998, **107**, 46–9.]

Eigenvalues and eigenvectors: Terms encountered primarily when using principal components analysis, with the eigenvalues giving the variances of each component and the eigenvectors the sets of coefficients defining each component. [Everitt, B. S. and Dunn, G., 2010, *Applied Multivariate Data Analysis*, 2nd ed., Wiley, Chichester.]

Electronic mail (email): The use of computer systems to transfer messages between users. It is usual for messages to be held in a central store for retrieval at the user's convenience. *See also* **Internet** and **network**.

Eligibility and exclusion criteria: Criteria for including and excluding patients from participating in a clinical trial. The choice of these criteria can influence greatly both the results and the interpretation of the trial. For example, very narrow eligibility criteria lead to a more homogeneous trial population and, consequently, greater power but a more limited ability to generalize the results to a wider population. [Everitt, B. S. and Wessely, S., 2008, *Clinical Trials in Psychiatry*, 2nd ed., John Wiley & Sons, Chichester.]

Empirical: Based on observation or experiment rather than deduction from basic laws or theory.

Empirical logits: The logistic transformation of an observed proportion y_i/n_i, adjusted so that finite values are obtained when y_i is equal to either zero or n_i. Commonly, 0.5 is added to both y_i and n_i. [Collett, D., 2003, *Modelling Binary Data*, 2nd ed., Chapman & Hall/CRC, Boca Raton, FL.]

End-aversion bias: A term that refers to the reluctance of some people to use the extremes of a scale. *See also* **acquiescence bias**. [*Medical Care*, 2002, **40**, 113–28.]

Endpoint: A clearly defined outcome or event associated with an individual in a medical investigation. A simple example is the death of a patient. Other examples are blood pressure and quality of life. The choice of endpoints in, for example, clinical trials, needs to be set out clearly in the study protocol. *See also* **surrogate endpoints**.

Entropy: A measure of the amount of information received or output by some system.

Environmental epidemiology: A wide variety of topics and procedures for determining how quality of life, occurrence of disease, etc. are affected by environmental factors such as air and water pollution, the use of hazardous substances, diet and drugs, occupation, lifestyle and so on. [Talbot, E. and Grauin, G., 1995, *Introduction to Environmental Epidemiology*, CRC, Boca Raton, FL.]

Epidemic: The occurrence of significantly more cases of some disease than past experience would have predicted for a location, time and population. [Rothman, K. J., 2012, *Epidemiology: An Introduction*, 2nd ed., Oxford University Press, Oxford.]

Epidemic chain: *See* **chains of infection**.

Epidemic curve: A plot of time trends in the occurrence of a disease or other health-related event for a defined population and time period. A large and sudden rise in excess of what would be expected based on past experience often corresponds to an epidemic. An example is shown in Figure 38. *See also* **back-calculation**. [*Science*, 1991, **253**, 37–42.]

Epidemic models: Models for the spread of an epidemic in a population. Can be deterministic or contain a random component, and often have to account for

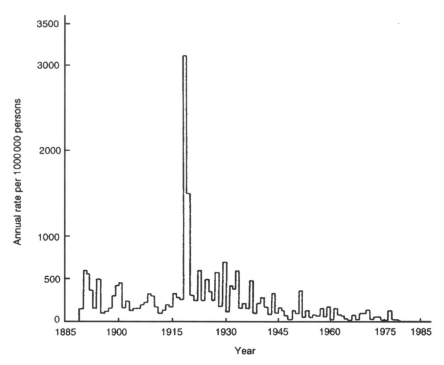

Figure 38 Epidemic curve of influenza mortality in England and Wales 1885–1985.

development within a spatial framework. [Mollison, D., 1995, *Epidemic Models: Their Structure and Relation to Data*, Cambridge University Press, Cambridge.]

Epidemic thresholds: A concept arising from `epidemic models` and specifying that an epidemic can become established in a population only if the initial susceptible population size is larger than some critical value that depends on the parameters controlling the spread of the disease. Of great practical importance since it gives a value from the proportion of susceptibles that need to be vaccinated in order to prevent the occurrence of an epidemic. [Mollison, D., 1995, *Epidemic Models: Their Structure and Relation to Data*, Cambridge University Press, Cambridge.]

Epidemiology: The study of the distribution and size of disease problems in human populations, in particular, to identify aetiological factors in the pathogenesis of disease and to provide the data essential for the management, evaluation and planning of services for the prevention, control and treatment of disease. *See also* **incidence rate**, **prevalence**, **prospective study** and **retrospective study**. [Woodward, M., 2005, *Epidemiology: Study Design and Data Analysis*, 2nd ed., Chapman & Hall/CRC, Boca Raton, FL.]

Epi Info: Free software for performing basic sample size calculations, developing a study questionnaire, performing statistical analyses, etc. The software can be downloaded from the website **www.cdc.gov/epiinfo/**.

Episodic hormone data: Data arising from endocrinology studies involving repeated measurements of blood hormone concentrations over time. Such data usually display a characteristic pattern of episodic pulses, which are produced in response to a burst of neural activity in the hypothalamus. *See also* **Harris and Stevens forecasting**. [*Biometrics*, 1988, **44**, 339–53.]

Epistatic genetic variance: The variance of a characteristic that can be explained by the interaction between genes at different loci.

Epstein test: A test for assessing whether a sample of survival times arises from an exponential distribution with a constant failure rate against the alternative hypothesis that the failure rate is not constant but increasing. [*Technometrics*, 1960, **2**, 83–101.]

Equipoise: A state of perfect balance regarding treatment preference implying that a clinician is as willing to treat their next patient with one treatment as with another. Equipoise is a precondition for any clinical trial, and the aim of the trial is to deliberately upset this equipoise by the time of its completion in order to make an impact on medical practice. [Senn, S., 2008, *Statistical Issues in Drug Development*, 2nd ed., John Wiley & Sons, Chichester.]

Equipotent dose: The dose of a new drug that leads to a response just as effective as the established dose of an old drug. [*Anesthetics and Analgesics*, 1995, **80**, 210–11.]

Equivalence trials: A clinical trial designed to evaluate whether an experimental treatment is sufficiently similar to an accepted or standard treatment to justify its use. [*British Medical Journal*, 1996, **313**, 36–9.]

Equivalent dose: Synonym for **equipotent dose**.

Error mean square: *See* **mean squares**.

Errors-in-variables problem: *See* **regression dilution**.

Errors of classification: A term used most often in the context of retrospective studies, where it is recognized that a certain proportion of the controls may be at an early stage of the disease and should have been diagnosed as cases. Additionally, misdiagnosed cases might be included in the disease group. Both errors lead to underestimates of the relative risk. [*American Journal of Public Health*, 1962, **52**, 1137–44.]

Errors of the third kind: Giving the right answer to the wrong question.

Estimate: Either a single number (*point estimate*) or a range of numbers (*interval estimate*) that are inferred to be plausible values for some parameter of interest.

Estimation: The process of providing a numerical value for a population parameter on the basis of information collected from a sample. If a single figure is calculated for the unknown parameter, then the process is called *point estimation*. If an interval is calculated within which the parameter is likely to fall, then the procedure is called *interval estimation*. *See also* **least squares estimation**, **maximum likelihood estimation** and **confidence interval**. [Altman, D. G., 2018, *Practical Statistics for Medical Research*, Chapman & Hall/CRC, Boca Raton, FL.]

Estimator: A statistic used to provide an estimate for a parameter. The sample mean, for example, is an unbiased estimator of the population mean. [Altman, D. G., 2018, *Practical Statistics for Medical Research*, Chapman & Hall/CRC, Boca Raton, FL.]

Ethical review committees: Formally constituted committees charged with vetting and approving (or otherwise) research protocols prior to study initiation to ensure sound ethics. The members of the committee must be independent of the investigator, the sponsor of any other kind of undue influence. [*British Medical Journal*, 1980, **281**, 1182–4.]

EU model: A model used in the investigation of the rate of success of in vitro fertilization (IVF), defined in terms of two probabilities: the probability of a viable embryo and the probability of a receptive uterus. *See also* **Barrett and Marshall model for conception**. [*Biostatistics*, 2002, **3**, 361–77.]

Evaluable patients: The patients in a `clinical trial` regarded by the investigator as having satisfied certain conditions and, as a result, retained for the purpose of analysis. Patients not satisfying the required conditions are not included in the final analysis.

Event history data: Observations on a collection of individuals, each moving among a small number of states. Of primary interest are the times taken to move between the various states, which are often observed only incompletely because of some form of censoring. The simplest kind of event history data involves `survival times`. `Multistate models` will often provide a relevant modelling framework for such data. [*Statistics in Medicine*, 1988, **7**, 819–42.]

Evidence-based medicine (EBM): Defined by its proponents as 'the conscientious, explicit, and judicious use of current best evidence in making decisions about the care of individual patients and integrating clinical experience with the best available external clinical evidence from systematic research'. Uncertainty regarding the evidentiary basis for many commonly accepted medical practices has led to the growth of EBM. *See also* **Cochrane Collaboration** and **CONSORT statement**. [*Evidence Based Medicine*, 1996, **1**, 98–9.]

Exact tests: Procedures that give exact `p-values` rather than values that can be justified only by asymptotic arguments. Particularly important in the analysis of `contingency tables` containing many cells with low or zero frequencies. *See also* **Fisher's exact test**. [*Statistical Science*, 1992, **7**, 131–77.]

> **Exact tests:** Allow the researcher to draw correct inferences from, for example, contingency tables even when the data are very sparse. Remove both the need for ad hoc rules of thumb about the minimal size of expected frequencies required and the need for Yates's correction.

Excess hazard models: Models for the excess mortality, that is, the mortality that remains when the expected mortality calculated from `life tables` is subtracted. [*Biometrics*, 1989, **45**, 523–35.]

Excess risk: The difference between the risk rate for a population exposed to some risk factor and the risk rate in an otherwise identical population without the exposure. Similar to `attributable risk`. [*Radiation Research*, 1996, **146**, 1–27.]

Expected frequencies: A term usually encountered in the analysis of `contingency tables`. Such frequencies are estimates of the values to be expected under the hypothesis of interest. In a two-dimensional table, for example, the values under the hypothesis of the independence of the two variables are calculated as the product of the appropriate row and column totals divided by the total number of observations. *See also* **exact tests**. [Everitt, B. S., 1992, *The Analysis of Contingency Tables*, 2nd ed., Chapman & Hall/CRC, Boca Raton, FL.]

Expected value: The theoretical mean of a random variable with a particular `probability distribution`. [Altman, D. G., 2018, *Practical Statistics for Medical Research*, Chapman & Hall/CRC, Boca Raton, FL.]

Experimental design: The arrangement and procedures used in an experimental study. Some general principles of good design are simplicity, avoidance of `bias`, the use of random allocation for forming treatment groups, replication and adequate sample size. [Ruxton, D. G. and Colegrave, N., 2016, *Experimental Designs for the Life Sciences*, Oxford University Press, Oxford.]

Experimental study: A general term for investigations in which the researcher can deliberately influence events and investigate the effects of the intervention. `Clinical trials` and many animal studies fall under this heading.

Experimenter-wise error rate: Synonym for per-experiment error rate.

Expert systems: Computer programs designed to mimic the role of an expert human consultant. Such systems are able to cope with the complex problems of medical decision-making because of their ability to manipulate symbolically, rather than just numerical, information and their use of judgemental or heuristic knowledge to construct intelligible solutions to diagnostic problems. Well-known examples include the *MYCIN* system, developed at Stanford University, and ABEL, developed at MIT. *See also* **computer-aided diagnosis**. [*Statistics in Medicine*, 1985, **4**, 311–16.]

Explanatory analysis: A term sometimes used for the analysis of data from a `clinical trial` in which treatments *A* and *B* are compared under the assumption that patients remain on their assigned treatment throughout the trial. In contrast, a *pragmatic analysis* of the trial would involve asking whether it would be better to start with *A* (with the intention of continuing this therapy if possible, but with the willingness to be flexible) or to start with *B* (with the same intention). With the explanatory approach, the aim is to acquire information on the true effect of treatment, while with the pragmatic analysis, the aim is to make a decision about the therapeutic strategy after taking into account the cost (e.g., withdrawal due to side effects) of administering treatment. *See also* **explanatory trials**, **pragmatic trials** and **intention-to-treat analysis**. [*Statistics in Medicine*, 1988, **7**, 1179–86.]

Explanatory trials: A term sometimes used to describe `clinical trials` that are designed to explain how a treatment works. To achieve this, the investigators set strict inclusion criteria that will produce highly homogeneous study groups. For example, investigators designing an explanatory trial of the effects of a new antihypertensive drug could decide to include only patients aged between 40 and 50 years with no coexisting diseases (e.g. diabetes) and to exclude those patients receiving other particular interventions (e.g. beta-blockers). *See also* **pragmatic trials**. [*Statistics in Medicine*, 1988, **7**, 1179–86.]

Explanatory variables: The variables appearing on the right-hand side of the equations defining, for example, `multiple linear regression` or `logistic regression` and that seek to predict or explain the response variable. Also known as *independent variables*, although this term is not recommended since they are rarely independent of one another.

Exploratory data analysis (EDA): An approach to data analysis that emphasizes the use of informal graphical procedures not based on prior assumptions about the structure of the data or on formal models for the data. The essence of this approach is that, broadly speaking, data are assumed to possess the following structure:

data = smooth + rough,

where 'smooth' is the underlying regularity or pattern in the data. The objective of the exploratory approach is to separate the 'smooth' from the 'rough' with minimal use of formal mathematics or statistical methods. *See also* **initial data analysis**. [Tukey, J. W., 1977, *Exploratory Data Analysis*, Addison-Wesley, Reading, MA.]

Exploratory factor analysis: *See* **factor analysis**.

Exponential distribution: The `probability distribution` of time intervals between consecutive random events. The shape of the distribution depends on the value of its single parameter. Figure 39 shows some examples of the distribution. The distribution is used to model highly skewed data. [Evans, M., Hastings, N. and Peacock, B., 2000, *Statistical Distributions*, 3rd ed., John Wiley & Sons, New York.]

Exponential family: A family of `probability distributions` that includes the `normal distribution`, the `binomial distribution` and the `Poisson distribution` as special cases. Used in `generalized linear` models. [Dobson, A. J., 2018, *An Introduction to Generalized Linear Models*, 4th ed., Chapman & Hall/CRC, Boca Raton, FL.]

Exposure effect: A measure of the impact of exposure on an outcome measure. Examples are **relative risk**, **excess risk** and **relative odds**. [*Journal of Clinical Oncology*, 2001, **19**, 3111–16.]

Exposure factor: Synonym for **risk factor**.

Exposure ratio: The ratio of the rates at which people in the case and control groups of a `retrospective study` are exposed to the risk factor. [*Journal of Aerosol Medicine*, 2001, **14**, 377–8.]

Extrabinomial variation: A type of `overdispersion`. [Collett, D., 2003, *Modelling Binary Data*, 2nd ed., Chapman & Hall/CRC, Boca Raton, FL.]

Extraim analysis: An analysis involving increasing the sample size in a `clinical trial` that ends without a clear conclusion, in an attempt to resolve the issue of, say, a group difference that is currently marginally nonsignificant. As in `interim`

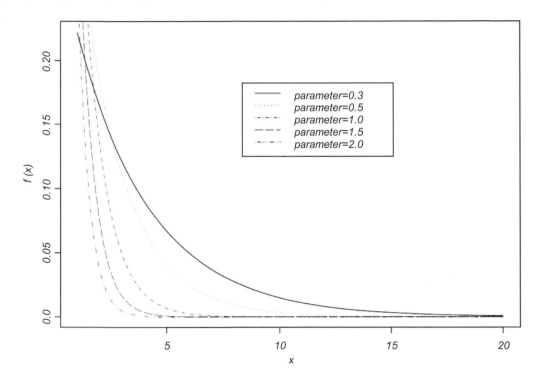

Figure 39 A number of exponential distributions.

analysis, significance levels need to be suitably adjusted. [*Statistical Science*, 2004, **19**, 175–87.]

Extrapolation: The process of estimating from a data set values lying beyond the range of the observed values. In regression analysis, for example, a value of the response variable may be estimated from the fitted equation for a new observation having values on one or more of the explanatory variables outside the range of values used in deriving the equation.

Extrapolation: Often a dangerous procedure since the model fitted for the range of variable values observed may not hold for other ranges.

Extremal quotient: Defined for non-negative observations as the ratio of the largest observation in a sample to the smallest observation. In medicine, usually used to compare the highest and lowest rates of some event or procedure of interest in different regions. [*Health Services Research*, 1989, **24**, 665–84.]

Extreme values: The largest and smallest values of a variable in a sample of observations.

Eyeball test: Informal assessment of data simply by inspection and mental calculation allied with the experience of the particular area from which the data arise.

Facets: *See* **generalizability theory**.

Factor: A term used in a variety of ways in statistics. Most commonly, it refers to a categorical variable with a small number of levels under investigation in an experiment as a possible source of variation in a response variable, that is, simply a categorical explanatory variable. Also used for the `latent variables`, which are the bases of `factor analysis`.

Factor analysis: A collection of techniques for investigating the `correlation matrix` or `variance-covariance matrix` between a set of variables to determine whether the correlation or `covariances` between the observed or `manifest variables` can be explained by assuming that the latter are related to a small number of underlying, unobservable `latent variables`, or *common factors*. More specifically, each measured variable is assumed to be a linear function of the common factors plus a residual term known in this context as a *specific factor*. The coefficients defining the common factors are known as *factor loadings*. A very early example of the application of the methodology postulated that the scores of individuals on a number of cognitive tests could be decomposed to a general factor common to all variables, which might be labelled general intelligence, and a specific factor, which was different for each variable. There are essentially two approaches to factor analysis that need to be differentiated carefully: the first, *exploratory factor analysis*, imposes no constraints on the structure of the common factors, whereas the second, *confirmatory factor analysis*, imposes constraints; in particular, it sets specific factor loadings to zero in line with some theoretical factor structure to be tested on the current data. *See also* **factor rotation** and **principal components analysis**. [Lewis-Beck, M. S., 1994, *Factor Analysis and Related Techniques*, Sage, London.]

Factor analysis: Often criticized by statisticians in the past, but nevertheless frequently a useful approach to understanding the patterns in correlation and covariance matrices.

Factorial designs: Designs that allow two or more questions to be addressed in an investigation. Although used for many years in agriculture and industrial research, such designs have been used only sparingly in medicine. The simplest factorial design is one in which each of two treatments or interventions are either present or absent, so that subjects are divided into four groups: those receiving neither treatment, those having only the first treatment, those having only the second treatment and those receiving both treatments. Such designs enable possible interactions between factors to be investigated. [*Journal of the American Medical Association*, 2003, **289**, 2545–53.]

Factor loadings: *See* **factor analysis**.

Factor rotation: The final stage of a factor analysis, in which the factors derived initially are transformed to make the interpretation simpler. In general, the aim of the process is to make the common factors defined more clearly by increasing the size of large factor loadings and decreasing the size of those that are small. Factors with a mixture of positive and negative loadings (*bipolar factors*) are generally split into two separate parts, one corresponding to those variables with positive loadings and the other corresponding to those variables with negative loadings. *See also* **varimax rotation**. [Lewis-Beck, M. S., 1994, *Factor Analysis and Related Techniques*, Sage, London.]

Faggot fallacy: The belief that multiple pieces of evidence, each independently being suspect or weak, provide strong evidence when bundled together. *See also* **meta-analysis**. [Skrabanek, P. and McCormick, J., 1992, *Follies and Fallacies in Medicine*, Tarragon Press, London.]

Faggot fallacy: A bundle of insecure evidence remains insecure.

Failsafe N: An estimate of the number of 'non-significant' articles remaining in researchers' file draws, and used as an indicator of possible publication bias in a meta-analysis. Failsafe N is prone to misinterpretation and misuse and no statistical criterion is available for interpretation of its values; its use is not recommended. [Rosenthal, R. and Rosnow, R. L. (eds.), 1969, *Artifact in Behavioral Research*, Academic Press, New York.]

Failure time: Synonym for **survival time**.

False discovery rate (FDR): An approach to controlling the error rate in an exploratory analysis where large numbers of hypotheses are tested, but where the strict control that is provided by multiple comparison tests controlling the family-wise error rate is not required. Suppose m hypotheses are to be tested, of which m_0 relate to cases where the null hypothesis is true and the remaining $m - m_0$ relate to cases where the alternative hypothesis is true; the FDR is defined as the expected proportion of incorrectly rejected null hypotheses. [*Journal of the Royal Statistical Society, Series B*, 1995, **57**, 289–300.]

False-negative rate: The proportion of cases in which a diagnostic test indicates that a disease is absent in patients who have the disease; usually expressed as a conditional probability or a percentage. [*New England Journal of Medicine*, 1988, **319**, 961–4.] *See also* **false-positive rate**.

False-positive rate: The proportion of cases in which a diagnostic test indicates that a disease is present in disease-free patients; usually expressed as a conditional probability or a percentage. [*New England Journal of Medicine*, 1988, **319**, 961–4.] *See also* **false-negative rate**.

Familial correlations: The correlation in some phenotypic trait between genetically related individuals. The magnitude of the correlation is dependent both on the heritability of the trait and on the degree of relatedness between the individuals. [Sham, P., 1998, *Statistics in Human Genetics*, Arnold, London.]

Familial disease: Disease that exhibits a tendency to familial occurrence due to a variety of possible reasons, for example, genetic, cultural or common environment. [*Arthritis and Rheumatism*, 2004, **50**, 1650–4.]

Family-wise error rate: The probability of making any error in a given family of inferences. *See also* **multiple comparison tests**, **per-comparison error rate** and **per-experiment error rate**. [*Statistical Applications in Genetics and Molecular Biology*, 2004, **3**, Article 15.]

Fan-spread model: A term sometimes applied to a model for explaining differences found between naturally occurring groups that are greater than those observed on some earlier occasion. Under this model, this effect is assumed to arise because individuals who are less unwell, less impaired, etc. and thus score higher initially, may have greater capacity for change or improvement over time. [*Applied Psychological Measurement*, 1994, **18**, 63–77.]

FDA: Abbreviation for **Food and Drug Administration**.

F-distribution: A statistical distribution with considerable practical importance, particularly in analysis of variance. Formally, the probability distribution of the ratio of two independent variables, each having a chi-squared distribution. The distribution is used in assessing the equality of two variances. [Evans, M., Hastings, N. and Peacock, B., 2000, *Statistical Distributions*, 3rd ed., John Wiley & Sons, New York.]

FDR: Abbreviation for **false discovery rate**.

Feasibility study: Essentially a synonym for **pilot study**.

Fecundability: The rate at which a sexually active, noncontracepting, ovulating woman conceives children. In the absence of direct observations on the biological determinants of fecundability, estimators of its distribution are derived from data on waiting times to first conception. *See also* **Barrett and Marshall model for conception** and **EU model**. [*Annals of New York Academy of Science*, 1994, **709**, 128–44.]

Fertility rate: The number of live births in a particular period expressed as a proportion of potentially fertile women in the population concerned. For example, in 2001 the rate for Chad was 6.56 per woman, for China it was 1.82 and for the United Kingdom it was 1.73.

Fertility ratio: A measure of the fertility of the population that restricts the denominator to the female population of appropriate age for childbearing. Defined explicitly as

$$\text{fertility ratio} = \frac{\text{number of girls under 15 years of age}}{\text{number of women in 15--49 age group}}.$$

[*Journal of Psychology*, 1973, **84**, 159--64.]

Fibonacci dose-escalation scheme: A scheme designed to estimate the maximum tolerated dose during a phase I study using as few patients as possible. Using the National Cancer Institute standards for adverse drug reactions, the procedure begins patient accrual with three patients at an initial dose level and continues at each subsequent dose level until at least one toxicity of grade 3 or above is encountered. Once the latter occurs, three additional patients are entered at that level, and six patients are entered into each succeeding level. The search scheme stops when at least two of six patients have toxicities of grade ≥ 3. [*Highlights in Oncology Practice*, 1994, **18**, 2--7.]

File draw problem: The problem that studies are not uniformly likely to be published in scientific journals since there is considerable evidence that statistical significance remains a major determining factor in both persuading editors to publish a paper and in authors deciding to submit their work for consideration. The existence of such a phenomenon implies that if the studies selected in a systematic review are all taken from the published literature, then there could be a degree of bias in the final results from the associated meta-analysis. *See also* **Failsafe N** and **publication bias**. [Everitt, B. S., 2003, *Modern Medical Statistics*, Arnold, London.]

Final-state data: A term often applied to data collected after the end of an outbreak of a disease and consisting of observations of whether each individual member of a household was infected at any time during the outbreak. [*Biometrics*, 1995, **51**, 956--8.]

Finite-mixture distribution: A probability distribution given by a linear function of a number of component probability distributions. An example of the use of this type of distribution was reported by Karl Pearson, who modelled measurements on a particular type of crab in terms of a weighted sum of two normal distributions. Such distributions are important for modelling variables in populations considered to consist of distinct groups of individuals; in medicine, for example, different diagnostic categories. Figure 40 shows the results of fitting a single normal distribution and a finite-mixture distribution with two normal components to the age of onset of schizophrenia in a sample of women and a sample of men to assess the evidence for a two-stage onset theory. [Everitt, B. S., Landau, S., Leese, M. and Stahl, D., 2011, *Cluster Analysis*, 5th ed., John Wiley & Sons, Chichester.]

Finite population: A population of finite size.

Finite population correction: A term sometimes used to describe the extra factor in the variance of the sample mean when n sample values are drawn without replacement

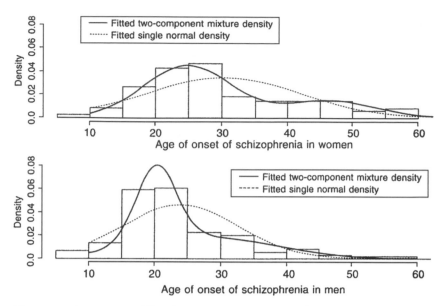

Figure 40 Histogram and fitted two-component (normal distributions) finite-mixture distributions for the age of onset of schizophrenia in men and women.

from a `finite population` of size N. The correction factor is simply the difference between N and n divided by $N − 1$. [Levy, P. S. and Lemeshow, S., 2008, *Sampling of Populations: Methods and Applications*, 4th ed., Wiley-Blackwell, Oxford.]

First-order Markov chain: *See* **Markov chain**.

Fisher's exact test: An alternative procedure to the use of the `chi-squared test` for assessing the independence of two variables forming a `two-by-two contingency table`, particularly when the `expected frequencies` are small. The method consists of evaluating the sum of the probabilities associated with the observed table and all possible two-by-two tables that have the same row and column totals as the observed data but exhibit more extreme departure from independence. The probability of each table is calculated from the `hypergeometric distribution`. *See also* **exact tests**. [Everitt, B. S., 1992, *The Analysis of Contingency Tables*, 2nd ed., Chapman & Hall/CRC, Boca Raton, FL.]

Fisher's linear discriminant function: *See* **discriminant analysis**.

Fisher's z-transformation: A transformation of `Pearson's product moment correlation coefficient` that leads to a normal variate, so enabling hypothesis about the size of the population correlation to be tested. [Altman, D. G., 2018, *Practical Statistics for Medical Research*, Chapman & Hall/CRC, Boca Raton, FL.]

Fishing expedition: Synonymous with **data dredging**.

Fitted values: Usually used to refer to the value of the response variable as predicted by some estimated model.

Five-number summary: A method of summarizing a set of observations using the minimum value, the lower quartile, the median, the upper quartile and the maximum value. Forms the basis of the `box-and-whisker plot`. [Altman, D. G., 2018, *Practical Statistics for Medical Research*, Chapman & Hall/CRC, Boca Raton, FL.]

Fixed effects: The effects attributable to a finite set of levels of a factor that are of specific interest. For example, the investigator may wish to compare the effects of three particular drugs on a response variable. *Fixed-effects models* are those that contain only factors with this type of effect. *See also* **mixed-effects models**.

Fixed-effects model: *See* fixed effects.

Fixed population: A group of individuals defined by a common fixed characteristic, such as all men born in Essex in 1944. Membership of such a population does not change over time by immigration or emigration.

Floating absolute risk: An alternative way of presenting `relative risk` for polychotomous risk factors. Instead of choosing a level of the risk factor as a reference category, each level is assigned a 'floated' variance which describes the uncertainty in risk without reference to another level. [*Statistics in Medicine*, 2004, **23**, 93–104.]

Floor effect: *See* **ceiling effect**.

Flow chart: A graphical display illustrating the interrelationship between the different components of a system. It acts as a convenient bridge between the conceptualization of a model and the construction of equations.

Foetal death rate: The number of foetal deaths in a year expressed as a proportion of the total number of births (live births plus foetal deaths) in the same year. For example, in 1997 the foetal death rate in the USA was 5.8 deaths per 1,000 live births. The rate has been decreasing steadily during the last 50 years. [*Obstetrics and Gynecology*, 1992, **79**, 35–9.]

Follow-back surveys: Surveys that use lists associated with vital statistics to sample individuals for further information. For example, the 1988 National Mortality Followback Survey sampled death certificates for 1986 decedents 25 years or older that were filed in the USA. Information was then sought from the next of kin or some other person familiar with the decedent and from healthcare facilities used by the decedent in the last year of life. Information was requested by emailed questionnaire, telephone or personal interview. The sample designs of this type are usually quite simple, involving a stratified selection of individuals from a list frame. [*American Journal of Industrial Medicine*, 1995, **27**, 195–205.]

Follow-up: Observation of an individual or group of individuals over a prolonged period of time, or the process of locating research subjects or patients sometime after they were subjected to an intervention to assess their current health status.

Food and Drug Administration (FDA): The US governmental agency responsible for the review and approval of all clinical studies and for food safety. The single-most important body influencing drug development. Its mission statement is as follows: 'The FDA is responsible for protecting the public health by assuring the safety, efficacy,

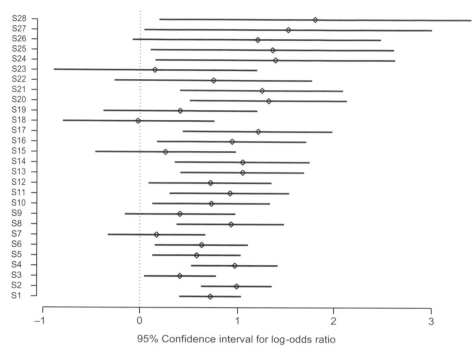

Figure 41 Forest plot of log-odds ratios and associated 95% confidence intervals from 28 case–control studies of *Chlamydia trachomatis* and oral contraceptive use.

and security of human and veterinary drugs, biological products, medical devices, our nation's food supply, cosmetics and products that emit radiation.' See **www.fda.gov**.

Force of mortality: Synonym for **hazard function**.

Forecast: An estimate of what may happen in the future in respect of some event or process, based on extrapolating existing trends. [*Journal of Business and Economic Statistics*, 1993, **11**, 121–44.]

Forest plot: A name sometimes given to a type of diagram commonly used in a `meta-analysis`, in which point estimates and `confidence intervals` are displayed for all studies selected. An example is shown in Figure 41. [Everitt, B. S., 2003, *Modern Medical Statistics*, Arnold, London.]

Forest plot: Often the most useful component of a systematic review.

Forward-looking study: An alternative term for `prospective study`.

Fourfold table: Synonym for **two-by-two contingency table**.

Fractal: A term used to describe a geometrical object that continues to exhibit detailed structure over a large range of scales. Snowflakes and coastlines are frequently quoted examples. A medical example is provided by electrocardiograms. [Mandelbroit, B. B., 1982, *The Fractal Geometry of Nature*, W. H. Freeman, San Francisco, CA.]

Fractal dimension: A numerical measure of the degree of roughness of a `fractal`. Need not be a whole number; for example, the value for a typical coastline is between 1.15 and 1.25. [Mandelbroit, B. B., 1982, *The Fractal Geometry of Nature*, W. H. Freeman, San Francisco, CA.]

Frailty: *See* **frailty model**.

Frailty model: A model for `survival time` data that allows for possible unobserved individual heterogeneity by the inclusion of random effect terms (known in this context as *frailties*). There are a number of possible sources of such heterogeneity, but most commonly it will reflect biological variation with, for example, some individuals having a weaker heart or a greater genetic disposition for cancer. [Everitt, B. S., 2003, *Modern Medical Statistics*, Arnold, London.]

Framingham study: A long-term investigation begun in Framingham, Massachusetts, in 1948, to identify the relation of possible `risk factors` to the occurrence of chronic circulatory disease and to characterize the natural history of the disease. [*American Journal of Public Health*, 1957, **47**, 4–24.]

Frequency distribution table: The division of a sample of observations into a number of classes, together with the number of observations in each class. Acts as a useful summary of the main features of the data, such as location, shape and spread. An example of such a table is given below: *See also* **histogram** and **cumulative frequency distribution**.

Hormone assay values (mmol/l)

Class limits	Observed frequency
75–79	1
80–84	2
85–89	5
90–94	9
95–99	10
100–104	7
105–109	4
110–114	2
$\geq$115	1

Frequency polygon: A diagram used to display graphically the values in a `frequency distribution`. The frequencies are graphed as ordinate against the class midpoints as abscissae. The points are then joined by a series of straight lines. Particularly useful in displaying a number of frequency distributions on the same diagram. Figure 42 gives an example.

Frequentist inference: An approach to statistics based on a frequency view of probability in which it is assumed that it is possible to consider an infinite sequence of independent repetitions of the same statistical experiment. Significance

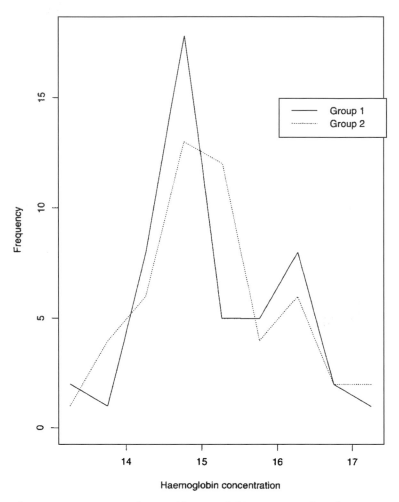

Figure 42 Frequency polygon of haemoglobin concentrations for two groups of men.

tests, hypothesis tests, and likelihood are the main tools of this form of inference. *See also* **Bayesian methods**. [Altman, D. G., 2018, *Practical Statistics for Medical Research*, Chapman & Hall/CRC, Boca Raton, FL.]

Frequentist inference: Still the form of inference used most commonly by clinical researchers, but increasingly challenged by Bayesian inference now that the latter can be applied almost routinely.

Friedman's two-way analysis of variance: A distribution-free method that is the analogue of the analysis of variance for a design with two factors. Can be applied to data sets that do not meet the assumptions of the parametric approach, namely normality and homogeneity of variance. Uses only the ranks of

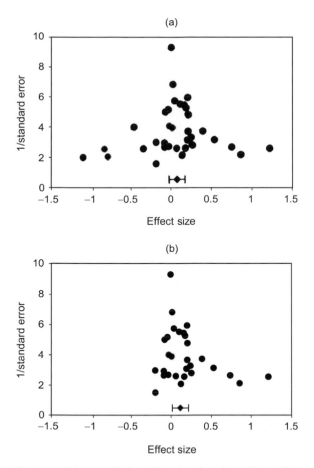

Figure 43 (a) Funnel plot of 35 simulated studies with true effect of zero; estimated effect size is 0.087 with a 95% confidence interval of [−0.018, 0.178]. (b) Funnel plot as in (a) with the five left-most studies suppressed; estimated effect size is now 0.124 with a 95% confidence interval of [0.037, 0.210].
(Taken with permission from S. Duval and R. Tweedie, *Journal of the American Statistical Association*, 2000, **95**, 89–98.)

the observations. [Hollander, M. and Wolfe, D. A., 2014, *Nonparametric Statistical Methods*, 3rd ed., Wiley-Blackwell, Oxford.]

***F*-test:** A test for the equality of the variances of two populations having `normal distributions`, based on the ratio of the variances of a sample of observations taken from each. Encountered most often in the `analysis of variance` where testing whether particular variances are the same also tests for the equality of a set of means. [Altman, D. G., 2018, *Practical Statistics for Medical Research*, Chapman & Hall/CRC, Boca Raton, FL.]

Functional data analysis (FDA): Data from many experiments arise as curves, for example, `growth curves`, hormone profiles and `biomarkers` measured over time. The curve can be used as a basic unit in the analysis of the data, for example, when we average across a group of curves, we can estimate the group-average curve. We can then test whether two group-average curves are the same. Such data analysis is labelled FDA. [Ramsey, J. O. and Silverman, B. W., 1997, *Functional Data Analysis*, Springer-Verlag, Berlin.]

Funnel plot: An informal method of assessing the effect of `publication bias` in the context of a systematic review. The effect sizes extracted from each study are plotted on the *x*-axis against the corresponding sample sizes (or measures of precision such as one over the standard error of the estimated effect) on the *y*-axis. Because of the nature of sampling variability, this plot should, in the absence of publication bias, have approximately the shape of a pyramid with a tapering funnel-like peak. Publication bias will tend to skew the pyramid by selectively excluding studies with small or nonsignificant effects. Such studies predominate when the sample sizes are small but are increasingly less common as the sample size increases. Therefore, their absence removes part of the lefthand corner of the pyramid. The effect is illustrated in Figure 43. *See also* **Begg's test** and **Egger's test**. [Everitt, B. S., 2003, *Modern Medical Statistics*, Arnold, London.]

Futility analysis: A type of `interim analysis` where the objective is to stop a clinical study if the interim data suggest lack of efficacy of the test treatment.

Future years of life lost: An alternative way of presenting data on mortality in a population, by using the difference between age at death and `life expectancy`. It has been estimated, for example, that the future years of life lost for white men aged 20–30 years with a severe level of obesity is 13. Future years of life lost is often used as a statistic in practical epidemiology when it is required to weight death at a young age more heavily compared with deaths at a higher age. [Alderson, M. A., 1983, *An Introduction to Epidemiology*, Macmillan, London.]

G

G²: Often used to denote `deviance`.

Galbraith plot: A graphical method for identifying `outliers` in a `meta-analysis`. The standardized `effect size` is plotted against precision (the reciprocal of the standard error). If the studies are homogeneous, then they should be distributed within $+/-2$ standard errors of the regression line through the origin. An example is given in Figure 44. [Ader, H. J. and Mellenberg, G. J., 1999, *Research Methodology*, Sage, London.]

GAM: Abbreviation for **geographical analysis machine** and for **generalized additive model**.

Gambler's fallacy: The belief that if an event has not happened for a long time, then it is bound to occur soon. [Everitt, B. S., 2009, *Chance Rules*, 2nd ed., Springer, New York.]

Game theory: The branch of mathematics that deals with the theory of contests between two or more players under specified sets of rules. The subject assumes a statistical aspect when part of the game proceeds under a chance scheme. [*International Journal of Game Theory*, 1979, **8**, 175–92.]

Gamma distribution: A `probability distribution` of which the shape depends on two parameters. Some examples are given in Figure 45. Often used to model heavily skewed data. [Evans, M., Hastings, N. and Peacock, B., 2000, *Statistical Distributions*, 3rd ed., John Wiley & Sons, New York.]

Gap time: The time between two successive events in `survival time` data in which each individual can potentially experience a series of events. An example is the time from the development of AIDS to death. [*Biometrika*, 1999, **86**, 59–70.]

Garbage in, garbage out (GIGO): A term that draws attention to the fact that sensible output follows only from sensible input. Specifically, if the data are originally of dubious quality, then so will be the results. Fancy statistical methods will not rescue garbage data.

Gaussian distribution: Synonym for **normal distribution**.

GEE: Abbreviation for **generalized estimating equation**.

Gehan's generalized Wilcoxon test: A `distribution-free` method for comparing the `survival times` of two groups of individuals. *See also* **Cox–Mantel test** and **log-rank test**. [*Statistics in Medicine*, 1989, **8**, 937–46.]

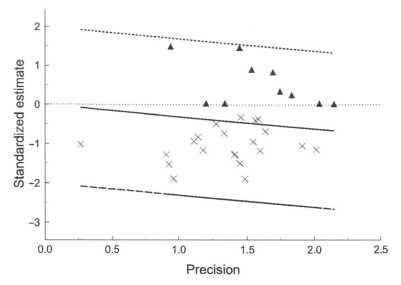

Figure 44 Example of a Galbraith plot.
(© Stephen Senn 2001.)

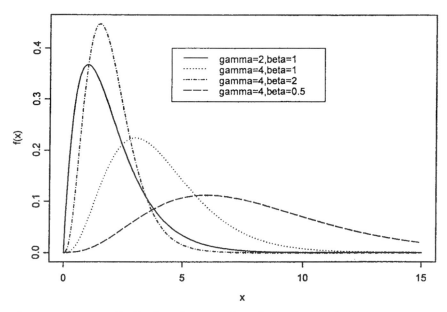

Figure 45 Gamma distributions for a number of parameter values.

Gene: A sequence of DNA that codes for a particular protein or that regulates other genes. Genes occur in pairs at locations along the pairs of chromosomes. Genes are the biological basis of heredity. [Sham, P., 1998, *Statistics in Human Genetics*, Arnold, London.]

Gene–environment interaction: An effect that arises when the joint effects of a genetic factor and an environmental factor are different from the sum of their individual effects. [Sham, P., 1998, *Statistics in Human Genetics*, Arnold, London.]

Gene frequency: For a given population, the number of loci at which a given `allele` is found divided by the total number of loci at which it could occur. [Sham, P., 1998, *Statistics in Human Genetics*, Arnold, London.]

Gene mapping: The placing of `genes` onto their positions on chromosomes. It includes both the construction of marker maps and the localization of genes that confer susceptibility to disease. [Sham, P., 1998, *Statistics in Human Genetics*, Arnold, London.]

General health questionnaire (GHQ): A self-administered questionnaire used for detecting individuals suffering from nonpsychotic psychiatric illness. Consists of 30 questions about current symptoms, abnormal feelings and thoughts, and aspects of observable behaviour. The 30 items are scored as `binary variables` and summed to provide an overall score. The properties of the instrument have been explored carefully and it has been used widely in `psychiatric epidemiology`. [Goldberg, D., 1972, *The Detection of Psychiatric Illness by Questionnaire*, Oxford University Press, Oxford.]

General Household Survey: A survey carried out in Great Britain on a continuous basis since 1971. Approximately 100,000 households are included in the sample each year. The main aim of the survey is to collect data on a range of core topics including household and family information, employment, education and income. The information is used by government departments and other organizations for planning, policy and monitoring purposes.

Generalizability theory (G theory): A theory or framework for conceptualizing, investigating and designing reliable observations that recognizes that in any measurement situation there are multiple (in fact, infinite) sources of variation (called *facets* in the theory), and that an important goal of measurement is to attempt to identify and measure `variance components` that are contributing error to an estimate. Strategies can then be implemented to reduce the influence of these sources on the measurement. [Cronbach, L. J., Gleser, G. C., Nanda, H. and Rajaratnam, N., 1972, *The Dependability of Behavioural Measurements*, John Wiley & Sons, New York.]

Generalized additive model (GAM): An extension to the usual `generalized linear model` in which the explanatory variables are represented in the model by smoothed functions (e.g. `locally weighted regression` fits) suggested by the empirical relationship between the response and the particular explanatory variable. Essentially allows the data to determine the form of the relationship between each explanatory variable and the response variable. [Everitt, B. S., 2003, *Modern Medical Statistics*, Arnold, London.]

Generalized distance: *See* **Mahalanobis D^2**.

Generalized estimating equations (GEEs): Models particularly for `longitudinal data` in which the response variable can be non-normal, for example binary, and that account for the nonindependence of the observations by the introduction of what is known as the *working correlation matrix*, essentially an acceptable approximation to the true `correlation matrix`, which is itself often too complex to model simply. [Diggle,P. J., Heagerty, P., Liang, K.-Y. and Zeger, S. L. 2013, *Analysis of Longitudinal Data*, 2nd ed., Oxford University Press, Oxford.]

Generalized estimating equations: A significant contribution to the methodology for analyzing longitudinal data from clinical trials, particularly when the response variable is non-normal.

Generalized linear mixed models: Models that extend the `generalized linear model` to deal with `clustered data`, in particular `longitudinal data`, by including random effect terms that introduce correlation structure between the repeated measures of the response variable. [Everitt, B. S., 2003, *Modern Medical Statistics*, Arnold, London.]

Generalized linear model (GLM): An elegant unifying framework that includes a wide range of seemingly disparate methods for modelling data, including `analysis of variance`, `multiple linear regression`, `logistic regression` and `Poisson regression`. The essential components of these models are:

- The *link function*, which specifies what function of the expected value of the response is to be modelled
- The *variance function*, which specifies how the mean and the variance of the response variable are related
- The error distribution, which is a distribution from the `exponential family` relevant for the type of response variable involved

Parameters in such models are generally estimated by `iteratively reweighted least squares`. [Everitt, B. S., 2003, *Modern Medical Statistics*, Arnold, London.]

Generalized linear model: Although now over three decades old, not as familiar to many clinicians and medical researchers as it should be.

Generalized odds ratio: Synonym for **Agresti's alpha**.

Genetic distance: A concept designed to indicate how dissimilar populations are with respect to their genetic compositions. The estimation of a genetic distance gives a relative estimate of the time that has passed since the populations have existed as single cohesive units. [*Evolution*, 1976, **30**, 851–3.]

Genetic epidemiology: The analysis of the familial distributions of traits, with a view to understanding any possible genetic basis by disentangling, as far as possible, environmental and genetic causes. [Morton, N. E., 1982, *Outline of Genetic Epidemiology*, Karger, New York.]

Genetic heritability: The proportion of the trait variance that is due to genetic variation in a population. [Sham, P., 1998, *Statistics in Human Genetics*, Arnold, London.]

Genetic liability model: A model for the probability of expressing a disorder based on the assumption that an individual's liability to develop a disease results from the additive effect of many genetic and environmental factors. An individual is then assumed to be infected when their liability exceeds some threshold value. [*British Medical Journal*, 1969, **25**, 58–64.]

Genome-wide association test: A test conducted to identify disease susceptibility markers when the genetic etiology is unclear. [*Nature Reviews Genetics*, 2005, **6**, 95–108.]

Genomics: The study of the structure, function and evolution of the deoxyribonucleic acid (DNA) or ribonucleic acid (RNA) sequences that comprise the genome of living organisms. [Sham, P., 1998, *Statistics in Human Genetics*, Arnold, London.]

Genotype: The genetic constitution of an organism, that is, what `alleles` it has, as distinguished from its physical appearance (its *phenotype*). [Sham, P., 1998, *Statistics in Human Genetics*, Arnold, London.]

Genotype assortment: *See* assortative mating.

Geographical analysis machine (GAM): A procedure designed to detect clusters of rare diseases in a particular region. Circles of fixed radii are created at each endpoint of a square grid covering the study region. Neighbouring circles are allowed to overlap to some fixed extent and the number of cases of the disease within each circle is counted. Significance tests are then performed based on the total number of cases and on the number of individuals at risk, both in total and in the circle in question, during a particular census year. *See also* **clustering** and **scan statistic**. [Draper, G., 1991, *The Geographical Epidemiology of Childhood Leukaemia and Non-Hodgkin Lymphomas in Great Britain, 1966–1983*. Studies on Medical and Population Subjects, No. 53, HMSO, London.]

Geographical correlations: The correlations between variables measured as averages over geographical units. *See also* **ecological fallacy**.

Geographical information systems (GIS): Software and hardware configurations through which digital georeferences are processed and displayed. Used to identify the geographic or spatial location of any known disease outbreak and, over time, to follow its movements as well as changes in `incidence rate` and `prevalence`. [*Computers and Geoscience*, 1997, **23**, 371–85.]

Geographic patterns of disease: The relation of mortality and/or morbidity rates to geographical areas. Variation in disease rates over different regions or countries may give important clues to aetiology. *See also* **disease mapping**. [Gardner, M. J., Winter, P. D. and Barker, D. J. P., 1984, *Atlas of Mortality from Selected Diseases in England and Wales, 1968–1978*, John Wiley & Sons, Chichester.]

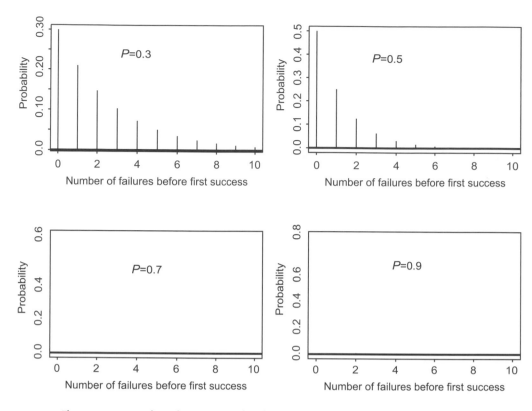

Figure 46 Examples of geometric distributions.

Geometric distribution: The probability distribution of number of trials before the first success in a Bernoulli sequence. The mean of the distribution is $1/p$ and its variance is $(1 - p)/p^2$, where p is the probability of a success on each trial. Figure 46 shows a number of examples. [Evans, M., Hastings, N. and Peacock, B., 2000, *Statistical Distributions*, 3rd ed., John Wiley & Sons, New York.]

Geometric mean: A measure of location suitable for skewed data. Given explicitly by the nth root of the product of the n observations. Only well defined for positive data. [*British Medical Journal*, 2002, **325**, 1387–91.]

GHQ: Abbreviation for **general health questionnaire**.

GIGO: Abbreviation for **garbage in, garbage out**.

Gini index: *See* **Lorenz curve**.

GLM: Abbreviation for **generalized linear model**.

Goal attainment scaling : An assessment instrument to evaluate interventions on the basis of individual, patient-specific goals. Typically, the choice of goals is a process in which both the patient and the investigator take part. Essentially a general tool to quantify the treatment benefit in a population with very heterogeneous symptoms. [*Communications in Mental Health Journal*, 1968, **4**, 443–53.]

Gold standard: A method, procedure or measurement that is widely accepted as being the best available. For example, gold-standard `clinical trials` are usually taken to be those involving random allocation of participants to treatments and `double-blinding`.

Gompertz curve: A curve used to describe the size of a population as a function of time when the relative growth rate declines at a constant rate. *See also* **growth curve**.

Goodman–Kruskal measures of association: A series of indices for measuring the association between two categorical variables forming a `contingency table`. Each measure is designed for a specific class of problem. In particular, different indices are used for unordered and ordered variables, and for situations in which one variable may be considered explanatory and the other the response. [Everitt, B. S., 1992, *The Analysis of Contingency Tables*, 2nd ed., Chapman & Hall/ CRC, Boca Raton, FL.]

Goodness-of-fit: Degree of agreement between an empirically observed distribution or data set and that predicted by some theoretical distribution or model. The most commonly used test of goodness-of-fit is the `chi-squared test`, which assesses the agreement between an observed set of frequencies and an expected set of frequencies. [D'Agostino, R. B. and Stephens, M. A., 1986, *Goodness-of-Fit Techniques*, Marcel Dekker, New York.]

Good's aphorism: Half-baked ideas of people are better than ideas of half-baked people.

Good's method: A procedure for combining independent tests of hypotheses. [Good, I. J., 1950, *Probability and the Weighting of Evidence*, Hafner, New York.]

Grand mean: Mean of all the values in a grouped data set, irrespective of groups.

Graphical deception: `Graphical displays` of data that may mislead the unwary either by design or by error. An example is shown in Figure 47(a) in which the death rate per million from breast cancer for several periods over the last three decades is plotted. The plot appears to show a rather alarming increase in the rate. But when the data are re-plotted with the vertical scale starting at zero as shown in Figure 47(b), the increase is much less disturbing. *See also* **lie factor**. [Tufte, E. R., 1983, *The Visual Display of Quantitative Information*, Graphics Press, Cheshire, CT.]

Graphical displays: Procedures for visually displaying measured quantities by means of the combined use of points, lines, a coordinate system, numbers, symbols, words, shading and colour. The greatest value of such displays is when they force the observer to notice the unexpected, although some graphical displays may deceive (*see* `Graphical deception`). Examples of graphical displays commonly used in medical research are `scatterplots`, `histograms` and `pie charts`. When constructing graphical displays, two points to bear in mind are: (1) captions must be complete and descriptions of the graphic as full as possible; and (2) line styles, colours and symbols are to be kept to a minimum. [Tufte, E. R., 1983, *The Visual Display of Quantitative Information*, Graphics Press, Cheshire, CT.]

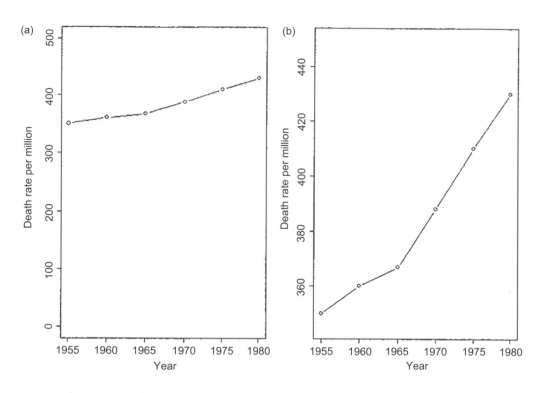

Figure 47 Death rates from cancer of the breast: Figure (a) includes the origin on the y-axis and Figure (b) does not.

Greenhouse–Geisser correction: A method for adjusting the degrees of freedom of the F-tests used in repeated-measures analysis of variance to allow for departures from the assumption of compound symmetry for the variance-covariance matrix of the repeated measures. [Everitt, B. S., 2001, *Statistics for Psychologists*, Lawrence Erlbaum Associates, Mahwah, NJ.]

Greenhouse–Geisser correction: The use of this correction term when analyzing repeated-measures data is less necessary than it once was because of the advances in the methodology available for the analysis of such data.

Greenwood's formula: A formula giving the variance of the product limit estimator of a survival function. [Collett, D., 2015, *Modelling Survival Data in Medical Research*, 3rd ed., Chapman & Hall/CRC, Boca Raton, FL.]

Gross reproduction rate: The average number of daughters born to a hypothetical cohort of 1,000 women if they experienced age-specific birth rates observed in a given year throughout their childbearing years and none of the cohort was to die during her childbearing years. [Everitt, B. S. and Palmer, C. R. (eds.), 2011, *Encyclopedic Companion to Medical Statistics*, 2nd ed., John Wiley & Sons, Chichester.]

Group average clustering: Synonym for **average linkage clustering**.

Group sequential design: *See* **sequential analysis**.

Grouped binary data: Observations of a binary variable tabulated in terms of the proportion of one of the two possible values for patients or subjects who, for example, have the same diagnosis, are the same sex, and so on.

Grouped data: Data recorded as frequencies of observations in particular intervals. *See also* **frequency distribution**.

Growth charts: Synonym for **centile reference charts**.

Growth curve: An expression giving either the size of a population or the size of an individual as a function of time. *See also* **Gompertz curve**. [Mirman, D., 2014, *Growth Curve Analysis and Visualization using R*, Chapman & Hall/CRC, Boca Raton, FL.]

Growth curve analysis: A general term for methods for analyzing observations involving the development of individuals over time. A classic example is that where recordings of height or weight are made on a group of children at different ages. Several types of models may be used in the analysis of such data, including mixed-effects models and low-degree polynomials. [Mirman, D., 2014, *Growth Curve Analysis and Visualization using R*, Chapman & Hall/ CRC, Boca Raton, FL.]

Growth rate: A measure of population growth, calculated as

$$\frac{\text{live births during the year} - \text{deaths during the year}}{\text{midyear population}} \times 100.$$

[*Annals of Human Biology*, 1986, **13**, 129–41.]

G theory: Abbreviation for **generalizability theory**.

Guttman scale: A scale based on a set of binary variables that attempts to measure an underlying latent variable, for example pain or wealth. The following is an example of the items used in such a scale used in social work research.

- Slapping a child's hand is an appropriate way to teach the meaning of 'No!'
- Spanking is sometimes necessary.
- Sometimes discipline requires using a belt or paddle. Some children need a good beating to keep them in line.

[Monette, D. R., Sullivan, T. J. and Dejing, C. R., 1994, *Applied Social Research*, 3rd ed., Harcourt Brace, Orlando, FL.]

Guyatt's responsiveness ratio: An index to assess the likelihood that a measuring instrument will detect a clinically important treatment effect. It is defined as the smallest change in score that patients consider important divided by the standard deviation of change scores in stable patients. [*Journal of Chronic Diseases*, 1987, **40**, 171–8.]

H_0: Symbol for **null hypothesis**.

H_1: Symbol for **alternative hypothesis**.

HALE: Abbreviation for **health-adjusted life expectancy**.

Halo effect: The tendency of a subject's performance on some task to be overrated because of the observer's perception of the subject doing well gained in an earlier exercise or when assessed in a different area. For example, a student who has made a good overall impression on a teacher may be rated as producing high-quality work and always meeting deadlines even when the work is relatively substandard. [*Journal of Applied Psychology*, 1920, **IV**, 25–9.]

Hanging rootogram: A diagram comparing an observed rootogram with a fitted curve, in which differences between the two are displayed in relation to the horizontal axis rather than to the curve itself. This makes it easier to spot large differences and to look for patterns. An example is shown in Figure 48. [Tukey, J. W., 1977, *Exploratory Data Analysis*, Addison-Wesley, Reading, MA.]

Haplotype: A combination of two or more alleles which are present in the same gamete. [Sham, P., 1998, *Statistics in Human Genetics*, Arnold, London.]

Haplotype analysis: The analysis of haplotype frequencies in one or more populations, with the aim of establishing associations between two or more alleles, or between a haplotype and a phenotypic trait, or establishing the genetic relationship between populations. [*American Journal of Human Genetics*, 1987, **41**, 356–73.]

HAQ: Abbreviation for **health assessment questionnaire**.

Hardy–Weinberg law: The law stating that both gene frequencies and genotype frequencies will remain constant from generation to generation in an infinitely large interbreeding population in which mating is at random and there is no selection, migration or mutation. In a situation where a single pair of alleles (A and a) are considered, the frequencies of germ cells carrying A and a are defined as p and q, respectively. At equilibrium, the frequencies of the genotype classes are $p^2(A\,A)$, $2\,pq\,(Aa)$ and $q^2(aa)$. [*Statistics in Medicine*, 1986, **5**, 281–8.]

Harmonic mean: The reciprocal of the arithmetic mean of the reciprocals of the observations. Essentially a form of weighted mean in which the probability that a

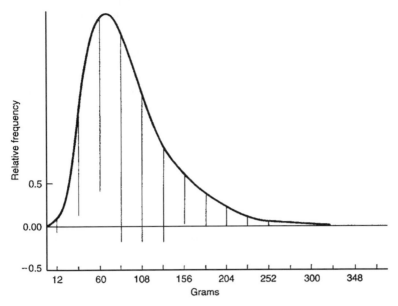

Figure 48 Example of a hanging rootogram.

unit is sampled is proportional to the variable of interest. For positive data, the harmonic mean is always less than or equal to the arithmetic mean.

Harris and Stevens forecasting: A method of making short-term forecasts in a `time series` that is subject to abrupt changes in pattern and transient effects. Examples of such series are those arising from measuring the concentration of certain biochemicals in biological organisms and from measuring the concentration of plasma growth hormone. [West, M. and Harrison, J., 1977, *Bayesian Forecasting and Dynamic Methods*, 2nd ed., Springer, New York.]

Hartley's test: A simple test of the equality of variances of several populations. Based on the ratio of the largest to the smallest sample variances of observations from each population. Often used in selecting optimal neighbourhood sizes in investigations of local geographic variation of health and social determinants. *See also* **Bartlett's test** and **Box's test**. [*International Journal of Health Geographics*, 2005, **4**, 12–15.]

Hat matrix: A matrix arising in `multiple linear regression`, the elements of which form the basis of a variety of `diagnostics` for detecting departures from model assumptions. [Lewis-Beck, M. S., 1993, *Regression Analysis*, volume 2, Sage, London.]

Hausdorf dimension: Synonym for **fractal dimension**.

Hawthorne effect: A term used for an effect produced simply from the awareness by the subjects in a study that they are participating in some form of scientific investigation. The name arises from study of industrial efficiency undertaken at the Hawthorne Plant in Chicago in the 1920s. The major finding of the study was that almost regardless of the experimental manipulation employed, the production of the workers seemed to improve. [*European Journal of Obstetrics*, 2008, **141**, 111–14.]

Hazard: A factor or risk or exposure that may affect health adversely.

Hazard function: The risk that an individual experiences an event (death, improvement, etc.) in a small time interval given that the individual has survived up to the beginning of the interval. It is a measure of how likely the individual is to experience an event as a function of the age of the individual. The conditional aspect of the hazard function is very important. For example, the probability of dying at age 100 years is very small because most people die before that age; in contrast, the probability of a person who has reached age 100 dying at age 100 is much greater. *See also* **bathtub hazard** and **Cox's proportional hazards model**. [Collett, D., 2015, *Modelling Survival Data in Medical Research*, 3rd ed., Chapman & Hall/CRC, Boca Raton, FL.]

Hazard ratio: The reduction of risk of death on treatment compared to control over the period of follow-up. A type of relative risk. [Altman, D. G., 2018, *Practical Statistics for Medical Research*, Chapman & Hall/CRC, Boca Raton, FL.]

Hazard regression: A procedure for modelling the hazard function that does not depend on the assumptions made in Cox's proportional hazards model, namely that the log of the hazard function is an additive function of both time and the explanatory variables. In this approach, smoothed functions of the explanatory variables are used to model the log-hazard function. [*Statistics in Medicine*, 1996, **15**, 1757–70.]

Health-adjusted life expectancy (HALE): An estimate of the expectation of life in 'full health' and an indicator of overall population health. Time expected to be spent in less than full health is subtracted from total life expectancy, after weighting by the severity of departure from full health. In Canada in the early 1990s the life expectancy for men aged 45 was 32.1 years; the corresponding value for HALE was 27.5 years. [*Health Policy*, 1990, **16**, 190–208.]

Health assessment questionnaire (HAQ): A multidimensional instrument developed by the Stanford Arthritis Centre that measures outcome in terms of mortality, disability, pain, iatrogenic events and economic impact. It is now used widely throughout the world, particularly for clinical trials in rheumatoid arthritis and some other diseases. *See also* **activities of daily living scale**. [*Arthritis and Rheumatism*, 1980, **23**, 137–45.]

Health technology assessment: Health technology is a term that can include drugs, devises and programs that can improve quality of life. Assessment of such technologies provides the evidence required to make better-informed decisions about how to help patients. [Hopkins, R. B. and Goeree, R. G., 2015, *Health Technology Assessment*, CRC Press, Boca Raton, FL.]

Healthy worker effect: The phenomenon whereby employed individuals tend to have lower mortality rates than unemployed individuals. The effect, which can pose a serious problem in the interpretation of industrial cohort studies, has two main components:

- Selection at recruitment to exclude the chronically sick, resulting in low `standardized mortality rates` among recent recruits to an industry. A secondary selection process by which workers who become unfit during employment tend to leave, again leading to lower standardized mortality ratios amongst long-serving employees.

[*Social Science and Medicine*, 1993, **36**, 1077–86.]

Hebdomadal mortality rate: The ratio of the number of infant deaths in the first week of life divided by the number of live births in a year. Usually expressed per 1,000 live births. For example, in Kansas in 1998 the rate was 3.4 per 1,000 and in 1999 it was 4.1 per 1,000. [*Maternal and Child Health Journal*, 1998, **2**, 211–21.]

Hello–goodbye effect: A phenomenon originally described in psychotherapy research but that may arise whenever a subject is assessed on two occasions with some intervention between the visits. Before an intervention, a person may present him/herself in as bad a light as possible, thereby hoping to qualify for treatment and impress staff with the seriousness of his/her problems. At the end of the study, the person may want to please the staff with his/her improvement, and so may minimize any problems. The result is to make it appear that there has been some improvement when none has occurred, or to magnify the effects that did occur. [*Journal of Clinical Psychology*, 2000, **56**, 853–9.]

Helmert contrast: A contrast often used in the analysis of variance, in which the mean of the response variable in each level of a factor is tested for equality against the average of the remaining levels. So, for example, if three groups are involved, of which the first is a control group and the other two are treatment groups, then the first contrast tests the control group against the average of the two treatments, and the second contrast tests whether the two treatment groups differ.

Helsinki Declaration: A set of principles to guide clinicians on the ethics of `clinical trials` and other clinical research. *See also* **Nuremberg Code**. [Fisher, L. D. and Van Belle, G., 2004, *Biostatistics*, 2nd ed., John Wiley & Sons, New York.]

Herd immunity: The resistance of a group to invasion and spread of an infectious agent based on the natural resistance to infection of a high proportion of individual members of the group, or as a result of vaccination among households or community contacts. [*Archives of Pediatrics and Adolescent Medicine*, 2001, **4**, 1–5.]

Heritability: A measure of the degree to which a `phenotype` is influenced genetically and can be modified by selection. For a quantitative trait, defined explicitly as the proportion of variation attributable to genetic factors. [Neel, J. V. and Schull, W. J., 1954, *Heredity*, University of Chicago Press, Chicago, IL.]

Heterogeneous: A term used in statistics to indicate the inequality of some quantity of interest (usually a variance) in a number of different groups, populations, etc. *See also* **homogeneous**.

Heuristic computer program: A computer program that attempts, in searching for solutions, to use the same sort of selectivity that human beings use. [101 Computing.net, 2018]

Hidden Markov models: Models useful for the characterization of `longitudinal data` in terms of a set of hidden states. In particular, such models have been applied to investigate disease progression to identify latent pathophysiological states, for example, in the progression of Alzheimer's disease. The models consist of two components, a transition model to describe the dynamic transition of hidden states and a conditional regression model to examine state-specific covariate effects on responses. *See also* **Markov chain**. [Bartolucci, F., Farcomeni, A. and Pennoni, F., 2013, *Latent Markov Models for Longitudinal Data*, Taylor & Francis, Boca Raton, FL.]

Hidden time effects: Effects that arise in data sets that may simply be a result of collecting the observations over a period of time. *See also* **cusum**.

Hierarchical models: A series of models for a set of observations, where each model results from adding or deleting parameters from other models in the series. Also used for a regression or `analysis of variance` model if the presence of an `interaction` term implies the inclusion of all lower-order interactions and main effects for the explanatory variables involved in the interaction. [*Journal of the Royal Statistical Society, Series A*, 1977, **140**, 48–77.]

High-throughput data: Data produced by modern biological assays and experiments which supply thousands of measurements per sample and where the sheer amounts of data increases the need for better models to enhance inference. [*Bioinformatics*, 2007, **23**, 906–9.]

Higgin's law: A 'law' that states that the `prevalence` of any condition is inversely proportional to the number of experts whose agreement is required to establish its presence.

High breakdown methods: Methods that are designed to be resistant to even multiple severe `outliers`. Such methods are an extreme example of `robust statistics`. [*Computational Statistics*, 1996, **11**, 137–46.]

Highest posterior density: *See* **Bayesian confidence interval**.

High–medium–low method: A method used in demographic forecasting to quantify uncertainty in projections. High, medium and low sets of assumptions are constructed and projections are based on each calculated. [*International Statistical Review*, 2004, **72**, 185–99.]

High-risk treatment trials: `Clinical trials` of treatments with major risks. Such trials are generally only used to prevent major outcomes such as mortality or serious morbidity, since potentially severe toxicity would usually not be acceptable for treatments addressing lesser health outcomes. [Ellenberg, S. S., Fleming, T. R. and DeMets, D. L., 2002, *Data Monitoring Committees in Clinical Trials*, Wiley, New York.]

Hill's criteria of causality: A statement of the necessary criteria that have to be satisfied to be able to make a reasonable claim of causality in `observational studies`, particularly in `epidemiology`. First given by a British medical statistician, Austin Bradford Hill. The details are as follows:

- *Consistency:* The observed association is consistent when results are replicated in different settings using different methods.
- *Strength:* Defined by the size of the risk as measured by appropriate statistical tests.
- *Specificity:* Established when a single putative cause produces a specific effect.
- *Dose–response relationship:* An increasing level of exposure (in amount and/or time) increases the risk.
- *Temporal relationship:* Exposure always precedes outcome. This is the only absolutely essential criterion.
- *Biological plausibility:* The association agrees with currently accepted understanding of pathobiological processes.
- *Coherence:* The observed association should be compatible with existing theory and knowledge.
- *Experiment:* The condition can be altered (e.g., prevented or ameliorated) by an appropriate experimental regimen.

[*Proceedings of the Royal Society of Medicine*, 1965, **58**, 295–300.]

Hinge: A more exotic (but less desirable) term for **quartile**.

HIPE: Abbreviation for **hospital in-patient enquiry**.

Histogram: A graphical representation of a set of observations, in which class frequencies are represented by the areas of rectangles centred on the class interval. If the latter are all equal, then the heights of the rectangles are also proportional to the observed frequencies. Figure 49 shows an example. [Altman, D., 2018, *Practical Statistics for Medical Research*, Chapman & Hall/CRC, Boca Raton, FL.]

Historical cohort study: Synonym for **noncurrent prospective study**. *See* **cohort study**.

Historical controls: A group of patients treated in the past with a standard therapy and used as the control group for evaluating a new treatment on current patients. Although used fairly frequently in medical investigations, the approach is not to be recommended since possible `biases` due to other factors that may have changed over time can never be eliminated satisfactorily. For example, past observations are unlikely to relate to a precisely similar group of patients. *See also* **literature controls**. [Everitt, B. S. and Pickles, A., 2004, *Statistical Aspects of the Design and Analysis of Clinical Trials*, revised ed., Imperial College Press, London.]

Historical controls: There is considerable evidence that treatment effects derived from historical control trials are often biased in favour of the new therapy.

Historical prospective study: A `prospective study` in which the cohort to be investigated and its subsequent disease history are identified from past records, for example from information of an individual's work history. [*American Journal of Independent Medicine*, 1983, **4**, 651–7.]

Hold-over effect: Synonym for **carry-over effect**.

Figure 49 Histogram of heights of 351 elderly women.

Homogeneous: A term that is used in statistics to indicate the equality of some quantity of interest (most often a variance) in a number of different groups, populations, etc. *See also* **heterogeneous**.

Hospital controls: *See* **control group**.

Hospital discharge rate: The number of discharges from hospital during a time period divided by the estimated midyear population for the hospital's catchment area. It is usually expressed per 1,000 people per year. The denominator for a discharge rate can be beds rather than the population, to give an indication of the use of beds, where the rate becomes the number of discharges per bed per year. [*British Medical Journal*, 2004, **328**, 1413–14.]

Hospital in-patient enquiry (HIPE): In England and Wales, the collection of data for every tenth patient discharged from a general hospital. In addition to the age, sex and marital status of the patient, information about date of admission, discharge, time on waiting list, diagnosis and operations undergone is recorded.

Hot deck: A method of imputation in which missing values are replaced by values selected from amongst existing cases. [Little, R. A. and Rubin, D. B., 2002, *Statistical Analysis with Missing Data*, 2nd ed., John Wiley & Sons, New York.]

Hotelling–Lawley trace: *See* **multivariate analysis of variance**.

Hotelling's T^2 test: A generalization of Student's t test to the multivariate situation. Used primarily for testing for between group differences on a set of correlated variables. *See also* **Mahalanobis D^2** and **simultaneous inference**. [Everitt, B. S. and Dunn, G., 2010, *Applied Multivariate Data Analysis*, 2nd ed., Wiley, Chichester.]

Household survey: A descriptive survey of illness and disability performed by interviewing people in their own homes, often by questioning a single informant about other members of the household.

Human capital model: A model for evaluating the economic implication of disease in terms of the economic loss of a person succumbing to morbidity or mortality at some specified age. Often, such a model has two components: the direct cost of disease, for example medical management and treatment, and the indirect cost of disease, namely the loss of economic productivity due to a person being removed from the labour force. [*Journal of Political Economy*, 1962, **70**, 9–49.]

Human height growth curves: The growth of human height is, in general, remarkably regular, apart from the pubertal growth spurt. A satisfactory longitudinal growth curve is extremely useful as it enables long series of measurements to be replaced by a few parameters and might permit early detection and treatment of growth abnormalities. Several such curves have been proposed. [*Annals of Human Biology*, 1978, **5**, 1–24.]

Huynh–Feldt correction: A correction term applied in the analysis of variance of repeated-measures data to ensure that the within-subject F-tests are approximately valid, even if the assumption of sphericity is invalid. *See also* **Greenhouse–Geisser correction** and **Mauchly test**. [Everitt, B. S., 2001, *Statistics for Psychologists*, LEA, Mahwah, FL.]

Huynh-Feldt correction: The use of this correction term when analyzing repeated-measures data is less necessary than it once was because of the advances in the methodology available for the analysis of such data.

Hypergeometric distribution: A probability distribution associated with sampling without replacement from a population of finite size. The basis of Fisher's exact test for two-by-two contingency tables. [Evans, M., Hastings, N. and Peacock, B., 2000, *Statistical Distributions*, 3rd ed., John Wiley & Sons, New York.]

Hypothesis testing: A general term for the procedure of assessing whether sample data are consistent or otherwise with statements made about the population. *See also* **null hypothesis, alternative hypothesis, composite hypothesis, significance test, significance level, type I error** and **type II error**. [Altman, D., 2018, *Practical Statistics for Medical Research*, Chapman & Hall/CRC, Boca Raton, FL.]

IBD: Abbreviation for **identical by descent**.

ICD: Abbreviation for **international classification of disease**.

IDA: Abbreviation for **initial data analysis**.

Identical by descent: A term used when two genes at a given locus have both been inherited from a common ancestor. For example, in a family without inbreeding, two siblings who have inherited the same gene from their father but two different genes from their mother have one gene (the paternal one) to which the term applies. [*American Journal of Human Genetics*, 1990, **47**, 842–53.]

Identification: The degree to which there is sufficient information in the sample observations to estimate the parameters in a proposed model. An *unidentified model* is one in which there are too many parameters in relation to the number of observations to make estimation possible. A *just identified model* corresponds to a *saturated model*. Finally, an *overidentified model* is one in which parameters can be estimated and there remain some degrees of freedom to allow the fit of the model to be assessed.

Immigration–emigration models: Models for the development of a population that is augmented by the arrival of individuals who found families independent of each other. [Jagers, P., 1975, *Branching Processes with Biological Applications*, John Wiley & Sons, New York.]

Immune proportion: The proportion of individuals who may not be subject to death, failure, relapse and so on. in a sample of censored survival times. The presence of such individuals may be indicated by a relatively high number of individuals with large censored survival times. Finite-mixture distributions that allow for such immunes can be fitted to such data and data analysis similar to that usually carried out on survival times can be performed. An important aspect of such analysis is to consider whether an immune proportion does in fact exist in the population. [*Biometrics*, 1995, **51**, 181–201.]

Imperfect detectability: A problem characteristic of many surveys of natural and human populations that arises because even when a unit is included in the sample, not all individuals in the selected unit are detected by the observer. For example, in a survey of homeless people, some individuals in the selected units may be missed. To estimate the population total in a survey in which this problem is likely to occur, both the `sampling design` and the detection probabilities must be taken into account. [*Biometrics*, 1994, **50**, 712–24.]

Imputation: The estimation of the `missing values` in a set of data. Many methods have been proposed; the most satisfactory is some form of `multiple imputation` in which the missing values are repeatedly estimated a small number of times and then each 'complete' data set analyzed. The results of these analyses are then combined appropriately. *See also* **hot deck** and **last observation carried forward**. [Everitt, B. S., 2003, *Modern Medical Statistics*, Arnold, London.]

> **Imputation:** Single imputation of missing values 'invents' data, which may lead to overstatements of precision, that is, standard errors that are underestimated, *p*-values of tests that are too small and confidence intervals that do not cover the true parameter at the stated rate. Multiple imputation overcomes some of these problems.

Incidence rate: A measure of the rate at which people without a disease develop the disease during a specific period of time. Calculated as

$$\text{incidence} = \frac{\text{incidence number of new cases of a disease over a period of time}}{\text{population at risk of the disease in the time period}}$$

it measures the appearance of disease. For example, the incidence rate of fetal alcohol syndrome in 1979 was 1 per 10,000 births; in 1992, it was 5 per 10,000 births. *See also* **prevalence**. [Altman, D., 2018, *Practical Statistics for Medical Research*, Chapman & Hall/CRC, Boca Raton, FL.]

Inclusion probability: *See* **simple random sampling**.

Incomplete block design: An experimental design in which not all treatments are represented in each `block`. *See also* **balanced incomplete block design**. [Cox, D. R., 1966, *Planning of Experiments*, John Wiley & Sons, New York.]

Incomplete contingency table: `Contingency tables` containing `structural zeros`. An example of such a table is shown below. The data involve health problems causing concern amongst a sample of teenagers. Since males are naturally not affected by menstrual problems, certain cells contain a priori zeros. Such tables can be investigated using appropriate `log-linear models`.[Everitt, B. S., 1992, *The Analysis of Contingency Tables*, 2nd ed., Chapman & Hall/CRC, Boca Raton, FL.]

Data on teenager's concern with health problems

Sex	Male	Male	Female	Female
Age	12–15	16–17	12–15	16–17
Sex reproduction	4	2	9	7
Menstrual problems	–	–	4	8
How healthy I am	42	7	19	10
Nothing	57	20	71	31

Incubation period: The time elapsing between the receipt of infection and the appearance of symptoms. For example, the mean incubation period for Creutzfeldt–Jakob disease (CJD) in human growth hormone recipients has been estimated to lie between 9 and 10 years. [Brookmeyer, R. and Gail, M. H., 1994, *AIDS Epidemiology: A Quantitative Approach*, Oxford University Press, New York.]

Independence: Two events are said to be independent if knowing that one has occurred does not help in predicting whether the other will occur. In terms of their probabilities, this means that the probability that both occur is the product of the individual event probabilities. *See also* **conditional probability**. [Altman, D., 2018, *Practical Statistics for Medical Research*, Chapman & Hall/CRC, Boca Raton, FL.]

Independent component analysis (ICA): A method for analyzing complex measured quantities thought to be mixtures of other more fundamental quantities, into their underlying components. Typical examples of the data to which ICA might be applied are:

- Electroencephalogram (EEG) signal, which contains contributions from many different brain regions
- Person's height, which is determined by contributions from many different genetic and environmental factors

[Hyvarinen, A., Karhunen, J. and Oja, E., 2001, *Independent Component Analysis*, Wiley, New York.]

Independent samples *t*-test: *See* **Student's *t*-test**.

Independent variable: A less satisfactory term for **explanatory variable**.

Index plot: A plot of some diagnostic quantity, for example a `residual`, calculated after fitting a statistical model to a set of observations against corresponding observation number. [Rawlings, J. O., Pantula, S. G. and Dickey, D. A., 2013, *Applied Regression Analysis: A Research Tool*, 2nd ed., Springer, New York.]

Indicator variable: Synonym for `manifest variable` as used when fitting `structural equation models`.

Indirect standardization: The process of adjusting a crude mortality or morbidity rate for one or more variables by using a known `reference population`. It might, for example, be required to compare cancer mortality rates of single and married women, with adjustment being made for the likely different age distributions in the two groups. `Age-specific death rates` in the reference population are applied separately to the age distributions of the two groups to obtain the expected number of deaths in each. These can then be combined with the observed number of deaths in the two groups to obtain comparable mortality rates. *See also* **direct standardization**. [*Statistics in Medicine*, 1987, **6**, 61–70.]

Individual patient data meta-analysis: Systematic reviews and `meta-analyses` that operate on the individual-level data obtained directly from the researchers responsible for the original studies. [*Journal of Pain Symptom Management*, 2002, **24**, 279–80.]

Infant mortality rate: A ratio of the number of deaths during a calendar year among infants under 1 year of age to the total number of live births during that year. Often considered as a particularly responsive and sensible index of health status of a country or geographical area. In the eighteenth century in the USA and the United Kingdom, infant mortality was about 500 per 1,000, but has now declined to about 10 per 1,000. The following table gives the rates per 1,000 births in England, Wales, Scotland and northern Ireland in both 1971 and 1992:

	1971	1992
England	17.5	6.5
Wales	18.4	5.9
Scotland	19.9	6.8
Northern Ireland	22.7	6.0

Infectious period: A term used in describing the progress of an epidemic for the time following the latent period during which a patient infected with the disease is able to discharge infectious matter in some way and possibly communicate the disease to other susceptibles. The period during which an infected person can transmit a pathogen to a susceptible host.

Infectivity: The probability of infection, given exposure to an infectious agent under specified conditions. [*Journal of Virology*, 2001, **75**, 2324–30.]

Inference: The process of drawing conclusions about a population on the basis of measurements or observations made on a sample of individuals from the population. There are two approaches to inference, frequentist inference and Bayesian methods. [Altman, D., 2018, *Practical Statistics for Medical Research*, Chapman & Hall/CRC, Boca Raton, FL.]

Infertile worker effect: The observation that working women may be relatively infertile since having children may keep women away from work. *See also* **healthy worker effect**. [*Journal of Occupational and Environmental Medicine*, 1996, **38**, 352–8.]

Influence: A term used primarily in regression analysis to denote the effect of each observation on the estimated regression parameters. One useful index of the influence of each observation is provided by the diagonal elements of the hat matrix. *See also* **residuals** and **diagnostics**. [Rawlings, J. O., Pantula, S. G. and Dickey, D. A., 2013, *Applied Regression Analysis: A Research Tool*, 2nd ed., Springer, New York.]

Influential observation: An observation that has a disproportionate influence on one or more aspects of the estimate of a parameter, in particular a regression coefficient. This influence may be due to differences from other subjects on the explanatory variables, an extreme value for the response variable, or a combination of these.

Outliers, for example, are often also influential observations. It may be necessary to reanalyze the data after removing observations with unduly large influence.

Informant: A person who provides a researcher with information. Distinguished from respondents or participants by the extent of their personal interaction with the researcher.

Information theory: A branch of applied probability theory applicable to many communication and signal-processing problems in engineering and biology. Information theorists devote their efforts to quantitative examination of the following three questions:

- What is information?
- What are the fundamental limitations on the accuracy with which information can be transmitted?
- What design methodologies and computational algorithms yield practical systems for communication and storing information that perform close to the fundamental limits mentioned previously?

[Abrahamson, N., 1968, *Information Theory and Coding*, McGraw-Hill, New York.]

Informative missing values: *See* **missing values**.

Informed consent: The voluntary consent given by a patient to participate in, usually, a clinical trial after being informed of its purpose, method of treatment, procedure for assignment to treatment, benefits and risks associated with participation, and required data-collection procedures and schedule. According to the Helsinki Declaration, potential participants in clinical research must be informed of their rights to withdraw their consent at any time. [*Journal of the American Medical Association*, 1997, **277**, 925–6.]

Initial data analysis (IDA): The first phase in the examination of a data set, which consists of a number of informal steps, including:

- Checking the quality of the data
- Calculating simple summary statistics and constructing appropriate graphs. The general aim is to clarify the structure of the data, obtain a simple descriptive summary, and perhaps get ideas for a more sophisticated analysis. [Chatfield, C., 1988, *Problem Solving: A Statistician's Guide*, Chapman & Hall/CRC, Boca Raton, FL.]

Instrumental variables: In situations where an explanatory variable in a multiple linear regression model is correlated with the error term in the model, then the model may give biased results. Such correlation may arise when changes in the dependent variable change the value of at least one of the explanatory variables, omitted variables affect both the dependent and the explanatory variables, and the explanatory variables are subject to non-random measurement error. Explanatory variables that suffer from one or more of these issues in the context of a regression are sometimes referred to as *endogenous*. To overcome the problem an instrumental variable is sought, which is a variable that is correlated with the true explanatory variable but uncorrelated with the measurement errors. An example is in the study of the causal effect of smoking on health, tax rate for smoking products might be used as an instrument for smoking. [*Econometrica*, 1994, **62**, 467–76.]

Instantaneous death rate: Synonym for **hazard function**.

Intention-to-treat analysis: A procedure in which all patients allocated randomly to a treatment in a `clinical trial` are analyzed together as representing that treatment, regardless of whether they completed the trial or even received the treatment after randomization. Here, the initial random allocation decides how the patient's data will be analyzed. This method is adopted to prevent disturbances to the prognostic balance achieved by randomization and to prevent possible `bias` from using `compliance`, a factor often related to outcome, to determine the groups for comparison. [*British Medical Journal*, 1999, **319**, 67–74.]

Integrity of blinding: To test the integrity of blinding in a randomized `clinical trial` requires a test of the null hypothesis, 'patients guess their treatment codes randomly'. For a two-group trial, the relevant test is either a `Fisher's exact test` or a `chi-square test` on the 2×2 `contingency table` of observed and expected frequencies resulting from the null hypothesis. [Shein-Chung Chow, 2011, *Controversial Statistical Issues in Clinical Trials*, Chapman & Hall/CRC, Boca Raton, FL.]

Intention-to-treat analysis: Never even consider using any other approach!

Interaction: A term applied when two (or more) explanatory variables do not act independently on a response variable. *See also* **additive effect**. [Everitt, B. S., 2001, *Statistics for Psychologists*, Lawrence Erlbaum Associates, Mahwah, NJ.]

Intercept: The parameter in an equation derived from a `regression analysis` corresponding to the expected value of the response variable when all the explanatory variables are zero. [Altman, D., 2018, *Practical Statistics for Medical Research*, Chapman & Hall/CRC, Boca Raton, FL.]

Interim analyses: Analyses made before the planned end of a `clinical trial`, usually with the aim of detecting treatment differences at an early stage and thus preventing as many patients as possible from receiving an inferior treatment. Such analyses are often problematical, particularly if carried out in a haphazard and unplanned fashion. *See also* **alpha spending function**. [Senn, S., 2008, *Statistical Issues in Drug Development*, 2nd ed., John Wiley & Sons, Chichester.]

Interlaboratory trials: Studies conducted to determine the accuracy of methods of laboratory measurements. In such trials, one or several samples of identical material are analyzed by a sample of laboratories. The main sources of variability are:

- The operator who performs the measurement
- The equipment used
- The environment in which the measurement takes place

In general, the `repeatability` and `reproducibility` of the measures are used as parameters in describing accuracy. *See also* **round robin study**. [Yosiden, W. J. and Steiner, A., 1975, *Statistical Manual of the Association of Official Analytic Chemists*, AOAC, Washington, DC.]

International classification of disease (ICD): A classification system designed to group together similar diseases, injuries and related health problems to facilitate statistical analysis of these conditions. The classification is determined by an internationally representative group of experts who advise the World Health Organization. Each disease category is given a three-digit code number, and almost all categories are subdivided further into categories with four-digit numbers. [World Health Organization, 1992, *International Statistical Classification of Diseases and Related Health Problems*, 10th revision ed., World Health Organization, Geneva.]

Internet: A computer network connecting millions of machines worldwide. Provides easy access to vast amounts of information. *See also* **electronic mail**.

Interpolation: The process of determining a value of a function between two known values without using the equation of the function itself.

Interquartile range (IQR): A measure of spread given by the difference between the first and third `quartiles` of a sample. The IQR has the advantage that it is little affected by the presence of extreme values. [Clark-Carter, D., 2004, *Quantitative Psychological Research: A Student's Handbook*, Psychology Press, Hove.]

Interval-censored observations: Observations that often arise in the context of studies of time elapsed to a particular event when subjects are not monitored continuously. Instead, the prior occurrence of the event of interest is detectable only at specific times of observation, for example at the time of medical examination. *See also* **censoring**. [*Statistics in Medicine*, 1996, **15**, 283–92.]

Interval estimate: *See* **estimate**.

Interval estimation: *See* **estimation**.

Interval scale: *See* **measurement scale**.

Interval variable: Synonym for **continuous variable**.

Intervention index: An estimate of the impact of a therapeutic or preventive intervention given by the ratio of the number of people whose risk level must change to prevent one premature death to the total number at risk. *See also* **number needed to treat**. [*Journal of Clinical Epidemiology*, 1992, **45**, 21–9; *Annals of Experimental Pediatrics*, 1987, **6**, 435–8.]

Intervention study: Synonym for **clinical trial**.

Interviewer bias: The `bias` that occurs in surveys of human populations because of the direct result of the action of the interviewer. This bias can arise for a variety of reasons, including failure to contact the right people and systematic errors in recording the answers received from the respondent. [*Journal of Occupational Medicine*, 1992, **34**, 265–71.]

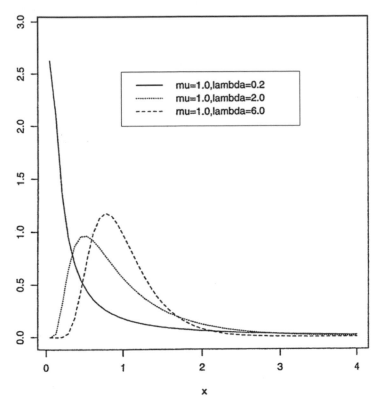

Figure 50 Examples of inverse normal distributions.

Intraclass correlation: The proportion of variance of an observation due to between-subject variability in the 'true' scores of a measuring instrument. The correlation can, for example, be estimated from a study involving a number of raters rating a number of subjects on some variable of interest. [Dunn, G., 2004, *Statistical Evaluation of Measurement Errors*, Arnold, London.]

Intrinsically nonlinear: *See* **nonlinear model**.

Intrinsic error: A term used most often in a clinical laboratory to describe the variability in results caused by the innate imprecision of each analytical step. [*International Journal of Cancer*, 2001, **96**, 320–5.]

Inverse normal distribution: A probability distribution that has been used to describe phenomena such as the length of time a particle remains in the blood, maternity data, and the length of stay in a hospital. Generally, a distribution that is skewed to the right as shown in Figure 50. [Chhikara, R. S. and Folks, J. L., 1989, *The Inverse Gaussian Distribution*, Marcel Dekker, New York.]

Ipsative scale: A rank order scale in which a particular rank can be used only once.

IQR: Abbreviation for **interquartile range**.

IRLS: Abbreviation for **iteratively reweighted least squares**.

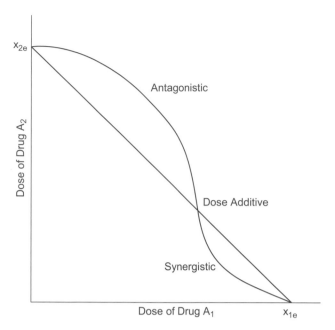

Figure 51 Example of an isobologram.

Isobole: *See* **isobologram**.

Isobologram: A diagram used to characterise the `interactions` between jointly administered drugs or chemicals. The contour of constant response (the *isobole*) is compared with the line of additivity, that is, the line connecting the single drug doses that yield the level of response associated with that contour. The interaction is described as synergistic, additive or antagonistic according to whether the isobole is below, coincident with, or above the line of additivity. See Figure 51 for an example. [*Statistics in Medicine*, 1994, **13**, 2289–310.]

Item non-response: A term used about data collected in a survey to indicate that particular questions in the survey attract refusals or responses that cannot be coded. Often, this type of `missing value` makes reporting of the overall response rate for the survey less relevant. *See also* **non-response**.

Item response theory (IRT): A class of models for `latent variables` that connects observed categorical item observations to an underlying construct, that is, the latent variable, which cannot be measured directly but is estimated from the observed item responses. The observed items are often the results of using questionnaires, for example, patient reported outcomes on questions about their current health issues. And the fitted models allow inferences about, for example, quality of life. [*Statistical Methods in Medical Research*, 2020, **29**, 959–61.]

Item-total correlation: A widely used method for checking the homogeneity of a scale made up of several items. It is simply the `Pearson's product moment correlation coefficient` of an individual item, with the scale total calculated from the remaining items. The usual rule of thumb is that an item should correlate with the total above 0.20. Items with lower correlation should be discarded. [Streiner, D. L. and Norman, G. R., 1989, *Health Measurement Scales*, Oxford Medical Publications, Oxford.]

Iteratively reweighted least squares (IRLS): A weighted least squares procedure in which the weights are revised or re-estimated at each iteration. In many cases, the result is equivalent to maximum likelihood estimation. Used widely in the fitting of generalized linear models. [Dobson, A. J., 2018, *An Introduction to Generalized Linear Models*, 2nd ed., Chapman & Hall/CRC, Boca Raton, FL.]

Iterative proportional fitting: A procedure for the maximum likelihood estimation of the expected frequencies in log-linear models, particularly for models where such estimates cannot be found directly from simple calculations using relevant marginal totals. [Agresti, A., 2013, *Categorical Data Analysis*, 3rd ed., Wiley-Blackwell, Oxford.]

Jackknife: A procedure for estimating bias and standard errors of parameter estimations when they cannot be obtained analytically. The principle behind the method is to omit each sample member in turn from the data, thus creating n samples each of size $n - 1$. The parameter of interest can now be estimated from each of these subsamples, thus enabling its standard error to be calculated. [Shao, J., 1995, *The Jackknife and Bootstrap*, Springer, New York.]

Jittering: A procedure for clarifying scatter diagrams when there is a multiplicity of points at many of the plotting locations, by adding a small amount of random variation to the data before graphing. Figure 52 shows a scatterplot before and after jittering. [Everitt, B. S. and Rabe-Hesketh, S., 2001, *The Analysis of Medical Data Using S-PLUS*, Springer, New York.]

Job-exposure matrix: A matrix whose elements provide information on exposures to each of many industrial agents in each of many finely subdivided categories of occupation. A small example of such a matrix is given below:

Job title	Number in survey	Proportion exposed to		
		S	LO	CO
Shoe factory worker	15	0.33	0.07	0.00
Stonemason	6	0.00	0.00	0.00
Maker of metal moulds	22	0.18	0.36	0.64

S = solvents, LO = lubricating oils, CO = cutting oils.

See also **occupational death rates**. [*Occupational and Environmental Medicine*, 2000, **57**, 635–41.]

Joint distribution: Essentially synonymous with multivariate distribution, although used particularly as an alternative to bivariate distribution when two variables are involved.

Joint modelling: Many medical studies involve the collection of longitudinal data along with an observation on a possibly censored time-to-event variable with, in addition, covariate information on each participant in the study. Interest

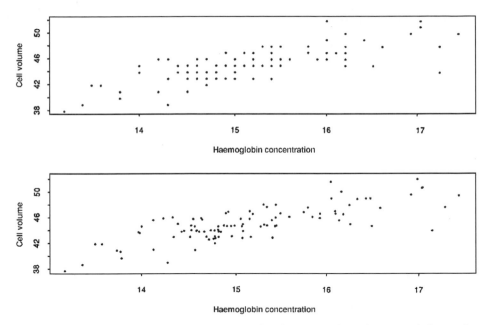

Figure 52 Example of jittering: the first scatterplot shows raw data; the second shows the same data after being jittered.

often focuses on interrelationships between these variables. An example of such a study would be a `clinical trial` of cancer treatment where the covariates would include treatment assignment, demographic information and physiological characteristics measured over time and the time-to-event variable might be `survival time` which would be censored for patients still alive at the closure of the study. Joint models are those that have been developed for dealing appropriately with such data. The most common such model involves two parts, the first a random effect model for the longitudinal measures followed by a `Cox proportional hazards model`. [*Biostatistics*, 2000, **4**, 465–80.]

Jonckheere's *k*-sample test: A `distribution-free method` for testing the equality of a set of location parameters against an ordered `alternative hypothesis`. [Lehman, E. L., 1975, *Nonparametric Statistical Methods Based on Ranks*, Holden-Day, San Francisco, CA.]

Jonckheere–Terpstra test: A test for detecting specific types of departures from independence in a `contingency table` in which both the row and column categories have a natural order. For example, suppose the *r* rows represent *r* distinct drug therapies at progressively increasing drug doses and the *c* columns represent *c* ordered responses. Interest in this case might centre on detecting a departure from independence, in which drugs administered at larger doses are more responsive than drugs administered at smaller doses. *See also* **linear-by-linear association test**. [Fisher, L. D. and Van Belle, G., 2004, *Biostatistics*, 2nd ed., John Wiley & Sons, New York.]

J-shaped distribution: An extremely `asymmetrical distribution` that is concentrated towards the larger values of the variable it describes, That is, an extreme case of negative `skewness`. A *reverse J-shaped distribution* (or *ski-jump distribution*) is one which is concentrated towards the smaller values of the variable, that is, an extreme case of positive skewness. An example of a J-shaped distribution is likely to be found for nicotine intake amongst patients with lung cancer. And a reverse J-shaped distribution is probable for age at death amongst children from birth to age 5 years. [*Journal of Hypertension*, 1990, **8**, 547–55.]

Just identified model: *See* identification.

Kaiser's rule: A rule often used in principal components analysis for selecting the appropriate number of components. When the components are derived from the correlation matrix of the observed variables, the rule advocates retaining only those components with variances greater than unity. *See also* **scree plot**. [Everitt, B. S. and Dunn, G., 2010, *Applied Multivariate Data Analysis*, 2nd ed., John Wiley & Sons, Chichester.]

Kaplan–Meier estimator: *See* **product limit estimator**.

Kappa coefficient: A chance-corrected index of the agreement between, for example, judgements or diagnoses made by two raters. Calculated as the ratio of the observed excess over chance agreement to the maximum possible excess over chance, the coefficient takes the value unity when there is perfect agreement and the value zero when observed agreement is equal to chance agreement. Chance agreement is agreement calculated according to the marginal totals of each rater for each diagnostic category. *See also* **Aickin's measure of agreement** and **weighted kappa**. [*Canadian Journal of Statistics*, 1999, **27**, 3–23.]

Karnofsky rating scale: A measure of the ability to cope with everyday activities. The scale has 11 categories ranging from 0 (dead) to 10 (normal, no complaints, no evidence of disease). *See also* **Barthel index**. [*Neurosurgery*, 1995, **36**, 270–4.]

Kendall's coefficient of concordance: Synonym for **coefficient of concordance**.

Kendall's tau statistic: A range of correlation coefficients that use only the ranks of the observations in a data set. *See also* **phi-coefficient**. [Everitt, B. S. and Palmer, C. (eds.), 2011, *Encyclopedic Companion to Medical Statistics*, 2nd ed., John Wiley & Sons, Chichester.]

Kermack and McKendrick's threshold theorem: A result concerned with the total size of an epidemic. It shows that the initial distribution of susceptible individuals is finally reduced to a point as far below some threshold value as it was originally above it. [*Proceedings of the Royal Society of London, Series A*, 1927, **115**, 700–21.]

K-means cluster analysis: A method of cluster analysis that partitions a set of multivariate data into a number of groups pre-specified by the user by seeking a solution that minimizes the within-group sum of squares calculated over all variables. [Everitt, B. S., Landau, S., Leese, M. and Stahl, D., 2011, *Cluster Analysis*, 5th ed., John Wiley & Sons, Chichester.]

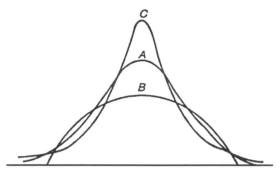

Figure 53 Curves with differing degrees of kurtosis.

Knox's tests: Tests designed to detect any tendency for patients with a particular disease to form a `disease cluster` in time and space. The tests are based on a `two-by-two contingency table`, formed from considering every pair of patients and classifying them as to whether the members of the pair were closer than a critical distance apart in space, and as to whether the times at which they contracted the disease were closer than a chosen critical period. *See also* **clustering** and **scan statistic**. [*Applied Statistics*, 1964, **13**, 25–9.]

Kolmogorov–Smirnov two sample method: A `distribution-free` method that tests for any difference between two population `probability distributions`. The test is based on the maximum absolute difference between the `cumulative frequency distribution` functions of the samples from each population. `Critical values` are available in many statistical tables. [Fisher, L. D. and Van Belle, G., 2004, *Biostatistics*, 2nd ed., John Wiley & Sons, New York.]

Kruskal–Wallis test: A `distribution-free` method that is the analogue of the `analysis of variance` of a one-way design, used to test whether a series of populations have the same median. [Hollander, M. and Wolfe, D. A., 2014, *Nonparametric Statistical Methods*, 3rd ed., Wiley-Blackwell, Oxford.]

Kuder–Richardson formulae: Measures of the internal consistency or reliability of tests in which items have only two possible answers, for example agree/disagree or yes/no. [Dunn, G., 2004, *Statistical Evaluation of Measurement Errors*, Arnold, London.]

Kurtosis: The extent to which the peak of a unimodal `probability distribution` departs from that of a `normal distribution`. More pointed distributions are known as *leptokurtic*; those that are flatter are *platykurtic*. Distributions that have the same kurtosis as the normal distribution are called *mesokurtic*. See Figure 53 for examples; curve A is mesokurtic, curve B is platykurtic and curve C is leptokurtic. [*The American Statistician*, 1970, **24**, 19–22.]

L

L'Abbé plot: A plot often used in the meta-analysis of clinical trials where the outcome is a binary variable. The event risk (number of events/number of patients in a group) in each treatment group is plotted against the risk for the controls for each selected study. If the studies are relatively homogeneous, then the points will form a 'cloud' close to a line, the gradient of which will correspond to the pooled treatment effect. Large deviations or scatter indicates possible heterogeneity amongst the effect sizes from the different trials. Figure 54 shows an example. [*Annals of Internal Medicine*, 1987, **107**, 224–33.]

Landmark analysis: A term applied to a form of analysis occasionally applied to survival time data in which a test is used to assess whether treatment predicts subsequent survival among subjects who survive to a landmark time (e.g. six months post-randomization) and who have, at this time, a common prophylaxis status and history of all other covariates. [*Statistics in Medicine*, 1996, **15**, 2797–812.]

Large sample method: Any statistical method based on an approximation to a normal distribution or other probability distribution that becomes more accurate as sample size increases. *See also* **asymptotic distribution**.

Large simple trials (LST): Clinical trials in which exceptionally large numbers of patients with minimally restrictive entry criteria are used and data are collected only on essential baseline characteristics and outcomes. Such a trial allows unprecedented discretion by both patients and clinicians; patients are randomized to a study treatment, but the rest of their care is left in their own hands. Such trials can provide reliable evidence on the balance of risk and benefit of treatments that have moderate effects on major clinical outcomes such as strokes. [*Journal of the Royal College of Physicians*, 1995, **29**, 96–100.]

Lasagna's law: States that once a clinical trial has started, the number of suitable patients dwindles to a tenth of what was calculated before the trial began. [*Family Practice*, 2004, **21**, 213–18.]

Last observation carried forward (LOCF): A method for replacing the observations of patients who drop out of a clinical trial carried out over a period of time. It consists of substituting for each missing value the subject's last available assessment of the same type. Although applied widely, particularly in the

At least 50% pain relief with rofecoxib 50 mg

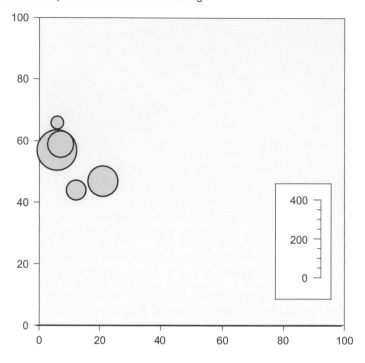

At least 50% pain relief with placebo

Figure 54 Example of a L'Abbé plot.

pharmaceutical industry, its usefulness is very limited since it makes very unlikely assumptions about the data, that is, that the (unobserved) post-dropout response remains frozen at the last value observed. *See also* **imputation** and **multiple imputation**. [Everitt, B. S., 2003, *Modern Medical Statistics*, Arnold, London.]

Last observation carried forward: Apart from its simplicity, this approach to replacing the missing values caused by dropouts in a longitudinal study has nothing to recommend it.

Latent class models: Models that have been developed as a flexible way of modelling the `correlation matrix` of `multivariate data`, as a method of discovering subpopulations with similar response profiles and as a dimension reduction tool. *See also* **structural equation modelling**. [*Statistical Methods in Medical Research*, 2007, **16**, 441–56.]

Latent period: A term used in describing an `epidemic` for the time during which the disease develops purely internally within the infected person. For some diseases, for example, yellow fever, the latent period is short and fairly constant; for others, such as cancer, it can be very long and can vary greatly between individuals. *See also*

infectious period. [*Journal of Environmental Pathology and Toxicology*, 1977, **1**, 279–86.]

Latent variable: A quantity that cannot be measured directly but that is assumed to relate to a number of observable or `manifest variables`. Examples include racial prejudice and social class. The common factors in a `factor analysis` are latent variables. In fact, latent variables can be used to represent a variety of phenomena such as true variables measured with error, hypothetical constructs and missing data. *See also* **indicator variable** and **structural equation modelling**. [Skrondal, A. and Rabe-Hesketh, S., 2004, *Generalized Latent Variable Modelling*, Chapman & Hall/CRC, Boca Raton, FL.]

Latent variable modelling: Any model that includes unobserved random variables. Examples include `factor analysis`, `structural equation models`, `mixed effects` and `frailty models`. Areas of application include `meta-analysis`, `disease mapping`, diagnostic testing and biometrical genetics. [Beaujean, A. A., 2014, *Latent Variable Modelling using R*, Routledge, New York.]

Latin square: An experimental design aimed at removing from the experimental error the variation from two extraneous sources (e.g. subjects and diagnostic category) so as to achieve a more sensitive test of the treatment effect. The rows and columns of the square represent the levels of the two extraneous factors, and the treatments are represented by Roman letters arranged so that no letter appears more than once in each row and column. The following is an example of a 4×4 Latin square:

A B C D
B C D A
C D A B
D A B C

Analysis of the data arising from such a design assumes that there are no `interactions` between the three sources of variation. [Cochran, W. G. and Cox, G. M., 1957, *Experimental Designs*, 2nd ed., John Wiley & Sons, New York.]

Law of large numbers: Essentially, the larger the sample, the more it will be representative of the population from which it is taken.

Law of truly large numbers: With a large enough sample, any outrageous thing is likely to happen. *See also* **coincidences**. [Everitt, B. S., 2008, *Chance Rules*, 2nd ed., Springer, New York.]

LD50: Abbreviation for **lethal dose 50**.

Lead time: An indicator of the effectiveness of `screening studies` for chronic diseases given by the length of time the diagnosis is advanced by the screening procedure, that is, the time between early diagnosis with screening and the time in which diagnosis would have been made without screening. [*Journal of the American Geriatrics Society*, 2000, **48**, 1226–33.]

Lead time bias: The difference in the time from when a tumour would have been detected by symptoms, in the absence of a screening programme, to when the detection occurred in the presence of a screening programme. For screen-detected cases, this time will vary from perhaps a month to several years. Statistical analysis comparing survival times in populations with and without screening, or comparing screening to symptomatic cases in a population to which screening is offered, will be subject to lead time bias if survival is estimated as the time from diagnosis to death in screen-detected cancer. *See also* **length bias**. [*Lancet*, 2013, **380**, 1778–86.]

Leaps-and-bounds algorithm: An `algorithm` used to find the optimal solution in problems that have a possibly very large number of solutions. Begins by splitting the possible solutions into a number of exclusive subsets and limits the number of subsets that need to be examined in searching for the optimal solution by a number of different strategies. Often used in `all-subsets regression` to restrict the number of models that have to be examined. [Rawlings, J. O., Pantula, S. G. and Dickey, D. A., 2013, *Applied Regression Analysis: A Research Tool*, 2nd ed., Springer, New York.]

Least absolute shrinkage and selection operator (LASSO): A method of `variable selection` for high-dimensional data that carries out variable selection and parameter estimation simultaneously. [*Journal of the Royal Statistical Society, Series B*, 1996, **58**, 267–88.]

Least significant difference (LSD) test: An approach to comparing a set of means that controls the `family-wise error rate` at some particular level, say *a*. The hypothesis of the equality of the means is tested first by an *a*-level `F-test`. If this test is not significant, then the procedure terminates without making detailed inferences on pairwise differences; otherwise each pairwise difference is tested by an *a*-level `Student's t-test`. [Fisher, R. A., 1935, *The Design of Experiments*, Oliver & Boyd, Edinburgh.]

Least squares estimation: A method of estimation due to Gauss in which parameters are estimated by minimizing the sum of squared differences between the observed values of the dependent variable and the values predicted by the model of interest. Used widely in statistics, particularly in simple `linear regression` and `multiple linear regression`. [Rawlings, J. O., Pantula, S. G. and Dickey, D. A., 2013, *Applied Regression Analysis: A Research Tool*, 2nd ed., Springer, New York.]

Ledermann model: A model for the `probability distribution` of alcohol consumption in the population of drinkers. Empirical data appear to indicate that alcohol consumption has a `log-normal distribution`. It has also been found that frequency of cannabis use by adolescents also conforms to this model. [*Quarterly Journal of Studies in Alcoholism*, 1974, **35**, 877–98.]

Length bias: The `bias` that arises in a sampling scheme based on patient visits, when some individuals are more likely to be selected than others simply because they make more frequent visits. In a `screening study` for cancer, for example, the sample of cases detected is likely to contain an excess of slow-growing cancers compared with the sample diagnosed positive because of their symptoms. Such a bias will result if `survival time` is associated with time a tumour is present in the body before being detected. [*Breast Cancer Research and Treatment*, 2009, **116**, 179–185.]

Leptokurtic: *See* kurtosis.

Lethal dose 50 (LD50): The administered dose of a compound that causes death of 50% of the animals during a specified period in an experiment involving toxic material. [Collett, D., 2003, *Modelling Binary Data*, 2nd ed., Chapman & Hall/CRC, Boca Raton, FL.]

Levene test: A test used for detecting heterogeneity of variance that consists of an analysis of variance applied to the differences between the observations and the group means. *See also* **Bartlett's test** and **Box's test**. [*Journal of the American Statistical Association*, 1974, **69**, 364–7.]

Leverage points: A term used in regression analysis for those observations that have an extreme value on one or more explanatory variables. The effect of such points is to force the fitted model close to the observed value of the response, leading to a small residual. *See also* **hat matrix** and **influence**. [Rawlings, J. O., Pantula, S. G. and Dickey, D. A., 2013, *Applied Regression Analysis: A Research Tool*, 2nd ed., Springer, New York.]

Lexis diagram: A diagram for displaying the simultaneous effects of two timescales (usually age and calendar time) on a rate. For example, mortality rates from cancer of the cervix depend upon age, as a result of the age-dependence of the incidence, and upon calendar time as a result of changes in treatment, population screening, and so on. The main feature of such a diagram is a series of rectangular regions corresponding to a combination of two time bands, one from each scale. Rates for these combinations of bands can be estimated by allocating failures to the rectangles in which they occur and then dividing the total observation time for each subject between rectangles according to how long the subjects spend in each. The diagram allows the researcher to see the pattern of age and period intervals traversed by different cohorts. An example of such a diagram is shown in Figure 55. *See also* **age–period–cohort analysis**. [*American Statistician*, 1992, **46**, 13–18.]

Lie factor: A quantity suggested by Tufte for judging the honesty of a graphical presentation of data. Calculated as

$$\frac{\text{apparent size of effect shown in graph}}{\text{actual size of effect in data}}$$

Values close to unity are desirable, but it is not uncommon to find values close to zero and greater than five. The example shown in Figure 56 has a lie factor of about 2.8. *See also* Graphical deception. [Tufte, E. R., 1983, *The Visual Display of Quantitative Information*, Graphic Press, Cheshire, CT.]

Life expectancy: The expected number of years remaining to be lived by people of a particular age. For example, for the year 2000, the life expectancy of all Americans at birth was 76.9 years and that at age 65 was 17.9 years. The life expectancy of a

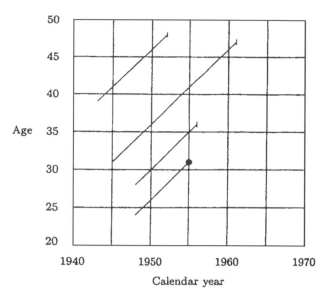

Figure 55 Lexis diagram.

THE SHRINKING FAMILY DOCTOR
In California

Percentage of Doctors Devoted Solely to Family Practice

1964	1975	1990
27%	16%	12%

1: 4,232
6.212

1: 3,167
6.694

1: 2,247 RATIO TO POPULATION

8.023 Doctors

Figure 56 Diagram with a lie factor of 2.8.

population is a general indication of the capability of prolonging life. It is used to identify trends and to compare longevity. Life expectancy at birth has increased substantially (at least in the West) over the last 100 years; for example, the life expectancy for all Americans at birth in 1929 was only 57.1 years. It is important to note that life expectancy is an average, with, for example, a life expectancy at birth of 70 in a particular year meaning that 50% of the people born in that year will live to be 70. [*Population and Development Review*, 1994, **20**, 57–80.]

Life history calendar data: A data collection tool for obtaining reliable retrospective data about life events. The method has the advantage that the order and proximity of important transitions in multiple life domains can be studied at the same time. As a data-collection tool, it encourages respondents to incorporate temporal changes as cues in the reporting of events. It has shown the ability to provide data of high quality. [Belle, R. F., Stafford, F. P. and Alwin, D. F., 2008, *Calendar and Time Diary: Methods in Life Course Research*, Sage, London.]

Life table: A procedure used to compute chances of survival and death and remaining years of life for specific years of age. An example of part of such a table is as follows: [Chiang, G. L., 1984, *The Life Table and Its Applications*, Krieger, Malabar, FL.]

Life table for white females, USA, 1949–51

1	2	3	4	5	6	7
0	23.55	100,000	2,355	97,965	7,203,179	72.03
1	1.89	97,465	185	97,552	7,105,214	72.77
2	1.12	97,645	109	97,406	7,007,662	71.90
3	0.87	97,351	85	97,308	6,910,256	70.98
4	0.69	97,266	67	97,233	6,812,948	70.04
⋮	⋮	⋮	⋮	⋮	⋮	⋮
100	388.39	294	114	237	556	1.92

1 = Year of age
2 = Death rate per 1,000
3 = Number surviving of 100,000 born alive
4 = Number dying of 100,000 born alive
5 = Number of years lived by cohort
6 = Total number of years lived by cohort until all have died
7 = Average future years of life.

Life-table analysis: A procedure often applied in prospective studies to examine the distribution of mortality and/or morbidity in one or more diseases in a cohort study of patients over a fixed period of time. For each specific increment in the follow-up period, the number entering the period, the number leaving during the period, and the number either dying from the disease (mortality) or developing the disease (morbidity) are all calculated. It is assumed that an individual not completing the follow-up period is exposed for half this period, thus enabling the data for those leaving and those staying to be combined into an appropriate denominator for the estimation of the percentage dying from or developing the disease. The advantage of this approach is that all patients, not only those who have been involved for an extended period, can be included in the estimation process. [Morton, K. G. and Stallard, E., 1984, *Recent Trends in Mortality Analysis*, Academic Press, New York.]

Lifetime tumour rate: A term encountered most often in animal research, and defined as the probability that an animal dies with a tumour at some time during its lifetime, or, during an experiment with a terminal sacrifice, at some particular time point. [*Biometrics*, 1991, **47**, 669–80.]

Likelihood: The probability of the observed data assuming a particular model. The likelihood function is the basis of `maximum likelihood estimation`. [Clayton, D. G. and Hills, M., 2013, *Statistical Models in Epidemiology*, Oxford University Press, Oxford.]

Likelihood ratio test: A test for comparing two competing models for a data set. The test statistics is −2 times the difference in the `log-likelihoods` of the two models. Under the hypothesis that the two models fit the data equally well, the test statistic has a chi-squared distribution with degrees of freedom equal to the difference in the two models. *See also* **deviance**. [Clayton, D. G. and Hills, M., 2013, *Statistical Models in Epidemiology*, Oxford University Press, Oxford.]

Likert scale: Scales often used in studies of attitudes in which the raw scores are based on graded alternative responses to each of a series of questions. For example, the subject may be asked to indicate his/her degree of agreement with each of a series of statements relevant to the attitude. A number is attached to each possible response, for example, 1: approve strongly; 2: approve; 3: undecided; 4: disapprove; 5: disapprove strongly. The sum of these is then used as the composite score.

A commonly used Likert-type scale in medicine is the *Apgar score*, which is used to appraise the status of newborn infants. This is the sum of the points (0, 1 or 2) allotted for each of five items:

- Heart rate (over 100 beats per minute: 2 points: slower: 1 point; no beat: 0 points)
- Respiratory effort
- Muscle tone
- Response to stimulation by a catheter in the nostril
- Skin colour

[Stewart, A. L. and Ware, J. E., 1992, *Measuring Functioning and Well-Being: The Medical Outcomes Study Approach*, Duke University Press, Durham, NC.]

Limits of agreement: A method of analyzing the way in which two ways of taking measurements agree and the extent to which they are compatible. The method gives an estimate of the interval where a proportion of the differences lies between measurements. Usually applied when interest lies in trying out a new measuring technique or method that may have advantages over the method currently in use. [*Statistical Methods in Medical Research*, 1999, **8**, 135–60.]

LIMS: Abbreviation for **laboratory information management system**.

Linear-by-linear association test: A test for detecting specific types of departure from independence in a `contingency table` in which both the row and column

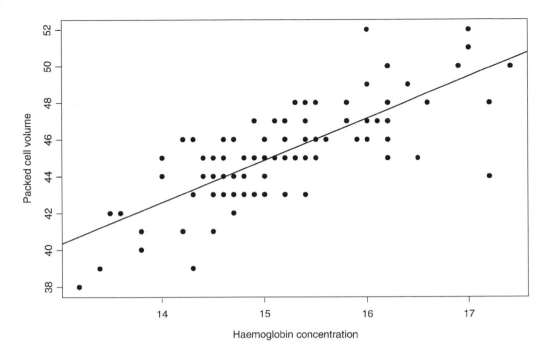

Figure 57 Scatter diagram of packed cell volume against haemoglobin concentration showing fitted linear regression.

categories have a natural order. *See also* **Jonckheere–Terpstra test**. [Everitt, B. S., 1992, *The Analysis of Contingency Tables*, 2nd ed., Chapman & Hall/CRC, Boca Raton, FL.]

Linear estimator: An estimator that is a linear function of the observations or of sample statistics calculated from the observations.

Linear logistic regression: Synonym for **logistic regression**.

Linear regression: A term usually reserved for the simple regression of a response variable on a single explanatory variable and involving just two parameters, the intercept of the line and its slope. Both intercept and slope are usually estimated from sample data by least squares estimation. Figure 57 shows a scatter diagram of two variables and the fitted regression line. [Altman, D. G., 2018, *Practical Statistics for Medical Research*, Chapman & Hall/CRC, Boca Raton, FL.]

Linear trend: A relationship between two variables in which the values of one change at a constant rate as the other increases.

Linkage analysis: A method used for testing the hypothesis that a genetic marker of known location is on a different chromosome from a gene postulated to govern susceptibility to a disease. [Ott, J., 1999, *Analysis of Human Genetic Linkage*, Johns Hopkins University Press, Baltimore, MD.]

Linkage map: A chromosome map showing the relevant positions of the known genes in the chromosomes of a given species.

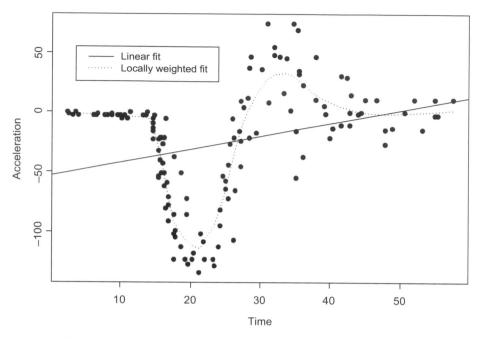

Figure 58 Time after impact and acceleration in a simulated motorcycle accident showing fitted linear and locally weighted regressions.

Link function: *See* **generalized linear model**.

Literature controls: Patients with the disease of interest who have received, in the past, one of two treatments under investigation, and for whom results have been published in the literature, now used as a control group for patients currently receiving the alternative treatment. Such a control group clearly requires careful checking for comparability. *See also* **historical controls**.

Loading dose: The dose of a drug needed to quickly bring a patient's serum concentration of the drug up to a desired level. For a drug that distributes equally into the entire body mass, the loading dose is simply the desired concentration times the patient's mass. [*Circulation*, 2005, **111**, 2099–106.]

Locally weighted regression: A method of regression analysis in which polynomials of degree one (linear) or two (quadratic) are used to approximate the regression function in particular 'neighbourhoods' of the space of the explanatory variables. Often useful for smoothing scatter diagrams to allow any structure to be seen more clearly, and for identifying possible nonlinear relationships between the response and explanatory variables. A robust estimation procedure (usually known as *lowess*) is used to guard against deviant points distorting the smoothed points. Essentially, the process involves an adaptation of iteratively reweighted least squares. The example shown in Figure 58 illustrates a situation in which the locally weighted regression differs considerably from the linear regression of y on x as fitted by least squares estimation. *See also* **generalized additive models**. [*Journal of the American Statistical Association*, 1979, **74**, 829–36.]

Local odds ratio: The odds ratio of the two-by-two contingency tables formed from adjacent rows and columns in a larger `contingency table`.

Location: The notion of central or typical value in a sample distribution. *See also* **mean**, **median** and **mode**.

LOCF: Abbreviation for **last observation carried forward**.

Lods: A term often used in `epidemiology` for the logarithm of an `odds ratio`. Also used in genetics for the logarithm of a `likelihood ratio`.

Logarithmic transformation: The transformation of a variable achieved by taking its logarithms. Often used when the frequency distribution of the variable suggests moderate to large `skewness` in order to achieve approximate normality.

Logistic regression: A form of `regression analysis` suitable for a binary response variable (e.g. 'occurs', 'does not occur'), in which the logarithm of the `odds` is modelled as a linear function of the explanatory variables. Using this form of regression avoids problems that might arise if, say, the probability of occurrence was modelled directly as a linear function of the explanatory variables. In particular, it avoids fitted probabilities outside the range zero to one. The estimated regression coefficients can be exponentiated to give estimated odds ratios. [Hosmer, D. and Lemenshow, S., 2013, *Applied Logistic Regression*, 3rd ed., Wiley-Blackwell, Oxford.]

Logit transformation: The logarithm of the odds of a categorical variable. The basis of `logistic regression`.

Log-likelihood: The logarithm of the `likelihood`. Generally easier to work with than the likelihood itself when using `maximum likelihood estimation`.

Log-linear models: Models for `count data` in which the logarithm of the expected value of a count variable is modelled as a linear function of parameters; the latter represent associations between pairs of variables and higher-order interactions between more than two variables. Estimated expected frequencies under particular models are found from `iterative proportional fitting`. Such models are, essentially, the equivalent for frequency data of the models for continuous data used in `analysis of variance`, except that interest usually now centres on parameters representing interactions rather than on those for main effects. *See also* **generalized linear model**. [Everitt, B. S., 1992, *The Analysis of Contingency Tables*, 2nd ed., Chapman & Hall/CRC, Boca Raton, FL.]

Log-normal distribution: The `probability distribution` of a variable whose logarithm has a `normal distribution`. Generally skewed, as shown by the examples in Figure 59. Useful for modelling data arising in a variety of medical studies, for example in cancer and biochemistry. [*Journal of Theoretical Biology*, 1996, **12**, 276–90.]

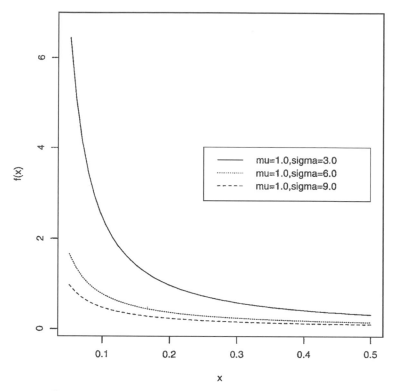

Figure 59 Some log-normal distributions.

Log-rank test: A method for comparing the survival times of two or more groups of subjects that involves the calculating of observed and expected frequencies of failures in separate time intervals. The relevant test statistic is, essentially, a comparison of the observed number of deaths occurring at each particular time point with the number to be expected if the survival experience of the two groups is the same. [Collet, D., 2015, *Modelling Survival Data in Medical Research*, 3rd ed., Chapman & Hall/CRC, Boca Raton, FL.]

Longini–Koopman model: A model describing the process underlying the transmission of an infectious disease in terms of household and community level transmission probabilities. [*Statistics in Medicine*, 1994, **13**, 1563–74.]

Longitudinal data: Data arising when each of a number of subjects or patients gives rise to a vector of measurements representing the same variable observed at a number of different time points. Such data combine elements of multivariate data and time series data. They differ from the former, however, in that only a single variable is involved, and differ from the latter in consisting of a (possibly) large number of short series, one from each subject, rather than a single long series. Such data can be collected either prospectively, following subjects forward in time, or retrospectively, by extracting measurements on each person from historical records. This type of data is also often known as *repeated-measures data*, particularly in the

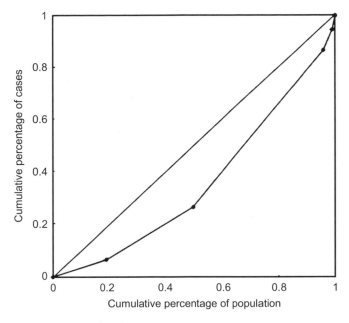

Figure 60 Example of a Lorenz curve.

social and behavioural sciences, although in these disciplines such data are more likely to arise from observing individuals repeatedly under different experimental conditions rather than from a simple time sequence. Special statistical methods are often needed for the analysis of this type of data because the set of measurements on one subject tend to be intercorrelated. This correlation must be taken into account to draw valid scientific inferences. *See also* **Greenhouse–Geisser correction, Huynh–Feldt correction, compound symmetry, generalized estimating equations, mixed-effects models** and **split-plot design**. [Diggle, P., Heagerty, P., Liang, K. Y. and Zeger, S., 2013, *Analysis of Longitudinal Data*, 2nd ed., Oxford University Press, Oxford.]

Longitudinal data: The last decade has seen major developments in methods for the analysis of this type of data, many of which are now available routinely in most major statistical software packages.

Longitudinal studies: Studies that give rise to `longitudinal data`. The defining characteristic of such a study is that subjects are measured repeatedly through time. [Diggle, P., Heagerty, P., Liang, K. Y. and Zeger, S., 2013, *Analysis of Longitudinal Data*, 2nd ed., Oxford University Press, Oxford.]

Lorenz curve: A plot of the cumulative percentage of cases against the cumulative percentage of the population for increasing exposure, used to indicate the level of exposure–disease association. A straight line rising at an angle of 45 degrees from the start of the graph would indicate a lack of association between the exposure and the disease. An example is shown in Figure 60. If the risks of disease are not

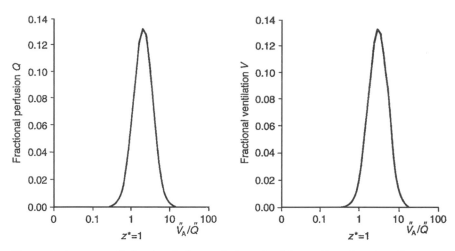

Figure 61 Lung ventilation/perfusion ratio for a healthy, well-perfused, well-ventilated lung.

increasing monotonically as the exposure becomes heavier, then the data have to be rearranged from the lowest to the highest risk before the calculation of the cumulative percentages. Associated with this type of curve is the *Gini index*, defined as twice the area between the curve and the diagonal line. This index takes values between zero and one, with larger values indicating greater variability and smaller ones suggesting greater uniformity. [*Economic Applications*, 1980, **33**, 327–67.]

Loss function: *See* **decision theory**.

Low-dose extrapolation: The process applied to the results from `bioassays` for carcinogenicity conducted in animals at doses that are generally well above human exposure levels, in order to assess risk in humans. Results are highly dependent on the shape of the `dose–response relationship` curve predicted by the extrapolation model. [*Radiation Effects*, 1992, **4**, 5–6.]

Lowess: *See* **locally weighted regression**.

LSD test: Abbreviation for **least significant difference test**.

LST: Abbreviation for **large simple trial**.

Lung ventilation/perfusion ratio: The ratio of airflow to blood flow in the lung, usually denoted by V_A/Q. A small value of the ratio corresponds to a portion of the lung where the airflow is severely restricted, while a large value corresponds to a part of the lung with little blood flow. The example shown in Figure 61 is for a healthy, well-perfused, well-ventilated lung. [*Journal of Applied Physiology*, 1960, **15**, 405–10.]

M

Mack–Wolfe test: A distribution-free method for one-way designs used to test a null hypothesis of equality of treatment effects against an alternative specifying an umbrella ordering. [Hollander, M. and Wolfe, D. A., 2013, *Nonparametric Statistical Methods*, 3rd ed., John Wiley & Sons, New York.]

Mahalanobis D²: A measure of the distance between two populations or two samples of individuals based on observations on a number of variables measured on each. The measure is based on the difference of the mean vectors of each group and on their assumed common variance-covariance matrix. *See also* **Hotelling's T² test**. [Everitt, B. S. and Dunn, G., 2010, *Applied Multivariate Data Analysis*, 2nd ed., Wiley, Chichester.]

Main effect: An estimate of the independent effect of (usually) a factor variable on a response variable in analysis of variance. [Altman, D. G., 2018, *Practical Statistics for Medical Research*, Chapman & Hall/CRC, Boca Raton, FL.]

Mainframe: High-speed, general-purpose computer with a very large storage capacity.

Majority rule: A requirement that the majority of a series of diagnostic tests are positive before declaring that a patient has a particular complaint. *See also* **unanimity rule**.

Malthusian parameter: The rate of increase that a population would ultimately attain if its age-specific birth rate and age-specific death rate were to continue indefinitely. *See also* **population growth model**. [*Proceedings of the National Academy of Sciences of the United States of America*, 1996, **93**, 15276–8.]

MAMS drop-the-losers design: *See* **Multi-arm multistage trials (MAMS)**.

Management trial: Synonymous with **pragmatic trial**.

Manifest variable: A variable that can be measured directly, in contrast to a latent variable. For example, blood pressure, weight, height, etc.

Mann–Whitney test: A distribution-free method used as an alternative to the Student's *t*-test for assessing whether two populations have the same location. Given a sample of observations from each population, all the observations are ranked as if they were from a single sample, and the test statistic is the sum of the ranks in the smaller group. Tables giving critical values of the test statistic are available, and for moderate and large sample sizes, a normal approximation can be used. [Hollander, M. and Wolfe, D. A., 2013, *Nonparametric Statistical Methods*, 3rd ed., John Wiley & Sons, New York.]

MANOVA: Acronym for **multivariate analysis of variance**.

Mantel–Haenszel estimator: An estimator of the assumed common odds ratio in a series of two-by-two contingency tables arising from different populations, for example, occupation, country of origin, etc. The estimator is essentially a type of weighted average of the individual odds ratios. [*Annual Review of Public Health*, 1988, **9**, 123–60.]

Marginal homogeneity: A term applied to square contingency tables when the probabilities of falling in each category of the row classification equal the corresponding probabilities for the column classification. *See also* **Stuart–Maxwell test**. [Everit, B. S., 1992, *The Analysis of Contingency Tables*, 2nd ed., Chapman & Hall/CRC, Boca Raton, FL.]

Marginal matching: The matching of treatment groups in terms of means or other summary characteristics of the matching variables. Has been shown to be almost as efficient as the matching of individual subjects in some circumstances.

Marginal models: Models for the data from longitudinal studies that are the direct analogues, for the repeated measurements encountered in such studies, of generalized linear models. With such models, interest focuses on the regression parameters of each response separately; the relationship of this marginal mean to the explanatory variables is modelled separately from the within-subject correlation. The term 'marginal' implies that interest lies with each response, conditional on the covariates, but not on the other responses, as in a transition model. For responses having a normal distribution, the parameters in such models can be estimated by maximum likelihood estimation. For non-normal response, generalized estimating equations can be used. *See also* **conditional regression models**. [Everitt, B. S., 2003, *Modern Medical Statistics*, Arnold, London.]

Marginal probability distribution: The probability distribution of a single variable, or combinations of variables, in a set of multivariate data. Obtained from the multivariate distribution by integrating over the other variables.

Marginal totals: A term often used for the total number of observations in each row and each column of a contingency table.

Markers of disease progression: Quantities that form a general monotonic sequence throughout the course of a disease and assist with its modelling. In general, such quantities are highly prognostic in predicting the future course. An example is CD4 cell count (cells per microlitre), which is generally accepted as the best marker of HIV disease progression. A further example is provided by selenium levels in HIV infection, where the evidence increasingly suggests that a selenium deficit is not only a correlate of disease progression but also a powerful predictor of mortality or survival in AIDS. [*Chemical and Biological Interactions*, 1994, **91**, 181–6.]

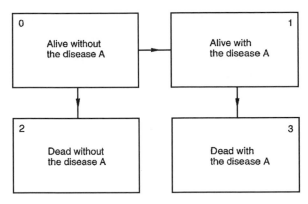

Figure 62 Markov illness–death model diagram.

Markov chain: A discrete `stochastic process` in which the probability that a system will be in a given state on the $(k + 1)$th trial depends only on the state of the system on the kth trial. (Sometimes known more specifically as a *first-order Markov chain*, to differentiate it from processes depending on more than the immediate previous state.) [Metcalfe, A. V., 1997, *Statistics in Civil Engineering*, Arnold, London.]

Markov chain Monte Carlo methods (MCMC): Powerful methods for indirectly simulating random observations from complex, and often high dimensional `probability distributions` and now widely used particularly in applications of `Bayesian methods` for evaluating `posterior distributions`. [Gamerman, D. and Lopes, H. F., 2006, *Markov Chain Monte Carlo: Stochastic Simulation for Bayesian Inference*, 2nd ed., CRC, Boca Raton, FL.]

Markov chain Monte Carlo: A procedure that has had, over the last ten years or so, a major impact on the ability to apply Bayesian inference routinely.

Markov illness–death model: A model in which live individuals are classified as either having or not having a disease, *A*, and then move between these possibilities and death as indicated in the diagram shown in Figure 62. An example of the use of such a model is in large-scale, community-based longitudinal dementia studies, where a significant source of `missing data` is death of elderly individuals. [*Mathematical Biosciences*, 1994, **122**, 95–125.]

Markov process: A `stochastic process` with the property that its state at any time in the future is dependent only on its present state and is unaffected by any additional knowledge of the past history of the system. *See also* **random walk**.

Masking: Synonym for **blinding**.

Matchability: A term used most often in kidney transplantation for the probability that a patient will be offered a well-matched kidney from a random donor. Depends on the patient's tissue type and also on the tissue type of other patients awaiting kidney transplantation. [*Transplantation Proceedings*, 1997, **29**, 1403–5.]

Matched pairs: A term used for observations arising from either two individuals who are individually matched on a number of variables, for example age or sex, or where two observations are taken on the same individual on two separate occasions. Essentially synonymous with **paired samples**. [Altman, D. G., 2018, *Practical Statistics for Medical Research*, Chapman & Hall/CRC, Boca Raton, FL.]

Matched-pairs *t*-test: A `Student's t-test` for the equality of the means of two populations when the observations arise as paired samples. The test is based on the differences between the observations on the matched pairs. [Altman, D. G., 2018, *Practical Statistics for Medical Research*, Chapman & Hall/CRC, Boca Raton, FL.]

Matched set: *See* **matching**.

Matching: The process of making a study group and a comparison group comparable with respect to extraneous factors. Often used in `retrospective studies` when selecting cases and controls to control variation in a response variable due to sources other than those immediately under investigation. Several kinds of matching can be identified, the most common of which is when each case is matched individually with a control subject on the matching variables, such as age, sex or occupation. When the variable on which the matching takes place is continuous, it is usually transformed into a series of categories (e.g., age), but a second method is to say that two values of the variable match if their difference lies between defined limits. This method is known as *caliper matching*. *See also* **paired samples**. [Altman, D. G., 2018, *Practical Statistics for Medical Research*, Chapman & Hall/CRC, Boca Raton, FL.]

Maternal mortality rate: A measure of the risk of dying from causes associated with child birth. Usually measured as

$$\text{maternal mortality rate} = \frac{\text{number of deaths from puerperal causes during a year}}{\text{number of live births in year}}$$

According to the World Health Organization, a maternal death (i.e., one due to puerperal causes) is defined as the death of a woman while pregnant or within 42 days of the termination of pregnancy, irrespective of the duration and site of the pregnancy, from any cause related to or aggravated by the pregnancy or its management, but not from accidental or incidental causes. Some figures for 1990 per 100,000 live births are:

- Bangladesh: 850
- India: 570
- Japan: 18
- Nepal: 1500
- Sri Lanka: 140

[*World Health Statistics Quarterly*, 1996, **49**, 77–87.]

Mathematical model: A description of the assumed structure of a set of observations that can range from a fairly imprecise verbal account to, more usually, a formalized mathematical expression of the process assumed to have generated the observed data. The purpose of such a description is to aid in understanding the data. *See also* **deterministic model**, **logistic regression**, **multiple linear regression** and **generalized linear models**.

Mauchly test: A test that the `variance–covariance matrix` of a set of `multivariate data` is a scalar multiple of the identity matrix, a property known as *sphericity*. Of importance in the analysis of `longitudinal data`. [Field, A. P., 2017, *Discovering Statistics Using SPSS*, 5th ed., Sage Publications, London.]

Maximum life span: The oldest age attainable by a member of the species. For humans, the maximum life span is considered by most experts to be about 115 years.

Maximum likelihood estimation: A method of estimating the parameters in a model by finding the values that maximize the `likelihood` of the model. The procedure is particularly important since it produces estimators with desirable properties such as consistency and asymptotic relative efficiency. [Everitt, B. S. and Palmer, C. (eds.), 2011, *Encyclopedic Companion to Medical Statistics*, 2nd ed., John Wiley & Sons, Chichester.]

Maximum tolerated dose (MTD): The highest possible dose of a drug that can be given with acceptable patient toxicity. This dose is usually determined in a `phase I study` and is the dose recommended for future studies. The standard method employed is a rule-based dose-escalation scheme in which escalation depends on the number of patients at a dose level that have dose-limiting toxicity. *See also* **Fibonacci dose-escalation scheme**. [*Journal of the National Cancer Institute*, 1993, 85, 217–23.]

MCAR: Abbreviation for **missing completely at random**.

MCMC: Abbreviation for **Markov chain Monte Carlo**.

McNemar's test: A test for comparing proportions in data involving paired samples. The `test statistic` is based on the difference between the counts of the number of pairs for which the individual receiving treatment *A* has a positive response and the individual receiving treatment *B* does not, and the number of pairs for which the reverse is the case. [Everitt, B. S., 1992, *The Analysis of Contingency Tables*, 2nd ed., Chapman & Hall/CRC, Boca Raton, FL.]

Mean: A measure of location or central value for a continuous variable given for a sample of observations by the sum of the observations divided by the number of observations (*arithmetic mean*). The usefulness of the mean as a summary statistic depends on the implicit assumption that the observations are distributed approximately symmetrically around a central value. *See also* **expected value**. [Altman, D. G., 2018, *Practical Statistics for Medical Research*, Chapman & Hall/CRC, Boca Raton, FL.]

Mean range plot: A graphical tool useful in selecting a transformation in `time series` analysis. The range is plotted against the mean for each seasonal period, and a suitable transformation is chosen according to the appearance of the plot. If the range appears to be independent of the mean, for example, then no transformation is needed. If the plot displays random scatter about a straight line, then a logarithmic transformation is appropriate.

Mean square contingency coefficient: The square of the `phi-coefficient`.

Mean squared error: The sum of the squared `bias` plus the variance of a parameter estimator. If the estimator is unbiased, then it is the same as the variance. In general, however, reflects both the bias and the precision of the estimator.

Mean square ratio: The ratio of two `mean squares` in an `analysis of variance`. [Altman, D. G., 2018, *Practical Statistics for Medical Research*, Chapman & Hall/ CRC, Boca Raton, FL.]

Mean squares: The name used in the context of `analysis of variance` for estimators of particular variances of interest. For example, in the analysis of a `one-way design`, the *within-groups mean square* estimates the assumed common variance in the k groups (this is often referred to as the *error mean square*). [Altman, D. G., 2018, *Practical Statistics for Medical Research*, Chapman & Hall/CRC, Boca Raton, FL.]

Mean vector: A vector containing the mean values of each variable in a set of `multivariate data`.

Measurement error: Errors in reading, calculating or recording a numerical value. The difference between observed values of a variable recorded under similar conditions and some fixed true value. [Altman, D. G., 2018, *Practical Statistics for Medical Research*, Chapman & Hall/CRC, Boca Raton, FL.]

Measurement scale: The range of possible values that a variable can take. Many different classifications of variable type have been proposed, the most common of which has the following four categories:

- *Nominal:* simply classifies observations into unordered qualitative categories, for example diagnosis, race or country of birth.
- *Ordinal:* a classification into ordered qualitative categories, for example, moderate, mild or severe rating for a certain condition.
- *Interval:* an ordinal scale with the additional property that equal differences between category levels on any part of the scale reflect equal difference in the characteristic being measured, for example temperature in degrees centigrade.
- *Ratio:* an interval scale with the addition of a true zero point, for example temperature in degrees Kelvin.

[*American Statistician*, 1993, **47**, 365–72.]

Median: The value in a set of ranked observations that divides the data into two parts of equal size. When there is an odd number of observations, then the median is the middle value. When there is an even number of observations, then the median is calculated as the mean of the two central values. Provides a measure of location of a sample that is suitable for `asymmetrical distributions` and is also relatively insensitive to the presence of `outliers`. *See also* **mean** and **mode**.

Median effective dose (ED50): A quantity used to characterize the potency of a stimulus. Given by the amount of the stimulus that produces a response in 50% of the cases to which it is applied. [Collet, D., 2002, *Modelling Binary Data*, 2nd ed., Chapman & Hall, London.]

Median lethal dose: Synonym for **lethal dose 50**.

Median survival time: A useful summary of a survival curve. Approximately 50% of the population under study could be expected to survive beyond this value. A more suitable summary statistic for survival times than the mean because of the censoring that occurs in such data. [*Biometrics*, 1982, **38**, 29–41.]

Medical audit: The examination of data collected from routine medical practice with the aim of identifying areas where improvements in efficiency and/or quality might be possible. *See also* **audit trail**.

Medical ethics and statistics: For healthcare professionals to be able to behave ethically, they must be aware of what effects their interventions have on the people they treat. Statistics provide the optimal methods for designing studies to gain knowledge and for making inferences from empirical data. Consequently, doctors need to work with statisticians. [Altman, D. G., 1982, Misuse of Statistics Is Unethical, in Sheila M. Gore and Douglas G. Altman (eds.), *Statistics in Practice*, British Medical Association, London.]

Medicines Control Agency (MCA): An executive agency of the Department of Health in the United Kingdom responsible for the promotion of public health through the regulation of the safety, quality and efficacy of human medicines. [www.gov.uk/ government/organisations/medicines-and-healthcare-products-regulatory-agency]

Medico-legal cases and statistics: Statistical reasoning has an important role in legal cases involving a variety of medical issues, for example, occupational health and safety laws, the safety and efficacy of drugs and medical devices, medical malpractice and exposure to potentially toxic chemicals. [Finkelstein, M. O., 2013, *Statistics for Lawyers*, 2nd ed., Springer-Verlag, New York.]

MEDLINE: Medical Literature Analysis Retrieval System online. Now available on the PubMed database: PubMed.gov.

MedWatch program: A program introduced by the FDA in 1993 to improve the detection of previously unknown serious adverse drug reactions and knowledge about the regulatory action taken in response to these reports. The program involves databases that contain over two million reports of serious adverse reactions. [Gibbons, R. D. and Amatya, A. K., 2016, *Statistical Methods for Drug Safety*, CRC, Boca Raton, FL.]

Mega-trial: Essentially synonymous with **large simple trial**.

Mendelian randomization: A method of using information in genes to examine the causal effect of exposure to some possible disease-causing agent as a method for obtaining unbiased estimates of the effects of the putative causal variable without conducting a randomized clinical trial. [*Statistics in Medicine*, 2008, **27**, 1133–63.]

Mesokurtic: *See* kurtosis.

Meta-analysis: A collection of techniques whereby the results of two or more independent studies are statistically combined to yield an overall answer to a question of interest. Essentially the quantitative component of a `systematic review` of the relevant literature. The rationale behind this approach is to provide a test with more `power` than is provided by the separate studies themselves. Either a `fixed-effects` or `random-effects` model is used in reaching an overall estimate of `effect size`. The procedure has become increasingly popular in the last decade or so, but it is not without its critics, particularly because of the difficulties of knowing which studies should be included and to which population final results actually apply.

See also **forest plot**. [Borestein, M., Hedges, L. V., Higgings, J. P. T. and Rothstein, H. R., 2009, *Introduction to Meta-Analysis*, John Wiley & Sons, New York.]

Meta-analysis: Perhaps the greatest growth area in medical research. Although the combination of the results from the studies selected is often seen as the main objective of a meta-analysis, it may be more sensible and productive to see the approach as giving an opportunity to explore heterogeneity between the studies.

Meta-regression analysis: A procedure for investigating sources of heterogeneity amongst the studies included in a meta-analysis. Techniques such as `logistic regression` or `multiple linear regression` are used to explore the relationship between study characteristics, for example, timing of the intervention, country in which a study was performed etc., and study results, that is, the magnitude of the effect observed in each study. [*Statistics in Medicine*, 2002, **21**, 1559–73.]

MetaWin: Software for `meta-analysis` able to create both `forest plots` and `Funnel plots`. [**www.metawinsoft.com**]

Michaelis–Menten equation: An equation that describes the theoretical relationship between the initial velocity of a simple enzymatically catalyzed reaction and the substrate concentration. [*Biochemical Journal*, 1974, **139**, 715–20.]

Microarrays: A novel technology that facilitates the simultaneous measurement of thousands of gene expression levels. A typical microarray experiment can produce millions of data points, and the statistical task is to efficiently reduce these numbers to simple summaries of the genes' structures. [*Journal of the American Statistical Association*, 2001, **96**, 1151–60.]

Micromaps: Graphics that link statistical information to an organized set of small maps. The aim of such maps is to highlight geographic patterns and associations among the variables in a data set and to use the maps to explore the data. Figures 63 and 64 show two examples. [Carr, D. B. and Williams-Pickles, Linda, 2010, *Visualizing Data Patterns with Micromaps*, Chapman & Hall, Boca Raton, FL.]

Figure 63 NCI State Cancer Profiles web implementation of linked micromaps with added features. Data are age-adjusted rates of mortality due to any type of cancer among white males, 2005.

(Copyright (© 2010) from *Visualizing Data Patterns with Micromaps* by Daniel B. Carr and Linda Williams Pickle. Reproduced by permission of Taylor & Francis Group, LLC, a division of Informa plc.)

Please refer to www.cambridge.org/9781108826464 for colour versions of these images.

Female Lung Cancer Mortality Rates
2000–2004 and Change

Figure 64 Linked micromap plot of average annual female lung cancer mortality rates plus confidence intervals in 2000–4 by state. Rate changes 1995–9 and 2000–4 are shown as arrows, and box plots display the distribution of county rates within each state. (Copyright (© 2010) from *Visualizing Data Patterns with Micromaps* by Daniel B. Carr and Linda Williams Pickle. Reproduced by permission of Taylor & Francis Group, LLC, a division of Informa plc.)

Please refer to www.cambridge.org/9781108826464 for colour versions of these images.

Mid-range: The mean of the smallest and largest values in a sample of observations. Sometimes used as a rough estimate of the mean of a `symmetrical distribution`.

Mid-variance: A `robust estimation` of the variation in a set of observations. Can be viewed as giving the variance of the middle of the distribution of the observations.

Mini mental state examination (MMSE): A test widely used to assess global cognition in older individuals. It consists of a set of questions devised to assess cognitive domains such as memory, language, attention and orientation for time and place. Each of the individual questions scores 1 if correctly answered and 0 if not, and the final score is an integer in the range 0–30. Scores below 10 are indicative of dementia. [*Journal of Psychiatric Research*, 1975, **12**, 189–98.]

Minimization: A method for allocating patients to treatments in `clinical trials`, which is usually an acceptable alternative to random allocation. The procedure ensures balance between the groups to be compared on prognostic variables by allocating with high probability the next patient to enter the trial to whatever treatment would minimize the overall imbalance between the groups on the prognostic variables at that stage of the trial. *See also* **biased coin method** and **block randomization**. [*British Medical Journal*, 1999, **319**, 947–8.]

Minimum therapeutically effective dose: The lower limit of the dose range of a drug product that provides effective and safe treatment for a particular medical complaint, and which is also superior to the response affected by a placebo. [*Statistics in Medicine*, 1995, **14**, 925–32.]

Minnesota multiphasic personality inventory (MMPI): An empirically based test of adult psychopathology designed to assess the major symptoms and signs of social and personal maladjustment commonly indicative of disabling psychological dysfunction. The inventory is used by clinicians in hospitals to assist with diagnosis of mental disorders and the selection of an appropriate method of treatment. [Butcher, J. N. and Williams, C., 2001, *Essentials of MMPI-2 and MMPI-A Interpretation*, University of Minnesota, Minneapolis, MN.]

Misinterpretation of *p*-values: A `p-value` is commonly interpreted in a variety of ways that are incorrect. Most common misinterpretations are that it is the probability of the null hypothesis, and that it is the probability of the data having arisen by chance. And many scientists misinterpret smaller *p*-values as providing stronger evidence against a null hypothesis relative to larger *p*-values. For the correct interpretation, *see* **P-value**. [Everitt, B. S. and Palmer, C., 2011, *Encyclopedic Companion to Medical Statistics*, 2nd ed., John Wiley & Sons, Chichester.]

Missing at random (MAR): *See* **missing values**.

Missing completely at random (MCAR): *See* **missing values**.

Missing values: Observations missing from a set of data for some reason. Such values are of most concern in `longitudinal studies`, where they occur for a variety of reasons, for example because subjects drop out of the study completely or do not appear for one or more scheduled visits, or because of equipment failure. Common causes of subjects prematurely ceasing to participate include recovery, lack of improvement, unwanted signs or symptoms that may be related to the investigational treatment, unpleasant study procedures, and inter-current health problems. Missing values greatly complicate many methods of analysis, and simply dealing with those individuals for whom the data are complete can be unsatisfactory in many situations. Different approaches may be necessary for the analysis of data containing missing values depending on whether they are thought to be *missing completely at random (MCAR), missing at random (MAR)* or *informative*. The MCAR variety arise when individuals drop out of a study in a process that is independent of both the observed measurements and those that would have been available had they not been missing; here, the observed values effectively constitute a `simple random sample` of the values for all study subjects. Random dropout (MAR) occurs when the probability of dropping out depends on the previous response values but given these, it is conditionally independent of all future (unrecorded) values following dropout. Finally, in the case of informative dropout, the dropout mechanism depends on the unobserved values of the outcome variable. *See also* **Diggle–Kenward method for dropouts**, **last observation carried forward**, **attrition** and **imputation**. [Raghunathan, T., 2015, *Missing Data Analysis in Practice*, Chapman & Hall/CRC, Boca Raton, FL.]

Missing values: Clinical researchers need to be aware of the implications for analysis of the different types of missing values, particularly in a longitudinal study.

Misspecification: A term sometimes applied in situations where the wrong model has been assumed for a particular set of observations.

Mixed data: Data containing a mixture of continuous variables, ordinal variables and categorical variables.

Mixed-effects models: A class of regression and `analysis of variance` models that allows the usual assumption that the residual or error terms are independently and identically distributed to be relaxed. Such models can take into account more complicated data structures in a flexible way, by either modelling interdependence directly or by introducing *random effect* terms to induce correlations between the observations made on the same subject, for example. Such models are of particular importance in the analysis of `longitudinal data`. *See also* **conditional regression models**, **marginal models**, **multilevel models** and **random coefficients models**. [Everitt, B. S., 2003, *Modern Medical Statistics*, Arnold, London.]

Mixture experiments: Experiments that consist of varying the proportions of two or more ingredients and studying the change that occurs in the measured response that is assumed to be related functionally to ingredient composition. The controllable variables are proportionate amounts of the mixture in which the proportions are by volume, weight or mole fraction. [Cornell, J. A., 1990, *Experiments with Mixtures*, 2nd ed., John Wiley & Sons, New York.]

MLE: Abbreviation for **maximum likelihood estimation**.

MMPI: Abbreviation for **Minnesota multiphasic personality inventory**.

Mobility table: A table showing the social or occupational status of a sample of people at two different times. [Hout, M., 1983, *Mobility Tables*, Sage Publications, London.]

Mode: The most frequently occurring value in a set of observations. Occasionally used as a measure of location. *See also* **mean** and **median**.

Model: *See* **mathematical model**.

Model building: A procedure that attempts to find the simplest model for a sample of observations that provides an adequate fit to the data. *See also* **parsimony principle**.

Monotonic decreasing: *See* **monotonic sequence**.

Monotonic increasing: *See* **monotonic sequence**.

Monotonic sequence: A sequence of numerical values is said to be *monotonic increasing* if each value is greater than or equal to the previous one, and *monotonic decreasing* if each value is less than or equal to the previous one. *See also* **ranking**.

Monte Carlo methods: Techniques used in situations in which the analytic solution of a problem is either intractable or time consuming. Instead of calculating exact quantities, simulation is used to produce stochastic approximations to the solution. Such techniques are used in a wide range of problems such as the construction of Monte Carlo hypothesis tests, `bootstrap` distributions and for numerical integration in applying `Bayesian methods`. [*Annals of Statistics*, 1979, **7**, 1–26.]

Monthly fecundity rate: The chance of achieving a pregnancy in any given month. Among fertile couples attempting to conceive, it is approximately 20%. Clinical studies of couples having unexplained infertility have severely reduced monthly fecundity of about 2–5%. The appropriateness of any therapy for such couples (e.g. in vitro fertilization) must be judged by its ability to increase the rate above this baseline rate. [*Fertility and Sterility*, 2001, **75**, 656–60.]

Morbidity: A term used in epidemiological studies to describe sickness in human populations. The World Health Organization Expert Committee on Health Statistics noted in its sixth report that morbidity could be measured in terms of three units:

- People who were ill
- The illness (periods or spells of illness) that those people experienced
- The duration of these illnesses

Mortality: A term used in studies in `epidemiology` to describe death in human populations. Statistics on mortality are compiled from the information contained in death certificates. Virtually complete registration and medical certification of death exists for industralized countries, including Eastern Europe and the former USSR. Of the developing regions, medical certification of deaths is most advanced in Latin America and the Caribbean (43% of deaths), and least advanced in sub-Saharan Africa (1% of deaths). [Preston, S. N., 1976, *Mortality Patterns in National Populations*, Academic Press, New York.]

Mortality odds ratio: The ratio of the observed number of deaths from a particular cause to its expected value, based on an assumption of equal mortality rates in the putative and comparison populations. For example, the mortality odds ratio for male liver cancer has been estimated to be 2.57. [*American Journal of Cardiology*, 2002, **89**, 1248–52.]

Mortality rate: Synonym for **death rate**.

Most powerful test: A test of a null hypothesis that has greater power than any other test for a given alternative hypothesis.

Most probable number: *See* **serial dilution assay**.

Mover–stayer model: A generalization of a Markov chain. The basic idea is that there are two populations in the sample: stayers, who always remain in their initial state, and movers, whose transitions between states are governed by a Markov process. The model has been used to study the size and the dynamics of the HIV/AIDS epidemic. [*Biometrics*, 1999, **55**, 1252–7.]

Moving average: A method used primarily for the smoothing of time series, in which each observation is replaced by a weighted average of the observation and its near neighbours. Moving averages are often used to eliminate the seasonal variation or cyclic variation from time series and hence to emphasize the trend terms. *See also* **secular trend**. [Chatfield, C., 2019, *The Analysis of Time Series*, 7th ed., Routledge, London.]

MTD: Abbreviation for **maximum tolerated dose**.

Multi-arm multistage trial (MAMS): A clinical trial that allows the simultaneous assessment of a number of research treatments against a single control. Such trials provide earlier answers and are potentially more cost-effective than a series of traditionally designed trials. Such trials include interim analyses so that experimental treatments can be dropped if they are deemed to be ineffective. These trials are then labelled *MAMS drop-the-losers designs*. [*Statistical Methods in Medical Research*, 2017, **26**, 508–24.]

Multicentre study: A clinical trial conducted simultaneously in a number of participating hospitals or clinics, with all centres following an agreed-upon study protocol and with independent random allocation within each centre. The benefits of such a study include the ability to generalize results to a wider variety of patients and treatment settings than would be possible with a study conducted in a single centre, and the ability to enrol into the study more patients than a single centre could provide. The potential problems with such studies include that they are more complex to plan and to administer, and that it is often difficult to obtain consistency of measurements across centres. [*Controlled Clinical Trials*, 1995, **16**, 4S–29S.]

Multicollinearity: A term used in regression analysis to indicate situations where the explanatory variables are related by a linear function, making the estimation of the regression coefficients impossible. Including the sum of the explanatory variables in the regression analysis would, for example, lead to this problem. Approximate multi-collinearity can also cause problems when estimating regression coefficients. In particular, if the `multiple correlation coefficient` of a particular explanatory variable with the other explanatory variables is high, then the variance of the corresponding regression coefficient will also be high. *See also* **ridge regression**, **tolerance** and **variance inflation factor**. [Rawlings, J. O., Pantula, S. G. and Dickey, D. A., 2001, *Applied Regression Analysis: A Research Tool*, 2nd ed., Springer, New York.]

Multi-episode models: Models for `event history data` in which each individual may undergo more than one transition, for example lengths of spells of unemployment or time period before moving to another region. [*Journal of Nervous Mental Disorders*, 1995, **183**, 320–4.]

Multi-hit model: A model for a toxic response that results from the random occurrence of one or more fundamental biological events. A response is assumed to be induced once the target tissue has been "hit" by a number, k, of biologically effective units of dose within a specified time period. [*Communications in Statistics – Theory and Methods*, 1995, **24**, 2621–33.]

Multilevel models: Models for data that are organized hierarchically. Examples include:

- Children within families
- Patients within centres in a multicentre study
- Repeated measure designs, where measurements are nested within subjects.

Random-effect terms are used in the models to allow for correlations between the nested observations. *See also* **mixed-effects models**. [Goldstein, H., 2010, *Multilevel Statistical Models*, 4th ed., John Wiley & Sons, Chichester.]

Multimode distribution: A `probability distribution` or frequency distribution with several modes. Multimodality is often taken as an indication that the observed distribution results from the mixing of the distributions of relatively distinct groups of observations. An example is shown in Figure 65. *See also* **finite-mixture distribution**.

Multinomial distribution: A generalization of the `binomial distribution` to more than two possible discrete outcomes that describes the joint distribution of frequencies of the outcomes from n independent replications of the experiment.

Multinormal distribution: Synonym for **multivariate normal distribution**.

Multiphasic screening: A process in which tests in `screening studies` may be performed in combination. For example, in cancer screening, two or more anatomical sites may be screened for cancer by tests applied to an individual during a single screening session. [*American Journal of Public Health*, 1964, **54**, 741–50.]

Multiple comparison tests: Procedures for detailed examination of the differences between a set of means, usually after a general hypothesis that they are all equal has been rejected. No single technique is best in all situations, and a major distinction between techniques is how they control the possible inflation of the `type I error`. *See also* **Bonferroni correction**, **Scheffé's test** and **Dunnett's test**.

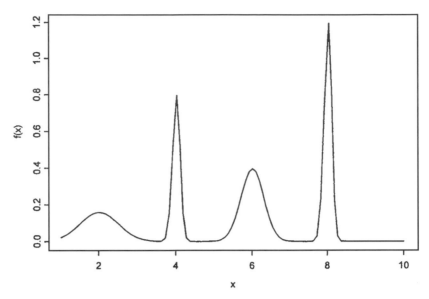

Figure 65 Probability distribution with four modes.

[Fisher, L. D. and Van Belle, G., 2004, *Biostatistics*, 2nd ed., John Wiley & Sons, New York.]

Multiple correlation coefficient: The `correlation coefficient` between the observed values of the dependent variable in a `multiple linear regression` and the values predicted by the estimated regression equation. Often used as an indicator of how useful the explanatory variables are in predicting the response. The square of the multiple correlation coefficient gives the proportion of variance of the response variable that is accounted for by the explanatory variables. *See also* **adjusted R^2**. [Rawlings, J. O., Pantula, S. G. and Dickey, D. A., 2001, *Applied Regression Analysis: A Research Tool*, 2nd ed., Springer, New York.]

Multiple-dose study: A `clinical trial` in which repeated administrations of a treatment are given, in order to examine the steady-state effects of a treatment. [*Chest*, 1980, **78**, 300–3.]

Multiple endpoints: A term used to describe the variety of outcome measures used in many `clinical trials`. Typically, there are multiple ways to measure treatment success, for example length of patient survival, percentage of patients surviving for two years, or percentage of patients experiencing tumour regression. The aim in using a variety of such measures is to gain better overall knowledge of the differences between the treatments being compared. The danger with such an approach is that the performance of multiple significance tests incurs an increased risk of a false positive result. *See also* **Bonferroni correction**. [*Statistics in Medicine*, 1995, **14**, 1163–76.]

Multiple imputation: A popular approach for handling the pervasive problem of `missing values` in medical studies. The method uses the distribution of the observed data to estimate a set of plausible values for the missing data, usually under the assumption that the missing values are missing at random. Extra variation and uncertainty are introduced by producing a small number (say three to five) of sets of missing values. Each 'complete' set of data is then analyzed in whatever way is of interest to the investigator and the results then combined to produce overall inferences, estimates, confidence intervals, etc. [Carpenter, J. and Kenward, M., 2012, *Multiple Imputation and Its Application*, John Wiley & Sons, New York.]

Multiple linear regression: A model for assessing the relationship between a continuous response variable and a set of explanatory variables. Conditional on the values of the explanatory variables, the response variable is assumed to have a `normal distribution` with constant variance. The parameters in the model, the regression coefficients, are usually estimated by `least squares`. The estimated regression coefficient for a particular explanatory variable gives the estimated change in the response variable corresponding to a unit change in the explanatory variable, conditional on the other explanatory variables remaining constant. [Rawlings, J. O., Pantula, S. G. and Dickey, D. A., 2001, *Applied Regression Analysis: A Research Tool*, 2nd ed., Springer, New York.]

Multiple time response data: Data arising in studies of episodic illness, such as bladder cancer and epileptic seizures. In the former, for example, individual patients may suffer multiple bladder tumours at observed times.

Multiplication rule for probabilities: For events *A* and *B* that are independent, the probability that both occur is the product of the separate probabilities. *See also* **addition rule for probabilities**.

Multiplicative model: A model in which the combined effect of a number of factors, when applied together, is the product of their separate effects. `Cox's proportional hazards model` is, for example, a multiplicative model for the `hazard function`. *See also* **additive model**.

Multiplicity in clinical trials: In many `clinical trials` the investigator may consider more than one endpoint. This multiple endpoint raises the issue of multiplicity, which is essentially the making of multiple inferences in simultaneous context. For valid inferences in this context the significance level of each test needs to be appropriately adjusted. [Chow, S.-C., 2018, *Encyclopedia of Biopharmaceutical Statistics*, 4th ed., Chapman & Hall/CRC, FL.]

Mutiple endpoints: *See* **Multiplicity in clinical trials**.

Multistage sampling: Synonym for **cluster sampling**.

Multistate models: Models that arise in the context of the study of `survival times`. The experience of a patient in such a study can be represented as a process that involves two (or more) states. In the simplest situation, at the point of entry to the study, the patient is in a state that corresponds to being alive. Patients then transfer from this 'live' state to the 'dead' state at some rate measured by the `hazard function` at a given time. More complex models will involve more states. For example, a three-state model might have patients alive and tumour-free, patients alive and tumour present, and the 'dead' state. *See also* **Markov illness–death model**. [*Statistics in Medicine*, 1988, **7**, 819–42.]

Multiregional clinical trial: The combination of patients from several countries/regions around the world under the same protocol. Such a clinical trial is seen as a useful means of accelerating the development of new drugs and abridging their approval time. [*Pharmaceutical Statistics*, 2010, **9**, 173–8.]

Multivariable analysis: A generic term for methods designed to determine the relative contributions of different causes to a single event or outcome. Multiple linear regression and logistic regression are two examples; indeed, the term is largely synonymous with regression analysis. Differentiated from multivariate analysis by the involvement of a response variable and a set of explanatory variables, with only the former being strictly considered a random variable. [Katz, M. H., 1999, *Multivariable Analysis*, Cambridge University Press, Cambridge.]

Multivariate analysis: A generic term for the many methods of analysis important in investigating multivariate data. Examples include cluster analysis, principal components analysis and factor analysis. [Everitt, B. S. and Dunn, G., 2010, *Applied Multivariate Data Analysis*, 2nd ed., Wiley, Chichester.]

Multivariate analysis of variance (MANOVA): An extension of analysis of variance procedures to situations involving related multiple measurements. Groups are now compared on all the variables simultaneously. In this multivariate case, no single test statistic can be constructed that is optimal in all situations and, consequently, a number of test statistics are generally quoted. The most commonly used are *Wilk's lambda*, *Roy's largest root*, the *Hotelling–Lawley trace* and the *Pillai–Bartlett trace*. It has been found that the differences in power between the various test statistics are quite small, so in most situations the statistic that is chosen will not affect conclusions greatly. [Bray, J. H. and Maxwell, S. E., 1985, *Multivariate Analysis of Variance*, Sage Publications, London.]

Multivariate data: Data for which each observation consists of values recorded on several variables, for example measurements of blood pressure, temperature, heart rate and gender for a sample of patients. Such data are usually arranged in a matrix with the number of rows equal to the number of observations, and the number of columns equal to the number of variables (*data matrix*); the elements in the rows of this matrix give the variable values for each individual in the sample. [Everitt, B. S. and Dunn, G., 2010, *Applied Multivariate Data Analysis*, 2nd ed., Wiley, Chichester.]

Multivariate distribution: The simultaneous probability distribution of a set of random variables. *See also* **multivariate normal distribution**.

Multivariate growth data: Data arising in studies investigating the relationships in the growth of several organs of an organism and how these relationships evolve. Such data enable biologists to examine growth gradients within an organism and to use these as an aid to understanding its form, function and biological niche, as well as the role of evolution in bringing it to its present form. [*Anatomia Embryologia*, 1992, **186**, 537–41.]

Multivariate normal distribution: An extension of the `normal distribution` to the multivariate situation of a set of correlated variables. The distribution depends on the population mean vector of the variables and their `variance–covariance matrix`. Such distributions are often central to the modelling and analysis of `multivariate data`. *See also* **bivariate normal distribution**. [Evans, M., Hastings, N. and Peacock, B., 2000, *Statistical Distributions*, 3rd ed., John Wiley & Sons, New York.]

Multivariate probit analysis: A method for assessing the effect of explanatory variables on a set of two or more correlated binary response variables. *See also* **probit analysis**. [*Statistics in Medicine*, 1991, **10**, 1391–403.]

Mutation distance: A distance measure for two amino acid sequences, defined as the minimal number of nucleotides that would need to be altered in order for the `gene` of one sequence to code for the other. [Jagers, P., 1975, *Branching Processes with Biological Applications*, John Wiley & Sons, New York.]

Mutation rate: The frequency with which mutations occur per `gene` or per generation.

Mutually exclusive events: See **addition rule for probabilities**.

MYCIN: An `expert system` developed at Stanford University to assist physicians in the diagnosis and treatment of infectious diseases. [Buchanan, B. G. and Shortliffe, E. H., 1985, *Rule-Based Expert Systems*, Addison-Wesley, Reading, MA.]

National Cancer Institute standards for adverse drug reactions: A five-category scale for assessing adverse drug reactions ranging from none (0) to mild (1), moderate (2), severe (3), life-threatening (4) and death (5). Both continuous variables, for example white blood count, and categorical variables, for example nausea, can be converted to this grading scale. [https://ctep.cancer.gov/protocoldevelopment/electronic_applications/docs/CTCAE_v5_Quick_Reference_8.5x11.pdf]

National Center for Health Statistics (NCHS): The principal health statistics agency of the USA, with responsibility for designing and maintaining a variety of general-purpose descriptive health surveys on a continuous basis and disseminating these data for widespread use. [NCHS, 1989, *Vital and Health Statistics*, volume 1, NCHS, Hyattsville, MD.]

National Institute for Health and Clinical Excellence (NICE): A government body responsible for making clinical recommendations and guidelines in practice in the United Kingdom. The recommendations made by this body often provide the basis of National Health Service Policy on what treatments it offers. [**www.nice.org.uk**]

National Institutes of Health (NIH): One of the world's foremost biomedical research centres and the federal focal point for biomedical research in the USA. [*Statistics in Medicine*, 1990, **9**, 903–6.]

Natural history of disease: The course of a disease when left untreated or when treated with the standard therapy. [*Transactions of the Royal Society of Tropical Medicine and Hygiene*, 1958, **52**, 152–68.]

Natural history studies: The use of data, often from hospital databases, to study the typical course of a disease, including the symptoms and patient characteristics that influence prognosis. Such studies help in the development of new treatments and in the design of clinical trials to evaluate them. [*Statistics in Medicine*, 1989, **8**, 1255–68.]

Natural pairing: *See* **paired samples**.

Natural response: A response of a subject or patient that is not due solely to the stimulus to which the individual has been exposed.

Nearest-neighbour clustering: Synonym for **single linkage clustering**.

Necessarily empty cells: Synonym for **structural zeros**.

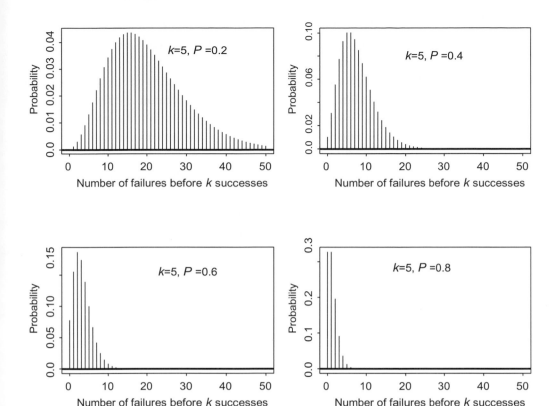

Figure 66 Examples of negative binomial distributions.

Negative binomial distribution: The probability distribution of the number of failures before the *k*th success in a Bernoulli sequence. Often used to model overdispersion in count data. Some examples of the distribution are shown in Figure 66. [Evans, M., Hastings, N. and Peacock, B., 2000, *Statistical Distributions*, 3rd ed., John Wiley & Sons, New York.]

Negative predictive value: The probability that a person having a negative result on a diagnostic test for a particular condition does not have the condition. For example, in a study of a screening tool for alcoholism, the negative predicted value was estimated to be 0.93. Consequently, 7% of patients with a negative result are actually likely to be alcoholic and so misclassified by the test. [*British Medical Journal*, 2001, **323**, 1159.]

Negative skewness: *See* **skewness.**

Negative study: A study that does not yield a statistically significant result.

Negative synergism: *See* **synergism.**

Neighbourhood controls: Synonym for **community controls.**

Neonatal mortality rate: The number of infant deaths in the first 28 days of life in a geographical area during a time period, divided by the number of live births. It is usually expressed per 1,000 live births per year. For example, the rate for mothers aged 16–19 in social class I in the United Kingdom in 1949 was 7.7 per 1,000 live births; in 1975, the corresponding rate was 2.1. [*International Journal of Epidemiology*, 1986, **15**, 188–96.]

Nested case–control study: A commonly used design in `epidemiology` in which a cohort is followed to identify cases of some disease of interest and the controls are selected for each case from within the cohort for comparison of exposures. The primary advantage of this design is that the exposure information needs to be gathered for only a small proportion of the cohort members, thereby considerably reducing the data-collection costs. *See also* **cohort component method**. [*Statistics in Medicine*, 1993, **12**, 1722–46.]

Nested design: A design in which levels of one or more factors are subsampled within one or more other factors so that, for example, each level of a factor *B* occurs at only one level of another factor *A*. Factor *B* is said to be nested within factor *A*. An example might be where interest centres on assessing the effect of hospital and doctor on a response variable, say patient satisfaction, with treatment. The doctors can practise at only one hospital, so they are nested within hospitals. *See also* **multilevel model**. [*Statistics in Medicine*, 1993, **12**, 1733–46.]

Nested model: Synonym for **hierarchical model**.

Net survival: A measure of cancer survival which can be interpreted as the survival that would be observed in a hypothetical situation where all the risks of dying from other causes than cancer have been removed. Net survival is used to compare cancer survivals in populations where the risks of dying from other causes are different, typically for comparisons between different regions or different periods. [*Statistical Methods in Medical Research*, 2020, **29**, 122–36.]

Network: A linked set of computer systems capable of sharing computer power and/or storage facilities. *See also* **Internet** and **electronic mail**.

Network meta-analysis: A method used to extend conventional `meta-analysis` by combining and summarizing direct and indirect evidence on multiple treatments for a given condition when the set of evaluated interventions differs among studies. By borrowing strength from the indirect evidence, there is a potential gain in precision of the estimates. In addition, the estimates may be less biased and more robust. [*Statistics in Medicine*, 1996, **15**, 2733–49.]

Network sampling: A type of sampling in which individuals can be associated with more than one of the types of sampling unit initially chosen by `simple random sampling`. For example, in a survey to estimate the prevalence of a rare disease, a random sample of medical centres might be selected first. From the records of each medical centre in the sample, records of the patients treated for the disease of interest can be extracted. A given patient may have been treated at more than one centre; the more centres from which treatment has been received, the higher the `inclusion probability` for the patient's records. [*AIDS*, 1996, **10**, 657–66.]

Neural networks: *See* **artificial neural network**.

Newman–Keuls test: A `multiple comparison test` used to investigate in more detail the differences between a set of group means indicated by a significant `F-test` in an `analysis of variance`. *See also* **Scheffe's test** and **least significant difference test.** [Altman, D., 2018, *Practical Statistics for Medical Research*, Chapman & Hall/CRC, Boca Raton, FL.]

NICE: Acronym for **National Institute for Health and Clinical Excellence**.

NNH: Abbreviation for **number needed to harm**.

NNT: Abbreviation for **number needed to treat**.

NOAEL: Abbreviation for **no-observed-adverse-effect level**.

NOEL: Abbreviation for **no-observed-effect level**.

N-of-1 trials: Trials in which patients are treated with two or more treatments on multiple occasions, with the objective of using these repeated episodes as a means of drawing controlled inferences about the effect of treatment. Such trials can be viewed as a special case of the `crossover design`. [*Statistical Methods in Medical Research*, 2019, **28**, 372–83.]

Noise: A `stochastic process` of irregular fluctuations. *See also* **white noise sequence**.

Nominal scale: *See* **measurement scale**.

Nominal significance level: The significance level of a test when its assumptions are valid. [*Journal of Pharmocokinetics and Pharmacodynamics*, 2001, **28**, 231–52.]

Nominal variable: Synonym for **categorical variable**.

Nomograms: Graphical methods that permit the representation of more than two quantities on a plane surface. The example shown in Figure 67 is of such a chart for calculating sample size or power. [Altman, D. G., 2018, *Practical Statistics for Medical Research*, Chapman & Hall/CRC, Boca Raton, FL.]

Non-compliance: *See* **protocol violations**.

Non-current cohort study: *See* **cohort study**.

Non-identified response: A term used to denote censored observations in `survival time` data that are not independent of the endpoint of interest. Such observations can occur for a variety of reasons, for example:

- Misclassification of the response, for example death from cancer, the response of interest, being misclassified as death from another unrelated cause
- Response occurrence causing prior censoring, for example relapse to heroin use causing a subject to quit a rehabilitation study to avoid chemical detection. [*Biometrics*, 1994, **50**, 1–10.]

Non-ignorable dropouts: *See* **missing values**.

Non-inferiority and superiority trials: A non-inferiority `clinical trial` is typically conducted to establish that the treatment effect of an experimental is not much worse than that of a 'standard' treatment or an active-control treatment. A superiority clinical trial is one conducted to establish that an experimental treatment is superior to a control treatment. *See also* **equivalence trials**. [*Federal Register*, 1998, **63**, 49583–98.]

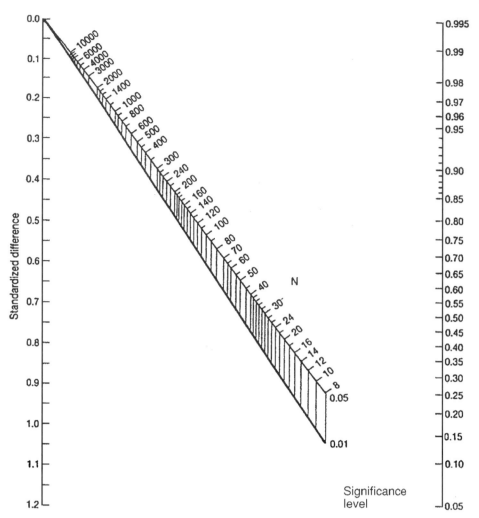

Figure 67 Nomogram for calculating sample size.

Non-informative censoring: Censored observations that can be considered to have the same probabilities of failure at later times as those individuals remaining under observation. The distribution of `survival times` provides no information about the distribution of censoring times and vice versa. [*Journal of the American Statistical Association*, 1988, **83**, 772–9.]

Nonlinear model: A model that is nonlinear in the parameters. Some of these models can be made linear by a suitable transformation. Those that cannot are often referred to as *intrinsically nonlinear*, although these can be approximated by linear equations in some circumstances. [Rawlings, J. O., Pantula, S. G. and Dickey, D. A., 2001, *Applied Regression Analysis: A Research Tool*, 2nd ed., Springer, New York.]

Non-masked study: Synonym for **open-label study**.

Non-orthogonal designs: Used most commonly in respect of `analysis of variance` designs with two or more factors, in which the number of observations in each cell are not equal. In such designs, the total sum of squares can no longer be partitioned into non-overlapping components associated with each main effect and interaction. Consequently, the order in which effects are considered becomes of importance. [Everitt, B. S., 2001, *Statistics for Psychologists*, Lawrence Erlbaum Associates, Mahwah, NJ.]

> **Non-orthogonal designs:** Far more complicated to analyze than their balanced design cousins. Researchers need to keep in mind that there is now an order effect when calculating sums of squares.

Non-parametric methods: *See* **distribution-free methods**.

Non-randomized clinical trials: `Clinical trials` in which new patients are all given the treatment under investigation, and the control group is formed in one of a variety of ways, including:

- `Historical controls`
- Patients from a computerized database
- From articles reported in the literature

In most cases, such trials would be considered greatly inferior to `randomized clinical trials`. [Pocock, S. J., 1985, *Clinical Trials: A Practical Approach*, John Wiley & Sons, New York.]

> **Non-randomized clinical trials:** Always inferior to their randomized cousins and often liable to give misleading and largely optimistic results about new therapies.

Non-response: A term generally used for failure to provide the relevant information being collected in a survey. Poor response can be due to a variety of causes. For example, if the topic of the survey is of an intimate nature, then respondents may not want to answer particular questions. Since it is quite possible that respondents in a survey differ in some of their characteristics from those who do not respond, a large number of non-respondents may introduce `bias` into the final results. To minimize the impact of nonresponse on the survey estimates, auxiliary data from respondents and groups of non-respondents can sometimes be used. *See also* **item non-response**. [*Sociological Methods and Research*, 1991, **20**, 139–81.]

No-observed-adverse-effect level: Greatest concentration or amount of a substance, found by experiment or observation, that causes no detectable adverse alteration of morphology, functional capacity, growth, development, or life span of the target organism under defined conditions of exposure.

No-observed-effect level (NOEL): The dose level of a compound below which there is no evidence of an effect on the response of interest. [*Food and Chemical Toxicology*, 1997, **35**, 349–55.]

No response level: Maximum dose of a substance at which no specified response is observed in a defined population under defined conditions of exposure.

Norm: Used most commonly to refer to what is usual, for example the range into which body temperatures of healthy adults fall, but also occasionally used for what is desirable, for example the range of blood pressures regarded as being indicative of good health.

Normal approximation: A normal distribution with mean np and variance np $(1 - p)$ that acts as an approximation to a binomial distribution as n, the number of trials, increases. The term p represents the probability of a success in any trial. [Altman, D. G., 2018, *Practical Statistics for Medical Research*, Chapman & Hall/CRC, Boca Raton, FL.]

Normal distribution: A probability distribution assumed by many statistical procedures. The distribution is bell-shaped and depends on two parameters, the population mean and the population variance. Several examples are shown in Figure 68. [Evans, M., Hastings, N. and Peacock, B., 2000, *Statistical Distributions*, 3rd ed., John Wiley & Sons, New York.]

Normality: A term used to indicate that some variable of interest has a normal distribution.

Normal range: Synonym for **reference interval**.

Novelty detection: Seeks observations among newly generated test data that are exceptional in some way compared with previously observed data in the same experimental situation. [*Signal Process*, 2014, **99**, 215–49.]

Notoriety bias: The public perception of the safety of a drug.

NS (ns): An abbreviation often used to denote that a result is non-significant at some particular significance level.

NS (ns): Not necessarily the end of the world!

Nuisance parameter: A parameter that is needed to specify a probability distribution, but is not of central importance compared with others. The presence of such parameters can make testing hypotheses about those of more interest difficult, and it is often necessary to find a test statistic that does not depend on them. *See also* **likelihood**. [Altman, D. G., 2018, *Practical Statistics for Medical Research*, Chapman & Hall/CRC, Boca Raton, FL.]

Null distribution: The probability distribution of a test statistic when the null hypothesis is true.

Null hypothesis: The no-difference or no-association hypothesis to be tested (usually by means of a significance test) against an alternative hypothesis that postulates

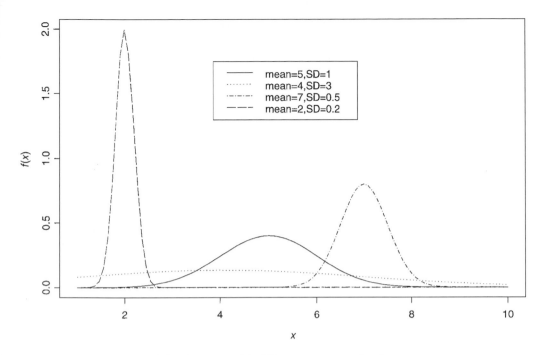

Figure 68 Normal distributions with different means and variances.

non-zero difference or association. [Altman, D. G., 2018, *Practical Statistics for Medical Research*, Chapman & Hall/CRC, Boca Raton, FL.]

Number needed to harm (NNH): *See* **number needed to treat**.

Number needed to treat (NNT): A measure of the impact of a treatment or intervention that is often used to communicate results to patients, clinicians, the public and policymakers. It states how many patients need to be treated in order to prevent an event that would occur otherwise (e.g., a death). Calculated as the inverse of the absolute risk reduction. An NNT can help in making a decision between treatment groups and in making choices for an individual patient. For example, in a study into the effectiveness of intensive diabetes therapy on the development and progression of neuropathy, 9.6% of patients randomized to usual care and 2.8% patients randomized to intensive therapy suffered from neuropathy, leading to an estimate of NNT of 1/6.4%, which rounded up gives the value 15. This means that 15 diabetic patients need to be treated with intensive therapy to prevent one patient from developing neuropathy. The concept of NNT can equally well be applied to harmful outcomes as well as beneficial ones, when instead it becomes *number needed to harm (NNH)*. [*Statistical Methods in Medical Research*, 2020, **29**, 2393–410.]

Number needed to treat: Although considered by many clinicians to be useful in communicating results to patients, NNT does not have such attractive statistical properties as the absolute risk reduction itself, properties that make it more suitable than NNT in analyses.

Numerical taxonomy: In essence, a synonym for **cluster analysis**.

Nuremberg Code: A list of 10 standards for carrying out clinical research involving human subjects, drafted after the trials of Nazi war criminals at Nuremberg. *See also* **Helsinki Declaration**.

Nutritional epidemiology: A branch of epidemiology that seeks to uncover the relationship between aspects of diet and the occurrence of human illness. [*American Journal of Epidemiology*, 1990, **132**, 999–1012.]

Nutritional table method: Procedure for evaluating the dietary intake of a large number of people. For each record of quantity of food consumed during a certain time period, the daily intake of a substance of interest is calculated by multiplying the substance concentration in the food item by the quantity of food consumed and dividing by the time of observation.

Oblique factors: A term used in `factor analysis` for `common factors` that are allowed to be correlated. [Everitt, B. S. and Dunn, G., 2010, *Applied Multivariate Data Analysis*, 2nd ed., Wiley, Chichester.]

O'Brien and Fleming boundaries: A method of `interim analysis` in a `clinical trial` in which very small `p-values` are required for early stopping of a trial, whereas later values for stopping are closer to conventional levels of significance. *See also* **alpha spending function**. [*Statistics in Medicine*, 1994, **13**, 1441–52.]

O'Brien two-sample tests: Extensions of the conventional tests for assessing differences between treatment groups that take account of the possible heterogeneous nature of the response to treatment, and that may be useful in the identification of subgroups of patients for whom the experimental therapy might have most (or least) benefit. [*Biometrics*, 1984, **40**, 1079–89.]

Observational study: A general term for investigations in which the researcher has little or no control over events, and the relationships between risk factors and outcome measures are studied without the intervention of the investigator. Surveys and most studies in `epidemiology` fall into this class. The classic example of such a study is that by Doll and Hill, which uncovered evidence of a causal relationship between smoking and lung cancer. *See also* **experimental study**, **prospective study** and **retrospective study**. [*New England Journal of Medicine*, 1953, **248**, 995–1001.]

Observational data: Data collected in an `observational study`. Such data are increasingly being used for comparative effectiveness research. In observational research, treatment selection is not assigned at random. Consequently, patients receiving a specific treatment or intervention frequently differ systematically from those receiving no treatment or from those receiving a comparator treatment or intervention. The statistical analysis of such data must reduce or minimize the effect of `confounding` if accurate estimates of treatment efficacy or safety are to be obtained. Methods based on the `propensity score` help to minimize the effects of confounding. [Altman, D. G., 2018, *Practical Statistics for Medical Research*, Chapman & Hall/CRC, Boca Raton, FL.]

Occam's razor: William of Occam's fourteenth-century dictum, '*entia non sunt multiplicanda praetor necessitatem*', that is, 'the assumptions introduced to explain a thing must not be multiplied beyond necessity'. In simple terms, 'given two equally predictive theories, choose the simpler'. An early statement of the `parsimony principle`.

Occupational death rates: Mortality rates calculated within occupational categories. For example, in the USA the two most lethal blue-collar jobs are timber cutting/logging (129 deaths per 100,000), and asbestos and insulation jobs (79 deaths per 100,000). For comparison, the two most dangerous white-collar jobs are airline pilots (97 deaths per 100,000) and office helpers/messengers (14 deaths per 100,000). *See also* experimental study, prospective **study** and **retrospective study**. [*Emergency Infectious Diseases*, 2005, **11**, 20–8.]

Occupational epidemiology: A branch of `epidemiology` concerned with the relationship between occupation and human illness and/or death. [Checkoway, H. A., Pearce, N. E. and Crawford-Brown, D. J., 1989, *Research Methods in Occupational Epidemiology*, Oxford University Press, New York.]

Occupational health: Procedures designed to protect the health of employees from harmful consequences arising out of their work. [Weindling, P., 1986, *The Social History of Occupational Health*, Croom Helm, London.]

Occupational risks: The probability of an adverse event, for example injury or illness, occurring as a result of hazards within the workplace. Some examples of safety hazards include the operation of moving parts or vehicles, working with explosive or toxic materials and exposures to asbestos. [Sadhra, S. S. and Rampal, K. G., 1999, *Occupational Health: Risk Assessment and Management*, Blackwell Publishing, Oxford.]

Odd–even technique: *See* **Split-half method**.

Odds: The ratio of the probabilities of the two possible states of a `binary variable`, for example the ratio of the probability of improving to not improving when given a particular treatment. *See also* **odds ratio** and **logistic regression**.

Odds ratio: The ratio of two `odds`, for example the odds of an event for males and the odds of the same event for females. *See also* **logistic regression**. [Everitt, B. S., 1992, *The Analysis of Contingency Tables*, 2nd ed., Chapman & Hall/CRC, Boca Raton, FL.]

Ogive: A graph in which cumulative relative frequency is plotted against the right end point of each class interval of a `frequency distribution table`. Useful for finding `percentiles` or the proportion of the data between two values.

O. J. Simpson paradox: A term arising from a claim made by the defence lawyer in the murder trial of O. J. Simpson. The lawyer stated that the statistics demonstrate that only 1/10th of 1% of men who abuse their wives go on to murder them, with the implication that one or two instances of alleged abuse provides very little evidence that the wife's murder was committed by the abusive husband. The argument simply reflects that most wives are not murdered and has no relevance once a murder has been committed and there is a body. What needs to be considered here is, given that a wife with an abusive partner has been murdered, what is the probability that the murderer is her abuser? It is this `conditional` probability that provides the relevant evidence for the jury to consider, and estimates of the probability range from 0.5 to 0.8. [Senn, S., 2003, *Dicing with Death*, Cambridge University Press, Cambridge.]

Omitted covariates: A term usually found in connection with generalized linear models, where the model has been specified incompletely by not including important covariates. In observational studies, for example, the omission may be due either to an incorrect conceptual understanding of the phenomena under study or to an inability to collect data on all the relevant factors related to the outcome under study. Mis-specifying generalized linear models in this way can result in seriously biased estimates of the effects of the covariates actually included in the model. [*Statistics in Medicine*, 1992, **11**, 1195–208.]

One-hit model: *See* multi-hit model.

One: *m* (1 : *m*) matching: A form of matching often used when control subjects are obtained more readily than cases. A number, $m(m > 1)$, of controls are attached to each case, these being known as the *matched set*. The theoretical efficiency of such matching in estimating, for example, relative risk is $m/(m + 1)$, so one control per case is 50% efficient, while four per case is 80% efficient. Increasing the number of controls beyond 5 to 10 brings rapidly diminishing returns. [*Biometrics*, 1969, **22**, 339–55.]

One-sided test: A significance test for which the alternative hypothesis is directional, for example that one population mean is greater than another. The choice between a one-sided and a two-sided test must be made before any test statistic is calculated. *See also* **critical region**. [Altman, D. G., 2018, *Practical Statistics for Medical Research*, Chapman & Hall/CRC, Boca Raton, FL.]

One-tailed test: Synonym for **one-sided test**.

One-way design: *See* **analysis of variance**.

Open-label trial: A clinical trial in which patient, investigator and peripheral staff are all aware of what treatment the patient is receiving. Most trials comparing different surgical interventions or comparing medication with surgery are of this type. [*International Journal of Geriatric Psychiatry*, 2002, **17**, 343–6.]

Open population: *See* **closed and open populations**.

Operational research: Research concerned with applying scientific methods to the problems facing executive and administrative authorities. [Hillier, F. S. and Luberman, G. J., 1967, *Introduction to Operations Research*, Holden-Day, San Francisco, CA.]

Opinion survey: A procedure that aims to ascertain opinions possessed by members of some population with regard to particular topics. A famous example is the Kinsey Report on sexual behaviour. *See also* **sample survey**. [*Trends in Neurosciences*, 2002, **25**, 166–7.]

Optimal treatment assignment: Treatment assignment based on individual covariate information for a patient and geared towards the 'best' outcome for a patient based on his/her genetic and genomic markers. [*Nature*, 2008, **452**, 564–70.]

Optimization methods: Procedures for finding the maxima or minima of functions of, generally, several variables. Most often encountered in statistics in the context of `maximum likelihood estimation`, where such methods are frequently needed to find the values of the parameters that maximize the `likelihood`. [Everitt, B. S., 1987, *An Introduction to Optimization Methods and Their Application in Statistics*, Chapman & Hall/CRC, Boca Raton, FL.]

Option-3 scheme: A scheme of measurement used in situations investigating possible changes over time in `longitudinal data`. The scheme is designed to prevent measurement `outliers` causing an unexpected increase in falsely claiming that a change in the data has occurred. Two measurements are taken initially and, if they are closer than a specified threshold, the average of the two is considered to be an estimate of the true mean, otherwise a third measurement is made, and the mean of the closest pair is considered to be the estimate. [*Statistics in Medicine*, 1998, **17**, 2607–15.]

Ordered alternative hypothesis: A hypothesis that specifies an order for a set of parameters of interest as an alternative to their equality, rather than simply that they are not all equal. For example, in an evaluation of the treatment effect of a drug at several different doses, it might be thought reasonable to postulate that the response variable shows either a `monotonic increasing` effect or a `monotonic decreasing` effect with dose. *See also* **umbrella hypothesis**. [*Statistics in Medicine*, 1994, **13**, 1583–96.]

Order statistics: Particular values in a ranked set of observations. The *r*th largest value in a sample, for example, is called the *r*th order statistic. Such statistics are used widely as the basis of estimators and assessment of fit. [David, H. A. and Nagaraja, H. N., 2003, *Order Statistics*, 3rd ed., John Wiley & Sons, New York.]

Ordinal scale: *See* **measurement scale**.

Ordination: The process of reducing the dimensionality of `multivariate data` by deriving a small number of new variables that contain much of the information in the original data. The reduced data set is often more useful for investigating possible structure in the observations. A commonly used technique here is `principal components analysis`. [Spencer, N. H., 2017, *Essential of Multivariate Analysis*, Chapman & Hall/CRC Press, Boca Raton, FL.]

Orthogonal: A term that occurs in several areas of statistics with different meanings in each case. Most commonly encountered in relation to two variables or two linear functions of a set of variables to indicate statistical independence. Literally means at right angles. *See also* **non-orthogonal designs**. [Altman, D. G., 2018, *Practical Statistics for Medical Research*, Chapman & Hall/CRC, Boca Raton, FL.]

Outcome variable: Synonym for **response variable**.

Outlier: An observation that appears to deviate markedly from the other members of the sample in which it occurs. In the set of systolic blood pressures, {125, 128, 130, 131, 198}, for example, 198 might be considered an outlier. Such extreme observations may be reflecting some abnormality in the measured characteristic of a patient, or they may result from an error in the measurement or recording. It is important to examine data for the presence of such observations, because in some cases a single undetected outlier can invalidate an entire analysis. [Barnett, V. and Lewis, T., 1994, *Outliers in Statistical Data*, John Wiley & Sons, Chichester.]

Outside observation: An observation that fall outside the limits defined by the lower `quartile` of the data minus 1.5 times the `interquartile` range and the upper quartile plus 1.5 times the interquartile range. Such observations are often regarded as potential `outliers`.

Overdispersion: A term used to describe the situation in which the empirical variance in a set of data exceeds the nominal variance under some presumed model. Observed most often in the analysis of discrete data, for example proportions under a `binomial distribution` assumption, or counts under a `Poisson distribution` assumption. Often the result of a lack of independence amongst the observations. For example, if the response variable is the proportion of family members who have been ill in the past year observed in a large number of families, then the individual binary observations that make up the observed proportions are likely to be correlated rather than independent. *See also* **extrabinomial variation** and **clustered data**. [Collett, D., 2003, *Modelling Binary Data*, 2nd ed., Chapman & Hall/CRC, Boca Raton, FL.]

Overfitted models: Models that contain more unknown parameters than can be justified by the data. [*Statistics in Medicine*, 1996, **15**, 361–87.]

Overidentified model: *See* **identification**.

Overmatching: A term applied to studies involving `matching` when the matching variable is related strongly to exposure but not to disease risk. Such a situation leads to a loss of efficiency. [*European Journal of Obstetrics, Gynecology and Reproductive Biology*, 1996, **69**, 73–5.]

Overview: Synonym for **systematic review**.

Paired availability design: A design that can reduce `selection bias` in situations where it is not possible to use random allocation of subjects to treatments. The design has three fundamental characteristics:
- The intervention is the availability of treatment, not its receipt.
- The population from which subjects arise is well defined with little in- or out-migration.
- The study involves many pairs of control and experimental groups.

In the experimental groups, the new treatment is made available to all subjects, although some may not receive it. In the control groups, the experimental treatment is generally not available to subjects, although some may receive it in special circumstances. [*Statistics in Medicine*, 1994, **13**, 2269–78.]

Paired Bernoulli data: Data arising when an investigator records whether a particular characteristic is present or absent at two sites on the same individual, for example the presence or absence of spots on the legs and arms. [*Biometrics*, 1988, **44**, 253–7.]

Paired samples: Two samples of observations with the characteristic feature that each observation in one sample has one and only one matching observation in the other sample. There are several ways in which such samples can arise in medical investigations. The first, *self-pairing*, occurs when each subject serves as his or her own control, as in, for example, therapeutic trials in which each subject receives both treatments, one on each of two separate occasions. Next, *natural pairing* can arise, particularly, for example, in laboratory experiments involving littermate controls. Lastly, *artificial pairing* may be used by an investigator to match the two subjects in a pair on important characteristics likely to be related to the response variable. *See also* **matched pairs *t*-test**. [Agresti, A., 2019, *An Introduction to Categorical Data Analysis*, Wiley-Blackwell, Oxford.]

Paired samples *t*-test: Synonym for **matched pairs *t*-test**.

Pandemic: An `epidemic` occurring over a very wide area and usually affecting a large proportion of the population. The spread of AIDS is a current example, and the influenza pandemic of 1918, which killed between 20 and 40 million people is a historical example. The coronavirus example is perhaps of more immediate concern. [*Statistics in Medicine*, 2021, **30**, In press.]

Panel study: A study in which a group of people, the panel, are interviewed or surveyed with respect to some topic of interest on more than one occasion. Essentially equivalent to a `longitudinal study`, although there may be many response variables observed at each time point. [Hsiao, C., 2015, *Analysis of Panel Data*, 3rd ed., Cambridge University Press, Cambridge.]

Parallel-dose design: *See* **dose-ranging trial**.

Parallel groups design: A simple experimental setup in which two different groups of patients, for example treated and untreated, are studied concurrently.

Parallel-line bioassay: A procedure for estimating equipotent doses of a standard and test preparation. [Finney, D. J., 1978, *Statistical Methods in Biological Assay*, 3rd ed., Arnold, London.]

Parameter: A numerical characteristic of a population or a model, for example the probability of a success in a `binomial distribution`, or the mean of a `normal distribution`. [Altman, D. G., 2018, *Practical Statistics for Medical Research*, Chapman & Hall/CRC, Boca Raton, FL.]

Parametric hypothesis: A hypothesis concerning the parameter(s) of a distribution. For example, the hypothesis that the mean of a population equals the mean of a second population, when the populations are each assumed to have a `normal distribution`. [Altman, D. G., 2018, *Practical Statistics for Medical Research*, Chapman & Hall/CRC, Boca Raton, FL.]

Parametric methods: Procedures for testing hypotheses about parameters in a population described by a specified distributional form, often a `normal distribution`. `Student's t-test` is an example of such a method. *See also* **distribution-free methods**. [Altman, D. G., 2018, *Practical Statistics for Medical Research*, Chapman & Hall/CRC, Boca Raton, FL.]

Parsimony principle: The general principle that amongst competing models, all of which provide an adequate fit for a set of data, the one with the fewest parameters is to be preferred. *See also* **Occam's razor**.

Partial correlation: The correlation between a pair of variables after adjusting for the effect of a third. Can be calculated from the sample `correlation coefficients` of each of the three pairs of variables. An example would be the calculation of a measure of the correlation between coronary heart disease and drinking coffee, after controlling for smoking behaviour. [Altman, D. G., 2018, *Practical Statistics for Medical Research*, Chapman & Hall/CRC, Boca Raton, FL.]

Partial questionnaire design: A procedure used in studies in `epidemiology` as an alternative to a lengthy questionnaire, which can result in lower rates of participation by potential study subjects. Information about the exposure of interest is obtained from all subjects, but information about secondary variables is determined for only a fraction of study subjects. [*Statistics in Medicine*, 1994, **13**, 623–34.]

Partner studies: Studies involving pairs of individuals living together. Such studies are often particularly useful for estimating the `transmission probabilities` of infectious diseases, and the effects of measured covariates on these probabilities.

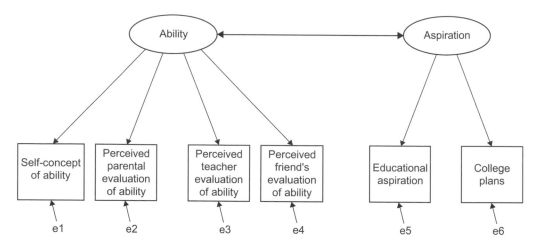

Figure 69 Path diagram for a correlated two-factor model.

Used widely for studying transmission of sexually transmitted diseases such as HIV. [*Annals of Epidemiology*, 1990, **1**, 117–28.]

Passenger variable: A term used occasionally for a variable, *A*, that is associated with another variable, *B*, only because of their separate relationship to a third variable, *C*. For example, coffee drinking is associated with increased coronary heart disease (CHD) only through the former's association with smoking and the well-known relationship of the latter to CHD. *See also* **partial correlation**.

Passing–Bulbok regression: A non-parametric linear regression procedure with no special assumptions regarding the distribution of the samples and the measurement errors. The approach is claimed to be less sensitive to outliers than its parametric counterparts. [*Journal of Clinical Chemistry and Clinical Biochemistry*, 1983, **21**, 709–20.]

Path analysis: A tool for evaluating the interrelationships among variables by analyzing their correlational structure. The relationships between the variables are often illustrated graphically by means of a *path diagram*, in which single-headed arrows indicate the direct influence of one variable on another, and curved, double-headed arrows indicate correlated variables. An example of a path diagram that depicts a simple confirmatory factor analysis model is shown in Figure 69. Originally introduced for simple regression models for observed variables, the method has now become the basis for more sophisticated procedures such as structural equation modelling involving both manifest variables and latent variables. [Sarwono, J., 2017, *Path Analysis: Data Analysis Application*, Independently published.]

Path diagram: *See* **path analysis**.

Patient-reported outcome (PRO): Any report of the status of a patient's health condition that comes directly from the patient without interpretation of the patient's response by a clinician or anyone else. Such PROs are often relevant in studying a variety of conditions, for example, pain, erectile dysfunction, fatigue, physical functioning and depression. [*Statistical Methods in Medical Research*, 2014, **23**, 398–408.]

Patient time: A term sometimes used for the period of time a patient spends in a study.

Pattern recognition: A technology that recognizes and analyzes patterns automatically by machine. *See also* **artificial intelligence** and **artificial neural network**. [Gregory, R. L., 1987, *The Oxford Companion to the Mind*, Oxford University Press, Oxford.]

Peak value: Synonymous with C_{max}.

Pearl rate: The standard method for comparison of effectiveness of contraceptive methods, given by the number of pregnancies that occur for each contraceptive method if used by 100 women for 1 year. Some recent figures are as follows:

- None (young women): 80–90
- None (age 45): 10–20
- Male condom: 2–15
- Rhythm methods: 6–25
- Diaphragm: 4–20
- Combined pill: 0.1–3

The range of values given reflects that failures are more likely in younger women, who may be more fertile and more sexually active. *See also* **discontinuation rate**. [*International Journal of Gynaecology and Obstetrics*, 1983, **21**, 139–44.]

Pearson's chi-squared statistic: *See* **chi-squared test**.

Pearson's product moment correlation coefficient: *See* **correlation coefficient**.

Pearson's residual: The difference between the observed frequency in a cell of a contingency table and the estimated expected value under independence, divided by the square root of the expected value. Such residuals have, if independence holds, an approximate normal distribution; consequently, values outside the range -2 to 2 suggest cells that do not satisfy independence. [Everitt, B. S., 1992, *The Analysis of Contingency Tables*, 2nd ed., Chapman & Hall/CRC, Boca Raton, FL.]

Penetrance function: The relationship between a phenotype and the genotype at a locus. For a categorically defined disease trait, it specifies the probability of disease for each genotype class. [Sham, P., 1998, *Statistics in Human Genetics*, Arnold, London.]

Percentile: The set of divisions that produce exactly 100 equal parts in a series of continuous values, such as blood pressure, weight, height, etc. Thus, a person with blood pressure above the 80th percentile has a greater blood pressure than 80% of the other recorded values. [Altman, D. G., 2018, *Practical Statistics for Medical Research*, Chapman & Hall/CRC, Boca Raton, FL.]

Per-comparison error rate: The significance level at which each test or comparison is carried out in an experiment. *See also* **per-experiment error rate** [Fisher, L. D. and Van Belle, G., 1993, *Biostatistics*, John Wiley & Sons, New York.]

Per-experiment error rate: The probability of rejecting at least one null hypothesis in an experiment involving one or more tests or comparisons, when the corresponding null hypothesis is true in each case. *See also* **per-comparison error rate**. [Fisher, L. D. and Van Belle, G., 1993, *Biostatistics*, John Wiley & Sons, New York.]

Perinatal mortality rate: The number of fetal and infant deaths between 28 weeks gestation and 1 week postnatal divided by the number of live births in a year. For example, in Texas in 1989, the rate was 11.8 per 1,000 live births; in 1994, the corresponding figure was 9.7. The major contributor to perinatal death, besides lethal malformations, is low birth weight. [*International Journal of Obstetrics and Gynaecology*, 2001, **108**, 1237–45.]

Periodic survey: Synonym for **panel study**.

Period prevalence: *See* **prevalence**.

Permutation tests: Synonym for **randomization test**.

Per protocol: A term used to describe a subset of participants in a randomized clinical trial who complied with the protocol. Also used to describe an analysis based on these patients. [*British Medical Journal*, 1996, **313**, 36–9.]

Personalised medicine: Synonym for **precision medicine**.

Personal probability: A radically different approach to allocating probabilities to events than, for example, the commonly used long-term relative frequency approach.

Now probability is taken to represent a degree of belief in a proposition, based on all the relevant information. Two people with different information and different subjective ignorance may therefore assign different probabilities to the same proposition. The only constraint is that a single person's probabilities should not be inconsistent. [*British Journal of General Practice*, 2001, **51**, 276–9.]

Personal risk model: A model that assigns to a patient a probability of developing an adverse outcome within some clinically relevant time period, based on the values taken by the patient for a number of covariates of interest. Examples include models for breast cancer development within 5 years, and prostate cancer within 10 years of diagnosis. [*Cancer*, 2008, **113**, 3075–99.]

Person-time: A term used in epidemiology for the total observation time added over subjects. [*Statistics in Medicine*, 1989, **8**, 525–38.]

Person-time incidence rate: A measure of the incidence of an event in some population given by the ratio of the number of events occurring during the interval to the number of person-time units observed during the interval.

Person-year: *See* **person-years at risk**.

Person-years at risk: Units of measurement that combine people and time by summing individual units of time (years and fractions of years) during which subjects in the study population have been exposed to the risk of the outcome under study.
A *person-year* is the equivalent of the experience of one individual for one year. [Rothman, K. J. and Greenland, S., 1998, *Modern Epidemiology*, 2nd ed., Lippincott-Raven Publishers, Philadelphia, PA.]

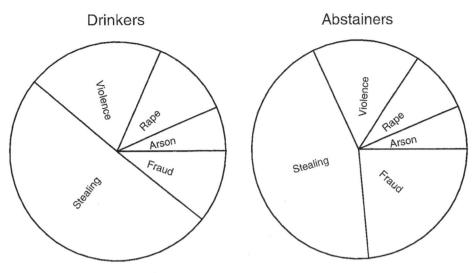

Figure 70 Examples of pie charts.

Person-years of life lost: For a particular cause of death, the difference between the expectation of life of the population and the expectation of life with the cause in question eliminated. [*International Journal of Cancer*, 1976, **17**, 429–35.]

Perspective plot: *See* **contour plot**.

Phase I study: *See* **clinical trial**.

Phase II study: *See* **clinical trial**.

Phase III study: *See* **clinical trial**.

Phase IV study: *See* **clinical trial**.

Phenotype: *See* **genotype**.

Phenotypic assortment: *See* **assortative mating**.

Phi-coefficient: A measure of the association of the two variables forming a `two-by-two` `contingency` `table` and given by the square root of the usual `chi-squared` `test` value after division by the sample size. [Everitt, B. S., 1992, *The Analysis of Contingency Tables*, 2nd ed., Chapman & Hall/CRC, Boca Raton, FL.]

Pickles charts: Day-by-day plots of new cases of infectious diseases according to their dates of onset. Used to demonstrate the progress of an epidemic in a relatively isolated population.

Pie chart: A widely used graphical technique for presenting the distributions associated with the observed values of a categorical variable. The chart consists of a circle subdivided into sectors whose sizes are proportional to the quantities (usually percentages) they represent. An example is given in Figure 70, which shows crime rates for drinkers and abstainers. *See also* **bar chart** and **dot plot**. [Everitt, B. S., 2001, *Statistics for Psychologists*, Lawrence Erlbaum Associates, Mahwah, NJ.]

Pillai–Bartlett trace: *See* **multivariate analysis of variance**.

Pill count: A count of the tablets taken by a patient in a `clinical trial` that is often used as a measure of `compliance`. The method is far from foolproof, and even when a subject returns the appropriate number of leftover pills at a scheduled visit, the question of whether the remaining pills were used accordingly remains largely unanswered. There is considerable evidence that the method can be unreliable and potentially misleading. [*Journal of Clinical Oncology*, 1993, **11**, 1189–97.]

Pilot study: A small-scale investigation designed either to test the feasibility of methods and procedures for later use on a large scale, or to search for possible effects and associations that may be worth following up in a subsequent larger study. [*Statistical Methods in Medical Research*, 2016, **25**, 1022–38.]

Pilot survey: A small-scale investigation carried out before the main survey, primarily to gain information and to identify problems relevant to the survey proper.

Pilot testing: An early phase in the development of a measuring instrument where the instrument is tested in a small sample of patients to assess the comprehensibility, relevance, acceptability and feasibility of the measurement instrument. [*Quality of Life Research*, 2003, **12**, 229–38.]

Pixel: A contraction of 'picture element'. The smallest element of a graphical display.

Placebo: The word *placebo*, literally 'I will please', has been defined as an inert substance given for its psychological effect to satisfy the patient. But nowadays the term is usually used for a treatment designed to appear exactly like a comparison treatment, but that is devoid of the active component. [Altman, D. G., 2018, *Practical Statistics for Medical Research*, Chapman & Hall/CRC, Boca Raton, FL.]

Placebo effect: A well-known phenomenon in medicine in which patients given only inert substances often show subsequent clinical improvement when compared with patients not so 'treated'. Often defined explicitly as the nonspecific effects of treatment attributable to factors other than the active drug, including physician attention, patient expectation, changes in behaviour, etc. It is the placebo effect that clinicians are relying on when, for example, prescribing antibiotics for a viral infection and indeed contributes to almost every therapeutic success. The placebo effect is a complex phenomenon which is still little understood. Such effects may also occur as a result of `regression to the mean`. [Shapiro, A. K. and Shapiro, E., 1997, *The Powerful Placebo: From Ancient Priest to Modern Physician*, Johns Hopkins University Press, Baltimore, MD.]

Placebo reactor: A term sometimes used for those patients receiving a placebo in a `clinical trial` who report side effects normally associated with the active treatment and sometimes used simply for an individual who gets benefit from placebos. Some people are more prone to influence than others and these differences may relate to the recipient's personality. [*Journal of Laboratory Medicine*, 1957, **49**, 837–41.]

Placebo run-in: A period before a `clinical trial` proper begins and during which all patients receive placebo. [Senn, S., 2008, *Statistical Issues in Drug Development*, 2nd ed., John Wiley & Sons, Chichester.]

Planned comparisons: Comparisons between a set of means suggested before data are collected. Usually more powerful than a general test for mean differences. *See also* **multiple comparison tests** and **post hoc comparisons**. [Everitt, B. S., 2001, *Statistics for Psychologists*, Lawrence Erlbaum Associates, Mahwah, NJ.]

Platykurtic: *See* **kurtosis**.

Play-the-winner rule: A data-dependent treatment-allocation rule sometimes used in `clinical trials` in which the response to treatment is either positive (a success) or negative (a failure). One of the two treatments is selected at random and used on the first patient; thereafter, the same treatment is used on the next patient whenever the response of the previously treated patient is positive, and the other treatment is used whenever the response is negative. The goal of using such a design is to place more study patients into the more successful treatment group, but still to gather reliable information about the treatment effects for the benefit of future patients. Such a rule is generally regarded as reasonable if a number of conditions hold, for example, that the therapies have been evaluated previously for toxicity, that sample sizes are moderate (at least 50 subjects), and the experimental therapy is expected to have significant benefits to public health if it proves effective. *See also* **two-armed bandit allocation**. [*Controlled Clinical Trials*, 1999, **20**, 328–42.]

PMR: Abbreviation for **proportionate mortality ratio**.

Point-biserial correlation: A special case of `Pearson's product moment correlation coefficient` used when one variable is continuous and the other is a binary variable representing a natural dichotomy. *See also* **biserial correlation coefficient**. [Altman, D. G., 2018, *Practical Statistics for Medical Research*, Chapman & Hall/CRC, Boca Raton, FL.]

Point estimate: *See* **estimate**.

Point prevalence: *See* **prevalence**.

Poisson distribution: A limiting form of the `binomial distribution` when the probability of the event is small but also important in its own right for the distribution of events taking place in time or space. Used in many areas of medical research to model data that arise in the form of counts. The shape of the

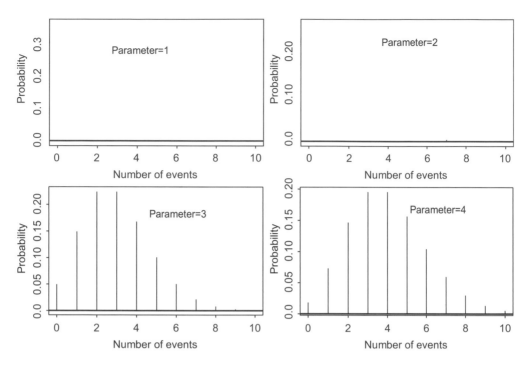

Figure 71 Examples of Poisson distributions.

distribution depends on its single parameter, the mean of the distribution. For a variable having the Poisson distribution, the mean and the variance are equal. Some examples of Poisson distributions are given in Figure 71. [Evans, M., Hastings, N. and Peacock, B., 2000, *Statistical Distributions*, 3rd ed., John Wiley & Sons, New York.]

Poisson regression: A method of regression appropriate for modelling the relationship between a response variable having a `Poisson distribution` and a set of explanatory variables. *See also* **generalized linear model**. [Clayton, D. and Hills, M., 2013, *Statistical Models in Epidemiology*, 3rd ed., Oxford University Press, Oxford.]

Politz–Simmons technique: A method for dealing with the not-at-home problem in household-interview surveys. The results are weighted in accordance with the proportion of days the respondent is ordinarily at home at the time he or she was interviewed. More weight is given to respondents who are seldom at home, who represent a group with a high nonresponse rate. [Cochran, W. G., 1977, *Sampling Techniques*, 3rd ed., John Wiley & Sons, New York.]

Polychotomous variables: Strictly, variables that can take more than two possible values. However, since this would include all but `binary variables`, the term is used conventionally for categorical variables with more than two categories, for example blood group. [Altman, D. G., 2018, *Practical Statistics for Medical Research*, Chapman & Hall/CRC, Boca Raton, FL.]

Polynomial regression: A linear model that includes powers of explanatory variables and also possible cross-products of these variables. [Altman, D. G., 2018, *Practical Statistics for Medical Research*, Chapman & Hall/CRC, Boca Raton, FL.]

Population: In statistics, this term is used for any finite or infinite collection of units, which are often people, but may be, for example, institutions, events, etc. *See also* **sample** and **target population**. [Altman, D. G., 2018, *Practical Statistics for Medical Research*, Chapman & Hall/CRC, Boca Raton, FL.]

Population-averaged models: Synonym for **marginal models**.

Population genetics: A discipline concerned with the analysis of factors affecting the genetic composition of a population. Centrally involved with evolutionary questions through the change in genetic composition of a population over time. [Sham, P., 1998, *Statistics in Human Genetics*, Arnold, London.]

Population growth model: Mathematical models for forecasting the growth of human populations. [*Demography*, 1971, **8**, 71–80.]

Population pyramid: A diagram designed to show the comparison of a human population by sex and age at a given time, consisting of a pair of histograms, one for each sex, laid on their sides with a common base. The diagram is intended to provide a quick overall comparison of the age and sex structure of the population. A population whose pyramid has a broad base and narrow apex has high fertility. Changing shape over time reflects the changing composition of the population associated with changes in fertility and mortality at each age. The example given in Figure 72 shows such diagrams for two countries with very different age/sex compositions. [*Human Biology*, 1994, **66**, 105–20.]

Positive predictive value: The probability that a person having a positive result on a diagnostic test for a particular condition actually has the condition. For example, in a study of a screening tool for alcoholism, the positive predictive value was estimated to be 0.85. Consequently, 15% of patients diagnosed by the test as suffering from alcoholism will be misclassified.

Positive skewness: *See* **skewness**.

Positive synergism: *See* **synergism**.

Posterior distributions: Probability distributions that summarize information about a random variable or parameter after having obtained new information from empirical data. Used almost entirely within the context of Bayesian methods. *See also* **prior distributions**.

Posterior probability: *See* **Bayes's theorem**.

Post hoc comparisons: Analyses not planned explicitly at the start of a study but suggested by an examination of the data. *See also* **multiple comparison tests**, **subgroup analysis** and **planned comparisons**. [Altman, D. G., 2018, *Practical Statistics for Medical Research*, Chapman & Hall/CRC, Boca Raton, FL.]

Post-licensure medical product safely surveillance: A process for detecting adverse events potentially not identified in pre-licensure studies which often lack

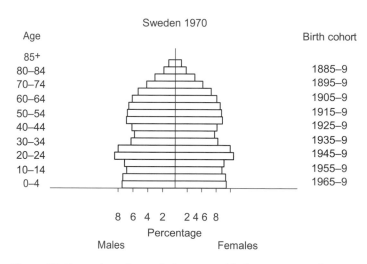

Figure 72 Examples of population pyramids for two countries.

power for rare outcomes and provide little information about longer-term effects. [*Statistical Methods in Medical Research*, 2015, **24**, 177–93.]

Post-mortem interval (PMI): Accurate estimation of the PMI is of obvious importance in the resolution of an investigation involving a corpse. The most common approach involves studying factors, such as temperature of various parts of the body, which vary with PMI. [*Journal of Forensic Science*, 1976, **7**, 56–81.]

Post-neonatal mortality rate: The number of infant deaths between the 29th day and the end of the first year of life, divided by the number of live births in the same time period. Usually expressed per 1,000 live births per year. For example, in the Republic of Ireland in 1995, the rate was 1.7 per 1,000 live births. [*Pediatrics*, 2005, **115**, 1247–53.]

Post-stratification: The classification of a simple random sample of individuals into strata after selection. In contrast to a conventional `stratified random sampling`, the stratum sizes are random variables. [*Statistician*, 1991, **40**, 315–23.]

Pothoff test: A conservative test for the equality of the locations of two distributions when the underlying distributions differ in shape. [*Biometrika*, 1966, **53**, 1183–90.]

Potthoff and Whitlinghill's test: A test of the existence of `disease clusters`. *See also* **clustering**. [*Biometrika*, 1966, **40**, 1183–90.]

Power: The probability of rejecting the null hypothesis when it is false. Power gives a method of discriminating between competing tests of the same hypothesis, the test with the higher power being preferred. It is also the basis of procedures for estimating the sample size needed to detect an effect of a particular magnitude, particularly in designing `clinical trials`. Realistic estimates of the minimally important effect of the intervention are required if trials are to be adequately powered. Similar considerations apply to estimating the likely loss to follow-up rate. [Altman, D. G., 2018, *Practical Statistics for Medical Research*, Chapman & Hall/CRC, Boca Raton, FL.]

Power: Beware of enthusiasm for a new disease prevention or health education programme leading to overestimating the likely effect of the estimation since the consequence may be a trial of the intervention that is underpowered.

Pragmatic analysis: *See* **explanatory analysis**.

Pragmatic trials: `Clinical trials` designed not only to determine whether a treatment works, but also to describe all the consequences of its use, good or bad, under circumstances as close as possible to clinical practice. Such trials use more lax criteria for inclusion than `explanatory trials`, and also tend to use active controls rather than placebo controls; they also involve more flexible treatment regimens. [*Health Policy*, 2001, **57**, 225–34.]

Precision: A term applied to the likely spread of estimates of a parameter in a statistical model. Measured by the standard error of the estimator, this can be decreased, and hence precision increased, by using a larger sample size. *See also* **accuracy**.

Precision medicine: This is an approach to patient care that allows doctors to select treatments that are most likely to help patients based on individual variability in genes, environment and lifestyle. In this way the method has the potential to provide significant benefits to patients and alter the way healthcare is delivered. [*Journal of the American Medical Association*, 2015, **313**, 2119–20.]

Prediction interval: The range of the predicted true treatment effect in a new study, given the realized (past) studies. [*Journal of the Royal Statistical Society, Series A*, 2009, **172**, 137–59.]

Predictor variables: Synonym for **explanatory variables**.

Prentice criterion: A procedure for assessing the validity of a `surrogate endpoint` in a `clinical trial`, that is, to determine whether the test based on the surrogate measure is a valid test of the hypothesis of interest about the true endpoint. [*Statistics in Medicine*, 1989, **8**, 431–40.]

Prescription sequence analysis: A procedure that uses pharmacy-based prescription drug histories to detect a subset of drug effects, those that are themselves indications for changes in the prescribing of another drug. Such an analysis can take only a few days and may be helpful in resolving certain of the controversies that often arise about adverse drug reactions. [*Statistics in Medicine*, 1988, **7**, 1171–5.]

Prevalence: The number of people who have a disease or condition at a given point in time in a defined population (*point prevalence*), or the total number of people known to have had the condition at any time during a specified period (*period prevalence*). The following are the HIV percentage prevalence rates for young people (age 15–24 years) in various countries:

- Ghana: females 2.4, males 0.8
- Kenya: females 11.1, males 4.3
- Thailand: females 1.5, males 0.5

See also **incidence rate**. [Altman, D. G., 2018, *Practical Statistics for Medical Research*, Chapman & Hall/CRC, Boca Raton, FL.]

Prevalence rate: The proportion of individuals with a disease or condition, that is, the `prevalence` divided by the number in the population at risk of having the disease.

Prevalent case: A subject with a given disease or condition who is alive in a defined population at a given time.

Preventable fraction: A measure that can be used to attribute protection against disease directly to an intervention. The measure is given by the proportion of disease that would have occurred had the intervention not been present in the population. *See also* **attributable risk**. [*American Journal of Epidemiology*, 1974, **99**, 325–32.]

Prevention trials: `Clinical trials` designed to test treatments preventing the onset of disease in healthy subjects. An early example of such a trial was that involving various whooping-cough vaccines in the 1940s. [*Controlled Clinical Trials*, 1990, **11**, 129–46.]

Principal components analysis: A procedure for analyzing `multivariate data`, which transforms the original variables into new variables that are uncorrelated and account for decreasing proportions of the variance in the data. The new variables, the principal components, are defined as linear functions of the original variables. The aim of the method is to reduce the dimensionality of the data. If the first few principal components account for a large percentage of the variance of the observations (say, above 70%), then they can be used both to simplify subsequent analyses and to display and summarize the data in a parsimonious manner. *See also* **factor analysis**. [Jolliffe, I. T., 2002, *Principal Components Analysis*, 2nd ed., Springer, New York.]

Principle of equipoise: For a clinician to have no ethical dilemmas with regard to taking part in a `clinical trial`, he or she must be truly uncertain about which of the trial interventions is superior at the start of the trial. [Everitt, B. S. and Wessely, S., 2008, *Clinical Trials in Psychiatry*, 2nd ed., John Wiley & Sons, Chichester.]

Prior distributions: `Probability distributions` that summarize information about a random variable or parameter known or assumed at a given time point before obtaining further information from empirical data. Used almost entirely within the context of `Bayesian methods`. In any particular study, a variety of such distributions may be assumed. For example, *reference priors* represent minimal prior information. *Clinical priors* are used to formalize opinion of well-informed specific individuals, often those taking part in the trial themselves. Finally, *sceptical priors* are used when large treatment differences are considered unlikely. *See also* **posterior distributions**.

> **Prior distributions:** An essential component of the increasingly popular Bayesian inference, and one that makes every Bayesian's approach to a problem potentially unique. But questions such as 'What will happen if the chosen prior is wrong?' and 'If I were a medical control agency, to what extent would I trust the chosen prior?' continue to make some people uneasy about the wider acceptance of this form of inference.

Probability: The quantitative expression of the chance that an event will occur. Can be defined in a variety of ways, of which the most common is still that involving long-term relative frequency:

$$P(A) = \frac{\text{number of times } A \text{ occurs}}{\text{number of times } A \text{ could occur}}$$

For example, if out of 100,000 children born in a region 51,000 are boys, then the probability of a boy is taken to be 0.51. *See also* **addition rule for probabilities**, **multiplication rule for probabilities** and **personal probability**. [Altman, D. G., 2018, *Practical Statistics for Medical Research*, Chapman & Hall/CRC, Boca Raton, FL.]

Probability density: *See* **probability distribution**.

Probability distribution: For a discrete random variable, a mathematical formula that gives the probability of each value of the variable. See, for example, `binomial distribution` and `Poisson distribution`. For a continuous random variable, a curve described by a mathematical formula that specifies, by way of areas under the curve, the probability that the variable falls within a particular interval. Examples include the `normal distribution` and the `exponential distribution`. In both cases, the term 'probability density' is also used.

(A distinction is sometimes made between density and distribution, when the latter is reserved for the probability that the random variable falls below some value.

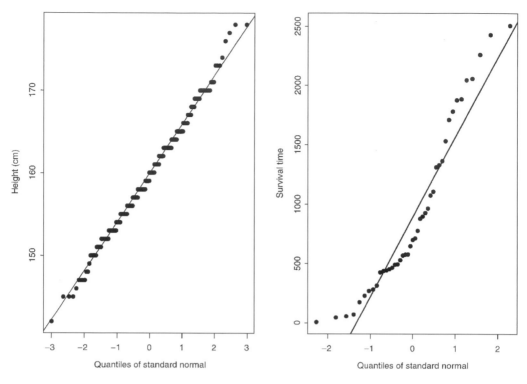

Figure 73 Examples of probability plots.

This distinction is not made in this book; here, `probability distribution` and probability density are used interchangeably.) [Altman, D. G., 2018, *Practical Statistics for Medical Research*, Chapman & Hall/CRC, Boca Raton, FL.]

Probability-of-being-in-response function: A method for assessing the response experience of a group of patients by using a function of time, $P(t)$, that represents the probability of being in response at time t. The purpose of such a function is to synthesize the different summary statistics commonly used to represent responses that are `binary variables`, namely the proportion who respond and the average duration of response. The aim is to have a function that will highlight the distinction between a treatment that produces a high response rate but generally with short-lived responses, and another that produces a low response rate but with longer response durations. [*Biometrics*, 1982, **38**, 59–66.]

Probability plot: A plot for assessing the distributional characteristics of a sample of observations, most often to see if the data have a `normal distribution`. The ordered sample values are plotted against the quantiles of a standard normal distribution; if the plot is roughly linear, then the data are accepted as being distributed normally. Figure 73 shows two such plots, the first for some data on heights and the second for some survival times. The first plot indicates that the data are probably normal, but the second suggests a degree of non-normality. [Everitt,

B. S. and Rabe-Hesketh, S., 2001, *The Analysis of Medical Data using S-PLUS*, Springer, New York.]

Probability sample: A sample obtained by a method in which every individual in a finite population has a known (but not necessarily equal) chance of being included in the sample.

Proband: The clinically affected family member through whom attention is first drawn to a pedigree of particular interest to human genetics. [Sham, P., 1998, *Statistics in Human Genetics*, Arnold, London.]

Probit analysis: A technique employed most commonly in bioassay, particularly toxicological experiments where sets of animals are subjected to known levels of a toxin, and a model is required to relate the proportion surviving at a particular dose to the dose. In this type of analysis, the probit transformation of a proportion is modelled as a linear function of the dose or, more commonly, the logarithm of the dose. Estimates of the parameters in the model are found by maximum likelihood estimation. [Collett, D., 2003, *Modelling Binary Data*, 2nd ed., Chapman & Hall/CRC, Boca Raton, FL.]

Probit transformation: A transformation of a proportion given by five plus the normal quantile corresponding to the proportion. The '5' in the equation was introduced by Sir Ronald Fisher to prevent the transformation leading to negative values, which the biologists of the day were unhappy with. The basis of probit analysis. [Collett, D., 2003, *Modelling Binary Data*, 2nd ed., Chapman & Hall/CRC, Boca Raton, FL.]

Product limit estimator: A procedure for estimating the survival function for a set of survival times, some of which may be subject to censoring. The idea behind the procedure is that of the product of a number of conditional probabilities, so that, for example, the probability of a patient surviving 2 days after a liver transplant can be calculated as the probability of surviving 1 day multiplied by the probability of surviving the second day given that the patient survived the first day. An example of two survival curves estimated in this way is shown in Figure 74. [Collett, D., 2015, *Modelling Survival Data in Medical Research*, 3rd ed., Chapman & Hall/CRC, Boca Raton, FL.]

Profiling: The process of comparing the quality of care or the use of medical services and cost with established standards. Often used to provide a comparison of institutions or procedures used, or as a comparison of quality assurance and improvement programmes. [*Statistical Science*, 2007, **22**, 206–26.]

Prognostic scoring system: A method of combining the prognostic information contained in a number of risk factors in a way that best predicts each patient's risk of disease. In many cases, a linear function of scores is used, with the weights being derived from, for example, a logistic regression. An example of such a system, developed in the British Regional Heart Study for predicting men aged 40–59 years to be at risk of ischaemic heart disease (IHD) over the next five years, is as follows:

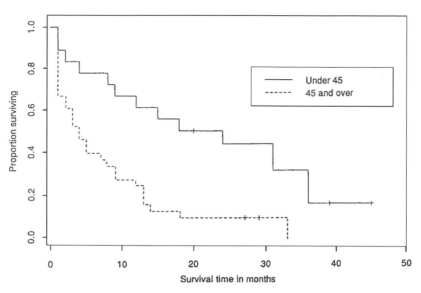

Figure 74 Survival curves estimated by product-limit estimator for two age groups.

51 × total serum cholesterol (mmol/l)

+ 5 × total time man has smoked (years)

+ 3 × systolic blood pressure (mm Hg)

+ 100 if man has symptoms of angina

+ 170 if man can recall diagnosis of IHD

+ 50 if either parent died of heart trouble

+ 95 if man is diabetic

[*Intensive Care Medicine*, 2002, **28**, 341–51.]

Prognostic survival model: A quantification of the survival prognosis of patients based on information at the start of follow-up. [*Statistics in Medicine*, 2000, **19**, 3401–15.]

Prognostic variables: In medical investigations, a synonym often used for **explanatory variables**.

Programming: The act of planning and producing a set of instructions to solve a problem by computer. *See also* **algorithm**.

Progressively censored data: Censored observations that occur in `clinical trials` where the period of the study is fixed and patients enter the study at different times during that period. Since the entry times are not simultaneous, the censored times are also different. *See also* **singly censored data**. [*Journal of Computational and Applied Mathematics*, 2018, **343**, 719–36.]

Projection: The numerical outcome of a specific set of assumptions regarding future trends. *See also* **forecast**.

Proof of concept trials: `Clinical trials` carried out to determine if a treatment is biologically active or inactive. [*Statistics in Medicine*, 2005, **24**, 1815–35.]

Propensity score: Randomized clinical trials are considered the gold standard for assessing the safety and efficacy of treatments and interventions. But they are not always feasible for ethical or practical reasons; for example, randomizing an intervention that may be harmful, cigarette smoking perhaps, or simply taking too long and being too expensive to provide evidence about a treatment of interest within a reasonable time frame. Consequently, observational data are increasingly used to estimate the effect of treatments, exposures and interventions, despite the oft quoted disadvantage of the possibility of systematic differences in baseline characteristics between treated and control subjects with the probable result that any observed differences in outcomes may not be due to treatment but simply reflect systematic differences in subject characteristics between treatment groups. Consequently, in order to obtain an unbiased estimate of the effect of treatment in an observational study a variety of statistical methods might be used. The most common is the use of the propensity score which is the probability of treatment selection conditional on observed baseline characteristics. Conditioning on the propensity score allows an experimenter to mimic the characteristics of the randomized clinical trial. Details of how the propensity score is used can be found in the reference for this entry. [*Multivariate Behavioral Research*, 2011, **46**, 399–424.]

Prophylactic trials: Synonym for **prevention trials**.

Proportional allocation: In stratified random sampling, the allocation of portions of the total sample to the individual strata, so that the sizes of these subsamples are proportional to the sizes of the corresponding strata.

Proportional hazards model: Synonym for **Cox's proportional hazards model**.

Proportional odds model: A model for investigating the dependence of an ordinal response variable on a set of explanatory variables. [*American Journal of Epidemiology*, 1989, **129**, 191–204.]

Proportionate mortality ratio (PMR): An index that may be used for comparing mortality rates for different diseases in different areas or regions of a country, or in different time periods. Calculated as the number of deaths assigned to the disease in a certain year divided by the total number of deaths in the year. For example, white males aged 20–24 years in the USA have a PMR due to motor vehicle accidents of 40%; the corresponding figure for white males aged 50–54 is 2.7%. [Morton, R. F., Hebel, J. R. and McCarter, R. J., 1990, *A Study Guide to Epidemiology and Biostatistics*, 3rd ed., Aspen, Gaithersburg, MD.]

Prosecutor's fallacy: A common error in the interpretation of evidence in which the probability of the evidence given the hypothesis, and the probability of the hypothesis given the evidence are interchanged. For example, there is often confusion in the media over crime reports where what is often stated is the probability of a DNA profile found at the scene of a crime, given that a suspect is innocent when of far more relevance (particularly for the suspect) is the probability that the suspect is innocent given the observed DNA match. *See also* **conditional probability**. [Everitt, B. S., 2008, *Chance Rules*, 2nd ed., Springer, New York.]

> **Prosecutor's fallacy:** Beware of jumping to conclusions when tabloid headlines about some gruesome murder or other talk about the one in a million chance for an observed DNA match with the obvious implication that the suspect who matches the profile, is guilty.

Prospective study: Study in which individuals are followed up over a period of time. A common example of this type of investigation is where samples of individuals exposed and not exposed to a possible risk factor for a particular disease are followed forward in time to determine what happens to them with respect to the illness under investigation. At the end of a suitable time period, a comparison of the incidence rate of the disease among the exposed and nonexposed is made. A classic example of such a study is that undertaken among British doctors in the 1950s to investigate the relationship between smoking and death from lung cancer. *See also* **retrospective study** and **cohort study**. [Morton, R. F., Hebel, J. R. and McCarter, R. J., 1990, *A Study Guide to Epidemiology and Biostatistics*, 3rd ed., Aspen, Gaithersburg, MD.]

Protective efficacy of a vaccine: The proportion of cases of disease prevented by the vaccine. For example, if the rate of the disease is 100 per 10,000 in a non-vaccinated group but only 30 per 10,000 in a comparable vaccinated group, then the protective efficacy is 70%. Essentially equivalent to attributable risk. [*Vaccine*, 2001, **20**, 853–7.]

Protocol: A formal document outlining the proposed procedures for carrying out a clinical trial. The main features of the document are study objectives, patient selection criteria, treatment schedules, methods of patient evaluation, trial design, procedures for dealing with protocol violations, and plans for statistical analysis. [Piantadosi, S., 1997, *Clinical Trials: A Methodological Perspective*, John Wiley & Sons, New York.]

Protocol violations: Patients who either deliberately or accidentally have not followed one or other aspect of the protocol for carrying out a clinical trial. For example, they may not have taken their prescribed medication. Such patients are said to show *non-compliance*.

Protopathic bias: A type of bias (also known as *reverse-causality*) that is a consequence of the differential misclassification of exposure related to the timing of occurrence.

Occurs when a change in exposure taking place in the time period following disease occurrence is incorrectly thought to precede disease occurrence. For example, a finding that alcohol has a protective effect for clinical gallstone disease might be explained by a reduction in alcohol use because of symptoms related to gallstone disease. [*Biological Psychiatry*, 1997, **41**, 257–8.]

Proximity measures: Measures that characterize the similarity or dissimilarity between the objects, items, stimuli or persons that are the basis of an empirical study. A variety of such measures exist. [Everitt, B. S. and Rabe-Hesketh, S., 1997, *The Analysis of Proximity Data*, Arnold, London.]

Psychiatric epidemiology: The study of the causes and consequences of mental illness.

Publication bias: The possible bias in published accounts of, for example, clinical trials, produced by editors of journals being more likely to accept a paper if a statistically significant effect has been demonstrated. A potential problem for systematic reviews. *See also* **funnel plot**. [Petitti, D. B., 1994, *Meta-Analysis, Decision Analysis and Cost-Effectiveness Analysis: Methods for Quantitative Synthesis in Medicine*, Oxford University Press, New York.]

Public Health Surveillance: Synonymous with **syndromic surveillance**.

Pulse data: A series of measurements of the concentration of a hormone or other blood constituent in blood samples taken from a single organism at regular time intervals. *See also* **episodic hormone data**.

P-value: The probability of the observed data (or data showing a more extreme departure from the null hypothesis) when the null hypothesis is true. When judging the size of an obtained p-value it has to be remembered that extremely small values might arise simply because of a large sample size and a large observed p-value may simply be due to a very small sample size. *See also* **misinterpretation of p-values**, **significance test** and **significance level**. [Altman, D. G., 2018, *Practical Statistics for Medical Research*, Chapman & Hall/CRC, Boca Raton, FL.]

> **P-value:** Researchers should avoid despair on finding a P-value of 0.051 and equally restrain from joy on finding a value of 0.049. P-values without accompanying confidence intervals are like Wise without Morecambe or Frasier without Nyles.

Q

QOL: Acronym for **quality of life**.

Quality-adjusted life-years (QALY): An adjustment of `life expectancy` that reduces the overall expectancy by amounts that reflect the existence of chronic conditions causing impairment, disability and handicap as assessed from health survey data. Useful in economic analyses as a measure of health outcomes that reflects both lives saved and patient's valuation of quality of life in alternative states. [*Quality of Life Research*, 2002, **11**, 37–45.]

Quality-adjusted survival analysis: A methodology for evaluating the effects of treatment and other covariates on `survival times` that allows consideration of both quality and quantity of life. [*Annals of Hematology*, 2005, **84**, 47–55.]

Quality-adjusted survival times: The weighted sum of different time episodes making up a patient's `survival time`, with the weights reflecting the quality of life of each period. [*Statistics in Medicine*, 1993, **12**, 975–88.]

Quality assurance: Any procedure or method for collecting, processing or analyzing data that is aimed at maintaining or improving the reliability or validity of the data.

Quality control procedures: Statistical procedures designed to ensure that the precision and accuracy of, for example, a laboratory test are maintained within acceptable limits. The simplest such procedure involves a chart (usually called a *control chart*) with three horizontal lines, one drawn at the target level of the relevant *control statistic*, and the others, called *action lines*, drawn at some pre-specified distance above and below the target level. The process is judged to be at an *acceptable quality level* as long as the observed control statistic lies between the two lines, and to be at a *rejectable quality level* if either of these lines is crossed. [Wadsworth, H. M. and Godfrey, A. B., 1986, *Modern Methods of Quality Control and Improvement*, John Wiley & Sons, New York.]

Quality-of-life (QOL) assessment: QOL is generally measured by means of a global physician's assessment or more generally by a broad range of items describing a patient's subjective reactions to perceptions of his or her environment. For a QOL instrument, the questions asked may be assessed by the patients themselves or by, for example, their spouses, nurses or social workers. Based on the collected data the health-related QOL is quantified. The measure is important for measuring the impact of disease, treatment, health and social policies. [Fairclough, D. L., 2010,

Design and Analysis of Quality of Life Studies in Clinical Trials, 2nd ed., CRC, Boca Raton FL.]

Quantal assay: An experiment in which groups of subjects are exposed to different doses of, usually, a drug to which a particular number respond. Data from such assays are often analyzed using the `probit transformation`, and interest generally centres on estimating the `median effective dose` or `lethal dose 50`. [Morgan, B. J. T., 1988, *Analysis of Quantal Response Data*, Chapman & Hall/CRC, Boca Raton, FL.]

Quantal variable: Synonym for **binary variable**.

Quantiles: Divisions of a `probability distribution` or frequency distribution into equal, ordered subgroups, for example `quartiles` or `percentiles`. [Altman, D. G., 2018, *Practical Statistics for Medical Research*, Chapman & Hall/CRC, Boca Raton, FL.]

Quantile regression: Situations frequently occur in medical studies where the use of `multiple linear regression` to examine the relationship between a continuous response variable and a set of explanatory variables does not answer the questions of most interest. For example, looking at how birth weight of babies relates to other variables of interest using multiple linear regression does not help because of most interest is the relationship between the lower `quantiles` of the response variable and the explanatory variables. Quantile regression provides a relevant model for such situations. [Furno, M. and Vistocco, D., 2018, *Quantile Regression*, John Wiley & Sons, Chichester.]

Quantitative health risk assessment: A tool for making predictions about the impact of substances in the environment on health. *See also* **comparative risk assessment**. [*Journal of Community Health*, 1989, **14**, 169–86.]

Quartiles: The values that divide a frequency distribution or `probability distribution` into four equal parts. [Altman, D. G., 2018, *Practical Statistics for Medical Research*, Chapman & Hall/CRC, Boca Raton, FL.]

Quasi-experiment: A term used for studies that resemble experiments but are weak on some of the characteristics, particularly if manipulation of subjects to groups is not under the investigator's control. For example, if interest centred on the health effects of a natural disaster, then those who experience the disaster can be compared with those who do not, but subjects cannot be deliberately assigned (randomly or not) to the two groups. *See also* **prospective study**, **experimental design** and **clinical trials**. [Campbell, D. T. and Stanley, J. C., 1963, *Experimental and Quasi-Experimental Designs for Research*, Houghton Mifflin, Boston, MA.]

Quasi-independence: A form of independence for a `contingency table`, conditional on restricting attention to only a particular part of the table. For example, in the following table showing the social classes of sons and their fathers, it might be of interest to assess whether once a son has moved out of his father's class, his destination class is independent of that of his father. This would entail testing whether independence holds in the table after ignoring the entries in the main diagonal. [Agresti, A., 2019, *An Introduction to Categorical Data Analysis*, 3rd ed., Wiley-Blackwell, Oxford.]

Father's social class	Son's social class		
	Upper	Middle	Lower
Upper	588	395	159
Middle	349	741	447
Lower	114	320	411

Quasi-likelihood: A function that is used as the basis for the estimation of parameters where it is not possible (and/or desirable) to make a particular distributional assumption about the observations, with the consequence that it is not possible to write down their likelihood. The function depends on the assumed relationship between the mean and the variance of the observations. Used when applying generalized linear models for overdispersion. [*Biometrika*, 1974, **61**, 439–47.]

Quantitative imaging: The extraction of quantifiable features from medical images for the assessment of normal or the severity, degree of change or status of a disease, injury, or chronic condition relative to normal. [*Statistical Methods in Medical Research*, 2015, **24**, 3–8.]

Quetelet's index: Synonymous with **body weight index (BMI).**

Queuing theory: A largely mathematical theory concerned with the study of various factors relating to queues such as the distribution of arrivals, the average time spent in the queue and so on. Used, for example, in medical investigations of waiting times for hospital beds. [Cooper, R. B., 1981, *Introduction to Queuing Theory*, North Holland, New York.]

Quick and dirty methods: A term once applied to many distribution-free methods, presumably to highlight their general ease of computation and their imagined inferiority to the corresponding parametric procedure.

Quintiles: The set of four variate values that divide a frequency distribution or a probability distribution into five equal parts.

Quitting ill-effect: A problem that occurs most often in studies of smoker cessation where smokers frequently quit smoking following the onset of disease symptoms or the diagnosis of a life-threatening disease, thereby creating an anomalous rise in, for example, lung cancer risk following smoking cessation relative to continuing smoking. Such an increase has been reported in many studies. [*Tobacco Control*, 2005, **14**, 99–105.]

Quorum: A group concerned with improving the quality of meta-analyses carried out in medicine. *See also* **CONSORT statement**. [*Lancet*, 1999, **354**, 1896–9.]

Quota sample: A sample in which the units are not selected completely at random but in terms of a certain number of units in each of a number of categories, for example, 10 men over age 40, or 25 women between ages 30 and 35. Used widely in opinion polls. *See also* **sample survey** and **random sample**. [Barnett, V. D., 1974, *Elements of Sampling Theory*, English Universities Press, London.]

Radical Statistics Group: A national network of social scientists in the United Kingdom committed to a critique of statistics as used in the policymaking process. The group attempts to build the competence of critical citizens in areas such as health and education. [Radical Statistics, 27/2, Hillside Crescent, Edinburgh.]

Radioimmunoassay: An assay performed in clinical and biomedical research laboratories to estimate the concentration of an antigen in a biological specimen. [*Clinical Chemistry*, 1977, **23**, 1624–7.]

Random: Governed by chance. Not determined completely by other factors. Non-deterministic.

Random allocation: A method for forming treatment and control groups, particularly in the context of a `clinical trial`. Subjects receive the active treatment or placebo on the basis of the outcome of a chance event, for example tossing a coin. The method provides an impartial procedure for allocation of treatments to individuals, free from personal biases, and ensures a firm footing for the application of significance tests and most of the rest of the statistical methodology likely to be used. Additionally, the method distributes the effects of covariates, both observed and unobserved, in a statistically acceptable fashion. *See also* **block randomization**, **minimization** and **biased coin method**. [Everitt, B. S. and Pickles, A., 2004, *Statistical Aspects of the Design and Analysis of Clinical Trials*, revised ed., Imperial College Press, London.]

Random allocation: One of Fisher's many contributions to scientific investigations.

Random coefficients models: A particular type of `mixed-effects model` for analyzing `longitudinal data`, in which random intercepts and possibly random slopes for each subject are included, to allow for different patterns in the `variance-covariance matrix` of the repeated measurements. *See also* **multilevel models**. [Brown, H. and Prescott, R., 2015, *Applied Mixed Models in Medicine*, 3rd ed., John Wiley & Sons, Chichester.]

Random digit dialling: A method of sampling households through the selection of telephone numbers by a random choice of the digits in the telephone numbers.

Initially developed as a sampling method for household surveys but now also used widely in epidemiological research for selecting controls in some case-control studies. [*American Journal of Epidemiology*, 1984, **120**, 825–33.]

Random effects: *See* **mixed-effects models**.

Random error: The amount by which the systematic part of a measurement differs from the true value of the quantity being measured.

Random events: Events that do not have deterministic regularity (e.g., the emission of a particle by a radioactive source) but do possess some degree of statistical regularity (such radioactive emissions may, for example, follow a Poisson distribution). [Altman, D. G., 2018, *Practical Statistics for Medical Research*, Chapman & Hall/CRC, Boca Raton, FL.]

Random forests: A non-parametric method for regression, classification and survival analysis which is particularly suitable for exploratory analysis with nonlinear influence on the response variable, in the presence of higher-order interactions and for high-dimensional data. [*Machine Learning*, 2001, **45**, 5–32.]

Randomization tests: Procedures for determining statistical significance directly from data, without recourse to some particular sampling distribution. For example, in a study involving the comparison of two groups, the data would be divided (permuted) repeatedly between treatments, and for each division (permutation) the relevant test statistic (e.g. a Student's t-test or F-test) calculated to determine the proportion of the data permutations that provide as large a test statistic as that associated with the observed data. If that proportion is smaller than some chosen significance level a, then the results are significant at the a level. [Edgington, E. S. and Onghena, P., 2007, *Randomization Tests*, 4th ed., Chapman & Hall, Boca Raton, FL.]

Randomized block design (RBD): An experimental design in which the treatments in each block are assigned to the experimental units in random order.

Randomized clinical trial (RCT): A clinical trial that involves formation of treatment groups by the process of random allocation. [Everitt, B. S. and Wessely, S., 2008, *Clinical Trials in Psychiatry*, 2nd ed., Wiley-Blackwell, Oxford.]

Randomized consent design: A design originally introduced to overcome some of the perceived ethical problems facing clinicians entering patients in randomized clinical trials. After the patient's eligibility is established, the patient is randomized to one of two treatments, *A* or *B* . Patients randomized to *A* are approached for patient consent. They are asked whether they are willing to receive therapy *A* for their illness. All potential risks, benefits and treatment options are discussed. If the patient agrees, then treatment *A* is given. If not, the patient receives treatment *B* or some other alternative treatment. Those patients assigned randomly to group *B* are similarly asked about treatment *B*, and transferred to an alternative treatment if consent is not given. *See also* **Zelen's single-consent design**. [*New England Journal of Medicine*, 1970, **300**, 1242–5.]

Randomized response technique: A procedure for collecting information on sensitive issues by means of a survey, in which an element of chance is introduced as to what question a respondent has to answer. In a survey about abortion, for example, a woman might be posed both the questions 'Have you had an abortion?' and 'Have you never had an abortion?', and instructed to respond to one or the other depending on the outcome of a randomized device under her control. The response is now not revealing since no one except the respondent is aware of which question has been answered. Nevertheless, the data obtained can be used to estimate quantities here, for example the proportion of women who have had an abortion, if the probability of selecting the question 'Have you had an abortion?' is known and is not equal to 0.5. [Chaudhuri, A. and Mukerjee, R., 1988, *Randomized Response Theory and Techniques*, Marcel Dekker, New York.]

Randomized stepped-wedge designs: Designs used to evaluate interventions targeting continuous outcomes measured at a number of fixed time points. At the start all patients are untreated and then randomly chosen patients switch to an intervention group at sequential time points until all patients are receiving the intervention. [*Journal of Clinical Epidemiology*, 2011, **64**, 936–48.]

Random model: A model containing random or probabilistic elements. *See also* **deterministic model**.

Random sample: Either a set of *n* independent and identically distributed random variables, or a sample of *n* individuals selected from a population in such a way that each sample of the same size is equally likely. [Everitt, B. S. and Palmer, C. (eds.), 2011, *Encyclopedic Companion to Medical Statistics*, John Wiley & Sons, Chichester.]

Random variable: A variable of which the values occur according to some specified probability distribution. A normal random variable, for example, has a normal distribution, and a Poisson random variable has a Poisson distribution. [Altman, D. G., 2018, *Practical Statistics for Medical Research*, Chapman & Hall/CRC, Boca Raton, FL.]

Random variation: The variation in a data set unexplained by identifiable sources.

Random walk: The motion of a particle that moves, with specific probabilities, from point to point in discrete jumps. As a concrete example, the position of the particle might represent the size of a population of individuals; a step to the left could represent a death, and a step to the right could represent a birth. Here, the process would stop if the particle ever reached the origin, which is, consequently, termed an *absorbing barrier*. *See also* **Markov chain**. [Chatfield, C., 2019, *The Analysis of Time Series*, 7th ed., Chapman & Hall/CRC, Boca Raton, FL.]

Range: The difference between the largest and smallest observations in a data set. Often used as an easy-to-calculate measure of the dispersion in a set of observations, but not recommended for this task because of its sensitivity to outliers. [Altman, D. G., 2018, *Practical Statistics for Medical Research*, Chapman & Hall/CRC, Boca Raton, FL.]

Range of equivalence: The range of differences between two treatments being compared in a `clinical trial`, within which it is not possible to make a definite choice of treatment. For example, if the true treatment difference is summarized by a parameter, δ, with large values of δ corresponding to superiority of the new treatment, then there may be a certain threshold level, δ_L, that the new treatment must achieve before it can be considered, with the values of $\delta < \delta_L$ being regarded as not providing sufficient evidence in favour of the new treatment.

Another value, δ_U, may also be postulated, where only values of δ such that $\delta > \delta_U$ provide evidence of the clinical superiority of the new treatment. The interval (δ_L, δ_U) is the range of equivalence of the two treatments. [*Statistics in Medicine*, 1998, **17**, 1691–701.]

Rank: The relative position of a member of a sample with respect to some characteristic.

Rank correlation coefficients: `Correlation coefficients` that depend only on the ranks of the variables, not on their observed values. Examples include `Kendall's tau statistic` and `Spearman's rank correlation`. [Kendall, M. and Gibbons, J. D., 1990, *Rank Correlation Methods*, 5th ed., Oxford University Press, New York.]

Ranking: The process of sorting a set of variable values into either ascending or descending order.

Rank order statistics: Statistics based only on the ranks of the sample observations, for example `Kendall's tau statistic`.

Rasch model: A `mathematical model` often used in psychology for analyzing the results of cognitive tests given to a set of individuals. Assumes an underlying, unobservable latent trait and allows the estimation of parameters associated with the ability of the individual and the difficulty of the terms in the test. [*American Journal of Epidemiology*, 1995, **142**, 1047–58.]

Ratchet scan statistic: A statistic that can be used to investigate whether there has been a sharp increase in the `incidence rate` of a disease during a particular time period, superimposed on a constant incidence over the entire year. For example, the statistics might be used to investigate whether there has been an increase in the incidence of AIDS in the summer period. *See also* **disease cluster** and **scan statistic**. [*Biometrics*, 1992, **48**, 1177–82.]

Rate: A measure of the frequency of some phenomenon of interest, given by

$$\text{Rate} = \frac{\text{number of events in specified period}}{\text{average population during the period}}$$

The resulting value is often multiplied by a power of 10 to convert it to a whole number. *See also* **crude death rate** and **age-specific birth rate**.

Ratio variable: A continuous variable that has a fixed rather than an arbitrary zero point. Examples are height, weight and temperature measured in Kelvin. *See also* **measurement scale** and **categorical variable**.

RBD: Abbreviation for **randomized block design**.

RCT: Abbreviation for **randomized clinical trial**.

Recall bias: A possible source of bias, particularly in a retrospective study, caused by differential recall among cases and controls, in general by under-reporting of exposure in the control group. Can seriously distort the results of such studies. For example, in an investigation of a possible link between abortion and breast cancer, breast cancer patients might be more likely to report honestly any abortions they may have had than are healthy women. *See also* **ascertainment bias**. [*American Journal of Epidemiology*, 2000, **151**, 1139–43.]

Receiver operating characteristic (ROC) curves: A plot of the sensitivity of a diagnostic test against one minus its specificity as the cut-off criterion for indicating a positive test is varied. Often used in choosing between competing tests, although the procedure takes no account of the prevalence of the disease being tested for. As an example, consider the following ratings from 1 (definitely normal) to 5 (definitely diseased) arising from 50 normal subjects and 50 diseased subjects:

	1	2	3	4	5	Total
Normal	4	17	20	8	1	50
Diseased	3	3	17	19	8	50

If the rating of 5 is used as the cut-off for identifying diseased cases, then the sensitivity is estimated as $8/50 = 0.16$, and the specificity is estimated as $49/50 = 0.98$. Now, using the rating of 4 as the cut-off leads to a sensitivity of $27/50 = 0.54$ and a specificity of $41/50 = 0.82$. The values of (sensitivity, $1 -$ specificity) as the cut-off decreases from 5 to 1 are (0.16, 0.02), (0.54, 0.18), (0.88, 0.58), (0.94, 0.92) and (1.00, 1.00). These points are plotted in Figure 75 to give the required receiver operating characteristic curve. [*Critical Reviews in Diagnostic Imaging*, 1989, **29**, 307–35.]

Recessive gene: A gene that is phenotypically manifest only when present in the homozygous state.

Reciprocal transformation: A transformation involving using one over a random variable. Particularly useful for certain types of variables; for example, resistances transformed in this way become conductances, and times become speeds. In some cases, the transformation can lead to achieving a linear relationship between variables; for example, airways resistance against lung volume is nonlinear, but airways conductance against lung volume is linear. [*British Medical Journal*, 1996, **312**, 1153.]

Recombination frequency: The number of recombinants divided by the total number of progeny. This frequency is used as a guide in assessing the relative distances between loci on a genetic map.

Record linkage: A method for assembling the information contained in two or more records on a patient that ensures that the same individual is counted only once. [*Medical Care*, 1994, **32**, 1004–18.]

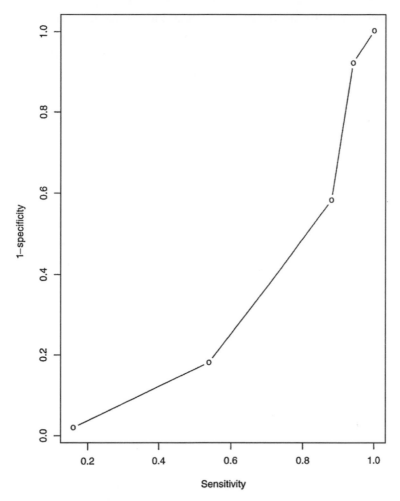

Figure 75 Example of an ROC curve for the normal/diseased ratings given in the text.

Rectangular distribution: Synonym for **uniform distribution**.

Recurrence risk: The probability of disease for an individual given that a relative is diseased. Important in genetic counselling. For example, trisomy 21 is the most common autosomal chromosome abnormality, with an incidence rate of 1/800 live births; it gives rise to Down's syndrome babies. The recurrence risk here depends on the aetiology and ranges from 2% to 15%. [*Archives of Internal Medicine*, 2004, **164**, 2266–72.]

Recurrent event data: Data in which recurrent events, for example tumours, are ordered and each event of interest is treated as being of the same nature. The primary research interest focuses on estimating and comparing the risk of recurrent clinical events. A variety of models have been proposed for analyzing such data. [*Statistical Methods in Medical Research*, 2010, **19**, 167–82.]

Reference-based error estimation: A method for estimating errors of a given measurement method by comparison with a reference method (the gold standard). Out of many methods to measure the same quantity the one that is considered to produce reasonably small errors is chosen as a substitute for the true value of the measurand. [*Statistical Methods in Medical Research*, 2019, **28**, 2196–209.]

Reference interval: A range of values for a variable that encompasses the values obtained from the majority of normal subjects. Generally calculated as the interval between two predetermined centiles (such as the 5th and the 95th) of the distribution of the variable of interest. For example, the reference interval for white blood cell count is 4.0–10.5×10^{-3}/ml. Often used as the basis for assessing the results of diagnostic tests in the classification of individuals as normal or abnormal with respect to a particular variable. [Harris, E. K. and Boyd, J. C., 1995, *Statistical Bases of Reference Values in Laboratory Medicine*, Marcel Dekker, New York.]

Reference population: The standard against which a population that is being studied can be compared. [*Archives of Disease in Childhood*, 2004, **89**, 843–4.]

Reference prior: *See* **prior distributions**.

Reference range: Synonymous with **reference interval**.

Regression analysis: A general term for methods of analysis that are concerned with estimating the parameters in some postulated relationship between a response variable and one or more explanatory variables. Particular examples are logistic regression and multiple linear regression. [Everitt, B. S. and Palmer, C. (eds.), 2011, *Encyclopedic Companion to Medical Statistics*, John Wiley & Sons, Chichester.]

Regression calibration: A method for adjusting point and interval estimates obtained from regression models for possible bias due to measurement error in the explanatory variables. [*American Journal of Clinical Nutrition*, 1997, **65**, 1179S–86S.]

Regression coefficient: *See* **multiple linear regression**.

Regression diagnostics: Synonymous with **diagnostics**.

Regression dilution: The term applied when a covariate in a model can be measured only with error. In general, if the model is specified correctly in terms of the true covariate, then a similar form of the model with a simple error structure will not hold for the observed values. In such cases, ignoring the measurement error will lead to biased estimates of the parameters in the model. Often also referred to as the *errors-in-variables problem*. *See also* **attenuation**, **latent variables** and **structural equation modelling**. [Rawlings, J. O., Pantula, S. G. and Dickey, D. A., 2013, *Applied Regression Analysis: A Research Tool*, 2nd ed., Springer, New York.]

Regression through the origin: In some situations, a relationship between two variables estimated by regression analysis is expected to pass through the origin, because the true mean of the dependent variable is known to be zero when the value of the explanatory variable is zero. In such situations, the linear `regression` model is forced to pass through the origin by setting the intercept parameter to zero and estimating only the slope parameter.

Regression to the mean: The process first noted by Sir Francis Galton that 'each peculiarity in man is shared by his kinsmen, but on the average to a less degree'. Hence, the tendency, for example, for tall parents to produce tall offspring but who, on average, are shorter than their parents. The term is now used generally to label the phenomenon that a variable that is extreme on its first measurement will tend to be closer to the centre of the distribution for a later measurement. For example, in a screening programme for hypertension, only people with high blood pressure are asked to return for a second measurement. On the average, the second measurement taken will be less than the first. [*Statistical Methods in Medical Research*, 1997, **6**, 103–14.]

> **Regression to the mean:** One reason for not using change scores.

Regression tree: *See* **classification and regression trees**.

Regression weight: Synonym for **regression coefficient**.

Reification: The process of naming `latent variables` and the consequent discussion of such things as quality of life and racial prejudice as though they were physical quantities in the same sense as, for example, length and weight are. [Everitt, B. S. and Dunn, G., 2010, *Applied Multivariate Data Analysis*, 2nd ed., John Wiley & Sons, Chichester.]

Rejectable quality level: *See* **quality control procedures**.

Relative efficiency: The ratio of the variances of two possible estimates of a parameter, or the ratio of the sample sizes required by two statistical procedures to achieve the same `power`.

Relative poverty statistics: Statistics on the properties of populations falling below given fractions of average income. Such statistics play an important role in the discussion of both the reasons for and the possible solutions to poverty. For example, the proportion below half national median income has been used as the basis of comparisons of poverty in different countries. In the United Kingdom, the figure for single parents is 40%; in Italy the corresponding figure is 25%, and in Finland it is 9%.

Relative reinforcing efficacy: A fundamental concept frequently used in substance abuse research that describes the reinforcing potency and abuse liability of a substance. Drug self-administration experiments are most often used to assess the abuse liability and reinforcing property of a compound, for example, hallucinogens, nicotine and alcohol. [*Statistical Methods in Medical Research*, 2018, **27**, 2401–12.]

Relative risk: A measure of the association between exposure to a particular factor and risk of a certain outcome, calculated as

$$\text{relative risk} = \frac{\text{incidence rate among exposed}}{\text{incidence rate among nonexposed}}$$

Thus, a relative risk of five, for example, means that an exposed person is five times as likely to have the disease than a person who is not exposed. Relative risk does *not* measure the probability that someone with the factor will develop the disease. The disease may be rare among both nonexposed people and the exposed people. For rare diseases, the odds ratio approximates the relative risk. *See also* **incidence rate** and **attributable risk**. *See also* **absolute risk.** [Altman, D. G., 2018, *Practical Statistics for Medical Research*, Chapman & Hall/CRC, Boca Raton, FL.]

Relative risk: An airline pilot probably has a much increased relative risk of dying in an aeroplane crash compared with the average airline passenger, but his/her probability of dying in this way remains (thankfully) extremely low.

Relative risk reduction: The proportional reduction in the relative risk amongst exposed and nonexposed individuals. For example, the results of the mammography trial described in the absolute risk reduction entry show a relative risk reduction of 20% compared to an absolute risk reduction of only 0.1%. Relative risk reduction is often more impressive than absolute risk reduction. Additionally, the lower the event rate in the nonexposed group, the larger the difference between relative risk reduction and absolute risk reduction.

Relative risk reduction: Potential benefits of treatments in medicine are often described in terms of relative risk reduction, but for the patient it is absolute risk reduction that really matters.

Relative standardized mortality rate: The ratio of the standardized mortality rate (SMR) for a particular cause of death, divided by the all-causes SMR. This index attempts to make an adjustment for overall differences in mortality due to healthy worker effects or other differences between the study and referent populations.

Relative survival rate: The ratio of the observed survival rate of a given group of patients to the expected survival rate for people in the general population similar to the patient group with respect to age, sex, race and calendar year of observation.

For example, the relative survival rate for kidney cancer patients five years following diagnosis is 58%. The five-year relative survival rate is often used to estimate the proportion of cancer patients who are potentially curable. [*Breast Cancer Research and Treatment*, 2001, **70**, 137–43.]

Release targets: A term used in the pharmaceutical industry for in-house limits for the average potency of a batch of some drug. These limits are calculated to give some degree of assurance that the average potency of a batch released is within the limits demanded by a regulatory body such as the Food and Drug Administration.

Reliability: The extent to which the same measurements of individuals obtained under different conditions yield similar results. *See also* **intraclass correlation** and **kappa coefficient**.

Repeatability: The closeness of the results obtained in the same test material by the same observer or technician using the same equipment, apparatus and/or reagents over reasonably short intervals of time.

Repeated-measures analysis of variance: The use of analysis of variance procedures to analyse longitudinal data. The basis of the analysis is a simple mixed-effects model. The approach is valid only if the variance-covariance matrix of the repeated observations satisfies sphericity and the matrix is the same in each treatment group. *See also* **Greenhouse–Geisser correction** and **Huynh–Feldt correction**. [Everitt, B. S., 2001, *Statistics for Psychologists*, LEA, Mahwah, FL.]

Repeated-measures data: *See* **longitudinal data**.

Replicate observation: An independent observation obtained under conditions as nearly identical to the original as the nature of the investigation will permit.

Reproducibility: The closeness of results obtained on the same test material under changes of reagents, conditions, technicians, apparatus, laboratories, and so on.

Reproduction rate: *See* **basic reproduction number**.

Research hypothesis: Synonym for **alternative hypothesis**.

Resentful demoralization: A possible phenomenon in clinical trials and intervention studies in which comparison groups not obtaining a perceived desirable treatment become aware of this potential inequity and become discouraged or retaliatory, and as a result perform worse on the outcome measures. [Cook, T. D. and Campbell, D. T., 1979, *Quasi-Experimentation: Design and Analysis Issues for Field Setting*, Rand-McNally, Chicago, IL.]

Residual: The difference between the observed value of a response variable and the value predicted by some model of interest. Examination of a set of residuals, usually by informal graphical techniques, allows the assumptions made in the model-fitting exercise, for example normality or homogeneity of variance, to be checked.

Generally, discrepant observations have large residuals, but some form of standardization may be necessary in many situations to allow identification of patterns among the residuals that may be a cause for concern. *See also* **diagnostics**, **influence** and **index plot**. [Cook, R. D. and Weisberg, S., 1994, *An Introduction to Regression Graphics*, John Wiley & Sons, New York.]

Residual sum of squares: *See* **analysis of variance**.

Responders versus non-responders analysis: A comparison of groups of patients according to whether there is some observed response to treatment. In general, such analyses are invalid because the groups are defined by a factor not known at the start of the treatment. [*European Respiratory Journal*, 2002, **19**, 664–71.]

Response-adaptive treatment allocation: Sequentially adaptive schemes for allocating treatments to groups in `clinical trials` that use past treatment assignments and patients' responses to select future treatment assignments. The aim is to assign more patients to the empirically better treatment. [*Journal of Biopharmaceutical Statistics*, 2012, **22**, 719–36.]

Response bias: The systematic component of the difference between information provided by survey respondent and the 'truth'.

Response feature analysis: An approach to the analysis of `longitudinal data` involving the calculation of suitable summary measures from the set of repeated measures on each subject. For example, the mean of the subject's measurements or the maximum value of the response variable over the repeated measurements might be calculated. Simple methods such as `Student's` `t-test` or the `Mann–Whitney test` are then applied to these summary measures to assess differences between treatments. Often a useful first step in the analysis of such data before fitting, for example, `mixed-effects models`. *See also* **area under curve**, C_{max} and T_{max}. [*British Medical Journal*, 1990, **300**, 230–5.]

> **Response feature analysis:** A simple but not simplistic approach to the analysis of longitudinal data from clinical trials.

Response rate: The proportion of subjects who respond to, usually, a postal questionnaire. Often response rates in survey research are calculated simply by dividing the number of completed interviews by the number of individuals who were selected to participate in the research. But this method is usually regarded as too simplistic and not to do justice to the complexity of research design, sampling process and the practical difficulties of contacting and assessing potential survey participants. The response rate is the single most important indicator of how much confidence can be placed in the results of a survey. A low response rate can undermine the results of any survey. [Lynn, P., Beerten, R., Laiho, J. and Martin, J., 2001, *Recommended Standard Final Outcome Categories and Standard Definitions of Response Rate for Social Surveys*, The Institute for Social and Economic Research, Colchester, Essex.]

Response variable: The variable of primary importance in medical investigations, since the major objective is usually to study the effects of treatment and/or other explanatory variables on this variable, and to provide suitable models for the relationship between it and the explanatory variables. May be continuous, for example blood pressure, or categorical, for example improved/not improved. The type of response variable generally determines the appropriate form of analysis. [Altman, D. G., 2018, *Practical Statistics for Medical Research*, Chapman & Hall/ CRC, Boca Raton, FL.]

Restricted randomization: A technique used to ensure that the groups formed by randomization in a `clinical trial` are allocated similar number of subjects, that is, are balanced. This is only really a problem in small samples where equal probability allocation can result in a large departure from balance. [Rosenberger, W. F. and Lachin, J. L., 2002, *Randomization in Clinical Trials: Theory and Practice,* John Wiley & Sons, New York.]

Retrospective cohort study: *See* **retrospective study**.

Retrospective study: A general term for studies in which all the events of interest occur before the onset of the study, and findings are based on looking backwards in time. Most common is the *case–control study*, in which comparisons are made between individuals who have a particular disease or condition (the cases) and individuals who do not have the disease (the controls). A sample of cases is selected from the population of individuals who have the disease of interest, and a sample of controls is taken from those individuals known not to have the disease. Information about possible risk factors for the disease is then obtained retrospectively for each person in the study by examining past records, by interviewing each person and/or interviewing their relatives, or by some other method. In order to make the cases and controls otherwise comparable, they are frequently matched on characteristics known to be related strongly to both disease and exposure, leading to a *matched case–control study*. Age, sex and socioeconomic status are examples of commonly used matching variables. Also commonly encountered is the *retrospective cohort study*, in which a past cohort of individuals is identified from previous information, for example, employment records, and their subsequent mortality or morbidity determined and compared with the corresponding experience of some suitable control group. [Hebel, J. R. and McCarter, R. J., 2011, *A Study Guide to Epidemiology and Biostatistics*, 7th ed., Jones & Bartlett, Boston, MA.]

Reverse causality: Synonym for **protopathic bias**.

Reverse J-shaped distribution: *See* **J-shaped distribution**.

Ridge regression: A method of `regression analysis` designed to overcome the possible problem of `multicollinearity` among the explanatory variables. Such multicollinearity makes it difficult to estimate the separate effects of variables on the response. By allowing regression estimates to be biased, this form of regression results in increased precision. [Rawlings, J. O., Pantula, S. G. and Dickey, D. A., 2013, *Applied Regression Analysis: A Research Tool*, 2nd ed., Springer, New York.]

Ridit analysis: A method of analysis for ordinal variables that proceeds from the assumption that the ordered categorical scale is an approximation to an underlying, but not directly measurable, continuous variable. The successive categories are assumed to correspond to consecutive intervals on the underlying continuum. Numerical values called *ridits* are calculated for each category, these values being estimates of the probability that a subject's value on the underlying variable is less than or equal to the midpoint of the corresponding interval. These scores are then used in subsequent analyses involving the variable. [Patrick, D. L. and Erickson, P., 1993, *Health Status and Health Policy: Allocating Resources to Health Care*, Oxford University Press, New York.]

Ridits: *See* **ridit analysis**.

Risk: The possibility of incurring misfortune or loss. Risk is synonymous with hazard. Quantifying and assessing risk in medicine involves the calculation and comparison of probabilities, although most expressions of risk are compound measures that describe both the probability of harm and its severity. Americans, for example, run a risk of about one in 4,000 of dying in an automobile accident. The probability is one out of 4,000 for lethally severe injuries. [Everitt, B. S., 2008, *Chance Rules*, 2nd ed., Springer, New York.]

Risk: It is very difficult to persuade the general public to be rational about risk.

Risk assessment: The qualitative or quantitative assessment of the risks to health and well-being associated with exposure to some hazard or from the absence of some benefit. [Royal Society Study Group, 1983, *Risk Assessment: Report of a Royal Society Study Group*, Royal Society, London.]

Risk–benefit analysis: The investigation as to whether a treatment of interest is worth the risk to a patient as compared to the possible benefits if the treatment is successful. Essentially an examination of the potential positive and negative results of undertaking a specific therapeutic course of action. [*Risk Analysis*, 2005, **25**, 161–8.]

Risk factor: An aspect of personal behaviour or lifestyle, an environmental exposure, or an inborn or inherited characteristic that is thought to be associated with a particular disease or condition. [Everitt, B. S., 2008, *Chance Rules*, 2nd ed., Springer, New York.]

Risk set: A term used in the analysis of survival times for those individuals who are alive and uncensored at a time just before some particular time point.

Robust estimation: Methods of estimation that work well not only under ideal conditions but also under conditions representing a departure from an assumed distribution or model. *See also* **high breakdown methods**. [Launer, R. and Wilkinson, G., 2014, *Robustness in Statistics*, Academic Press, New York.]

Robust regression: A general class of statistical procedures designed to reduce the sensitivity of the parameter estimates to failures in the assumption of the model. For example, `least squares estimation` is known to be sensitive to `outliers`, but the impact of such observations can be reduced by basing the estimation process not on a sum-of-squares criterion but on a sum-of-absolute-values criterion. [Huber, P. J. and Rouchetti, E. M., 2009, *Robust Statistics*, 2nd ed., John Wiley & Sons, New York.]

Robust statistics: An extension of classical parametric statistics that specifically takes into account the fact that the assumed parametric models used are only ever approximate. The approach provides statistical procedures and tests that still work reasonably well even when the assumptions on which they are based are mildly (or perhaps moderately) violated. `Student's t-test`, for example, is robust against departures from normality. *See also* **high breakdown methods**. [Launer, R. and Wilkinson, G., 2014, *Robustness in Statistics*, Academic Press, New York.]

Figure 76 A rug plot of percentage body fat in a number of individuals.

ROC curves: Abbreviation for **receiver operating characteristic curves**.

Rootogram: A diagram obtained from a histogram in which the rectangles represent the square roots of the observed frequencies rather than the frequencies themselves. The idea behind such a diagram is to remove the tendency for the variability of a count to increase with its typical size. *See also* **hanging rootogram**. [Tukey, J. W., 1977, *Exploratory Data Analysis*, Addison-Wesley, Reading, MA.]

Rosenbaum's test: A `distribution-free method` for the equality of the scale parameters of two populations known to have the same median. The `test statistic` is the total number of values in the sample from the first population that are either smaller than the smallest or larger than the largest values in the sample from the second population.

Rosenthal effect: The observation that investigators often find what they expect to find from a study unless stringent safeguards are instituted to minimize human `bias`. For example, in a reliability study in which auscultatory measurements of the foetal heart rate were compared with the electronically recorded rate, it was found that when the true rate was under 130 beats per minute the hospital staff tended to overestimate it, and when it was over 150 they tended to underestimate it. [*Psychological Bulletin*, 1985, **97**, 363–86.]

Rounding: The procedure used for reporting numerical information to fewer decimal places than used during analysis. The rule generally adopted is that excess digits are simply discarded if the first of them is less than five, otherwise the last retained digit is increased by one. So rounding 127.249341 to three decimal places gives 127.249, and rounding 138.256644 to three decimal places gives 138.257.

Round robin study: A term sometimes used for interlaboratory comparisons in which samples of a material manufactured to well-defined specifications are sent out to the participating laboratories for analysis. The results are used to assess differences between laboratories and to identify possible sources of incompatibility or other anomalies. *See also* **interlaboratory trials**. [*Clinical Chemistry*, 2003, **49**, 1672–5.]

Roy's largest root: *See* **multivariate analysis of variance**.

Rug plot: A method for displaying graphically a sample of values on a continuous variable by indicating their positions on a horizontal line. Figure 76 shows an example.

Rule of threes: A rule that states that if, in n trials, zero events of interest are observed, then a 95% confidence bound on the underlying rate is $3/n$. [*American Statistician*, 1997, **51**, 137–9.]

Run-in: A period of observation, before the formation of treatment groups by random allocation, during which subjects acquire experience with the major components of a study `protocol`. Those subjects who experience difficulty complying with the protocol are excluded, while the group of proven compliers are randomized into the trial. The rationale behind such a procedure is that, in general, a study with higher compliance will have higher `power` because the observed effects of the difference between treatment groups will not be subjected to the diluting effects of non-compliance. [Senn, S., 2008, *Statistical Issues in Drug Development*, 2nd ed., John Wiley & Sons, Chichester.]

Runs: In a series of observations, the occurrence of an uninterrupted sequence of the same value. For example, in the series 111224333333, there are four runs, the single value 4 being regarded as a run of length unity.

Runs test: A test used frequently to detect `serial correlations`. The test consists of counting the number of `runs`, or sequences of positive and negative residuals, and comparing the result with the expected value under the null hypothesis of independence. [Rawlings, J. O., Pantula, S. G. and Dickey, D. A., 2013, *Applied Regression Analysis: A Research Tool*, 2nd ed., Springer, New York.]

S

Sample: A selected subset of a population chosen by some process, usually with the objective of investigating particular properties of the parent population.

Sample size: The number of individuals to be included in an investigation.

Sample size estimation: The sample size to be used in a particular study is generally chosen so that the study has a particular power of detecting an effect of a particular size. Software is available for calculating sample size for many types of study. *See also* **nomograms**. [Chow, S.-C., 2017, *Sample Size Calculations in Clinical Research*, 3rd ed., Chapman & Hall/CRC, Boca Raton, FL.]

> **Sample size estimation** : According to Professor Stephen Senn, sample size estimation is generally a guess masquerading as mathematics. As usual, he is probably correct!

Sample survey: A study that aims to estimate population characteristics of interest by the answers to questions about these characteristics given by a sample of individuals from the population. *See also* **opinion survey** and **random sample**. [*Journal of Official Statistics (Sweden)*, 1985, **1**, 427–33.]

Sampling: The process of selecting some part of a population so as to estimate something of interest about the whole population, for example the prevalence of a particular disease. Some obvious questions are how to obtain the sample and make the observations, and, once the sample data are available, how best to use them to estimate the characteristic of the population under investigation. [Everitt, B. S. and Palmer, C. (eds.), 2011, *Encyclopedic Companion to Medical Statistics*, 2nd ed., John Wiley & Sons, Chichester.]

Sampling design: The procedure by which the sampling units are selected from the population when sampling. In general, a particular design is determined by assigning to each possible sample the probability of selecting that sample. *See also* **random sample**. [Lavrakas, P. J. (ed.), 2008, *Encyclopedia of Survey Research Methods*, Sage, Newbury Park, CA.]

Sampling distribution: The probability distribution of a statistic calculated from a random sample of a particular size. For example, the sampling distribution of the arithmetic mean of samples of size n, taken from a normal distribution with mean μ and standard deviation σ, is a normal distribution also with mean μ but with standard deviation $\sigma/\sqrt{n}$. The sampling distribution is an essential feature of statistical inference. [Altman, D. G., 2018, *Practical Statistics for Medical Research*, Chapman & Hall/CRC, Boca Raton, FL.]

Sampling error: The difference between the sample result and the population characteristic being estimated. In practice, the sampling error can rarely be determined because the population characteristic is not usually known. With appropriate sampling procedures, however, it can be kept small and the investigator can determine its probable limits of magnitude. *See also* **standard error**. [Cochran, W. G., 1977, *Sampling Techniques*, 3rd ed., John Wiley & Sons, New York.]

Sampling frames: The portion of the population from which a sample is to be selected. Usually defined by geographical listings, maps, directories, membership or other kinds of lists. [Wright, T., 1983, *Statistical Methods and the Improvement of Data Quality*, Academic Press, New York.]

Sampling units: The entities to be sampled by a `sampling design`. In many studies, these will be individual people, but often they will be larger groups of individuals, for example hospitals, schools and so on.

Sampling variation: The variation shown by different samples of the same size from the same population.

Sampling with and without replacement: Terms used to describe two possible methods of taking samples from a `finite population`. When each element is replaced before the next one is drawn, sampling is said to be *with* replacement. When elements are not replaced, then the sampling is referred to as *without* replacement. *See also* **bootstrap**, **jackknife** and **hypergeometric distribution**.

Sampling zeros: Zero frequencies that occur in the cells of `contingency tables` simply as a result of inadequate sample size. *See also* **structural zeros**. [Everitt, B. S., 1992, *The Analysis of Contingency Tables*, 2nd ed., Chapman & Hall/CRC, Boca Raton, FL.]

Saturated model: A model that contains all `main effects` and all possible `interactions` between factors. Since such a model contains the same number of parameters as observations, it results in a perfect fit for a data set. *See also* **identification**. [Altman, D. G., 2018, *Practical Statistics for Medical Research*, Chapman & Hall/CRC, Boca Raton, FL.]

Scalar: A single number, for example 4, 10 or 3.1, as opposed to a collection of numbers given in a vector or matrix.

Scale parameter: A general term for that parameter of a `probability distribution` that determines the scale of measurement, for example the parameter σ^2 in the `normal distribution`.

Scan statistic: A statistic for evaluating whether an apparent `disease cluster` in time is due to chance. The statistic employs a moving window of a particular length, and finds the maximum number of cases revealed through the window as it moves over the entire time period. Approximations for an upper bound to the probability of

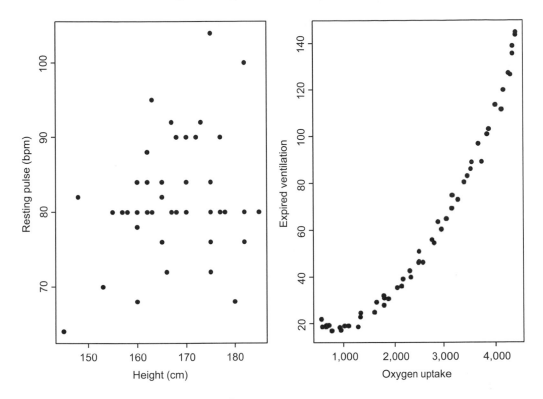

Figure 77 Examples of scatter diagrams.

observing a certain size cluster under the null hypothesis of a `uniform distribution` are available. The statistic has been applied to test for possible clustering of lung cancer at a chemical works, for rashes following injection of a varicella virus vaccine, and for trisomic spontaneous abortions. *See also* **geographical analysis machine** and **ratchet scan statistic**. [*Journal of Toxicology*, 1992, **30**, 459–65.]

Scatter: Synonym for **dispersion**.

Scatter diagram: A two-dimensional plot of a sample of bivariate observations. The diagram is an important aid in assessing what type of relationship links the two variables. Two scatterplots are shown in Figure 77. The first plot shows resting pulse rate plotted against height and indicates a tendency for taller people to have a higher resting pulse. The second plot involves expired ventilation and oxygen uptake, measures taken in an experiment in kinesiology; here, the diagram shows that there is a very strong, possibly nonlinear relationship between the two variables. *See also* **bubble plot**, **correlation coefficient** and **scatterplot matrix**. [Altman, D. G., 2018, *Practical Statistics for Medical Research*, Chapman & Hall/CRC, Boca Raton, FL.]

Scattergram: Synonym for **scatter diagram**.

Scatterplot: Synonym for **scatter diagram**.

Scatterplot matrix: An arrangement in the form of a square grid of the pairwise `scatter diagrams` of the variables in a set of `multivariate data`. Each panel of the grid is a scatter diagram for one pair of variables. The upper lefthand triangle of the grid contains all possible pairs of scatter diagrams, as does the lower righthand triangle of the grid. The reasons for including both the upper and lower triangles in the grid, despite the apparent redundancy, is that it enables a row or column to be scanned visually to see one variable against all others, with the scales for the one variable lined up along the horizontal or the vertical. Such a diagram is often helpful in an initial assessment of the data. An example is shown in Figure 78 for data collected in an investigation into the haematology of paint sprayers. The variables involved were haemoglobin concentration (HAEMO), packed cell volume (PCV), white blood cell count (WBC), lymphocyte count (LYMPHO), neutrophil count (NEUTRO), and serum lead concentration (LEAD). [Cleveland, W. S., 1993, *Visualizing Data*, Hobart Press, Summit, NJ.]

Sceptical priors: *See* **prior distributions**.

Scheffé's test: A multiple comparison test that protects against a large per-experiment error rate. [Fisher, L. R. and Van Belle, G., 1993, *Biostatistics*, John Wiley & Sons, New York.]

Screened-to-eligible ratio: The number of subjects that have to be examined in a clinical trial to identify one protocol-eligible subject. [*AIDS Supplement*, 1997, **11**, 13–19.]

Screening studies: Studies in which diagnostic tests are applied to a symptomless population in order to diagnose disease at an early stage. Such studies are designed both to estimate disease prevalence and to identify for treatment patients who have particular diseases. The procedure is usually concerned with chronic illness and aims to detect disease not yet under medical care. Such studies need to be carefully designed and analyzed in order to avoid possible problems arising because of lead time bias and length-biased sampling. Most suitable designs are based on random allocation. For example, in the *continuous screen design*, subjects are randomised either to a group that is given periodic screening throughout the study or to a group that does not get such screening but simply follows the usual medical care practices. One drawback of this type of design is that the cost involved in screening all the patients in the intervention arm of the trial for the duration of the trial may be prohibitive; if this is so, then an alternative approach can be used, namely the *stop screen design*, in which screening is offered for only a limited time in the intervention group. If screening is not conducted properly, then effectiveness and cost-effectiveness can easily be impaired. And it has to be remembered that all screening programmes do harm. Some do good as well and, of these, some do more good than harm at reasonable cost; see the reference for more detail. [Raffle, A. and Muir Gray, A. J., 2007, *Screening*, Oxford University Press, Oxford.]

Scree plot: A graphical procedure for determining the number of factors to retain in a factor analysis or principal components analysis. The plot consists of the variances of the factors against factor number. The critical feature looked for is an 'elbow', indicating a levelling-off after a steep decline. The example in

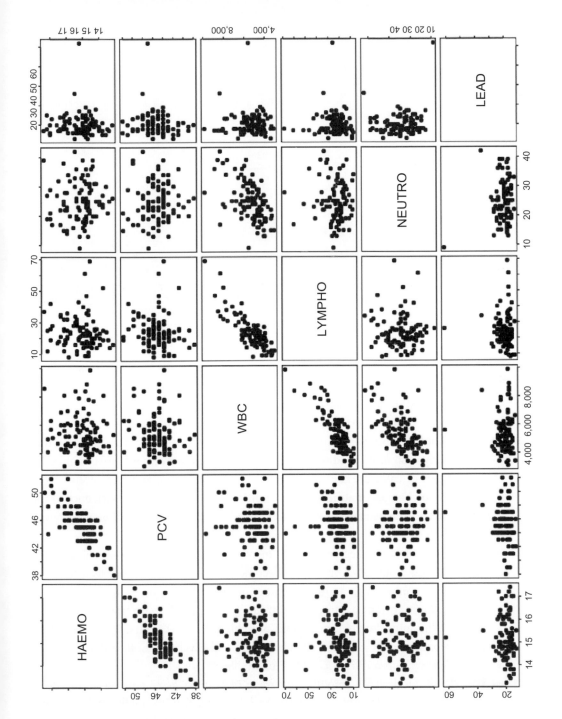

Figure 78 Example of scatterplot matrix.

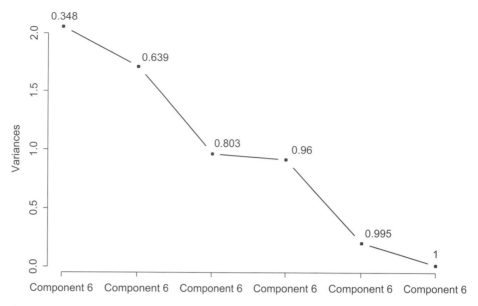

Figure 79 Scree plot showing an elbow indicating three factors.

Figure 79 shows a clear elbow corresponding to three factors. *See also* **Kaiser's rule**. [*Multivariate Behavioural Research*, 1966, **1**, 245–76.]

SD: Abbreviation for **standard deviation**.

SE: Abbreviation for **standard error**.

Seasonal variation: Although strictly used to indicate the cycles in a time series that occur yearly, also often used to indicate other periodic movements. Seasonal cycles of infectious diseases are the rule rather than the exception, and have been attributed to changes in atmospheric conditions, the prevalence or virulence of the pathogen, and the behaviour of the host. [*International Journal of Epidemiology*, 1982, **11**, 5–14.]

Secondary attack rate: The degree to which members of some collective or isolated unit, such as a household, litter or colony, become infected with a disease as a result of coming into contact with another member of the collective unit who became infected. An important parameter of infectious diseases that are transmitted by contact. Whooping cough, for example, is highly infectious, with a secondary attack rate approaching 100%. [Fox, J. P., Hall, C. E. and Elveback, L. P., 1970, *Epidemiology: Man and Disease*, Macmillan, New York.]

Secular trend: The underlying smooth movement of a time series over a fairly long period of time. For example, age at menarche has become gradually lower in many parts of the world over the last three decades. [*International Journal of Cancer*, 2005, **115**, 497.]

Segregation analysis: The statistical analysis of family data to determine the mode of inheritance. [Sham, P., 1998, *Statistics in Human Genetics*, Arnold, London.]

Selection bias I: The `bias` that may be introduced into `clinical trials` and other types of medical investigations whenever a treatment is chosen by the individual involved or is subject to constraints that go unobserved by the researcher. If there are unobserved factors influencing health outcomes and the type of treatment chosen, then any direct links between treatment and outcomes are confounded with unmeasured variables in the data. A classic example of this problem occurred in the Lanarkshire milk experiment of the 1920s. In this trial, 10,000 children were given free milk supplementation and a similar number received no supplementation. The groups were formed by random allocation. Unfortunately, however, well-intentioned teachers decided that the poorest children should be given priority for free milk rather than sticking to the original groups. The consequence was that the effects of milk supplementation were indistinguishable from the effects of poverty. A further example is provided by the recent demand that health services researchers obtain patient consent before examining personally identifiable data. A selection `bias` may result if consenting patients differ from those who do not give consent. [*Archives of Family Medicine*, 2000, **9**, 1111–18.]

Selection bias II: A term often used in the context of `multiple linear regression` when subsets of variables chosen by some procedure are optimal for prediction on the original data but perform poorly on future data.

Selection bias III: Sometimes used when individuals included in a study are not representative of the target population.

Selection methods in regression: Methods that attempt to select subsets of explanatory variables in a regression analysis that are of most importance in predicting the response variable. Three commonly used procedures are:

- *Forward selection:* This begins with none of the explanatory variables in the regression and then selects variables one by one according to some criterion measuring how well the particular variable predicts the response over and above the variables already selected.
- *Backward elimination:* This begins with all the explanatory variables in the regression and then eliminates variables one by one according to a criterion that assesses the effect that dropping a variable has on the predictive power of the current regression equation.
- *Stepwise regression:* Essentially a mixture of the previous two procedures.

  It should be stressed that none of these procedures is foolproof and they must be used with a certain amount of caution. *See also* **all-subsets regression**. [Rawlings, J. O., Pantula, S. G. and Dickey, D. A., 2013, *Applied Regression Analysis: A Research Tool*, 2nd ed., Springer, New York.]

Selection methods in regression: Need to be used with care and perhaps a little scepticism.

Self-pairing: *See* **paired samples**.

Semantic differential scale: A scale for eliciting ratings of a particular concept on a series of dimensions. For example:

My treatment is

Painful ——————————————————————————— Painless

Helpful ——————————————————————————— Not helpful

See also **adjectival scales** and **visual analogue scales**. [Osgood, E. C., Suci, G. J. and Tannenbaum, P. H., 1957, *The Measurement of Meaning*, University of Illinois Press, Urbana, IL.]

Semi-continuous data: Data generated from a response which is a mixture of true zeros and continually distributed positive values. Essentially synonymous with zero-inflated data. [*Journal of the American Statistical Association*, 2001, **96**, 730–45.]

Semi-interquartile range: Half the difference between the upper and lower quartiles. [Altman, D. G., 2018, *Practical Statistics for Medical Research*, Chapman & Hall/CRC, Boca Raton, FL.]

Semi-parametric regression: Regression models that are a compromise between parametric and non-parametric models, which aim to offer the flexibility of the latter whilst retaining a certain amount of the parsimony and structure of the former. The most widely used of such models is the semi-parametric Cox's proportional hazards model in which latent variables are used. [Rupert, D. and Wand, M. P., 2003, *Semiparametric Regression*, Cambridge University Press, Cambridge.]

Sensibility: A term used in the context of constructing scales for measuring clinical phenomena that relates to how appropriate or 'sensible' the proposed scale is likely to be. The qualitative judgements used in the evaluation of the sensibility of a scale include:

- The purpose and framework for which the scale is intended; what are its clinical function, clinical justification and clinical applicability?
- Is the scale comprehensible, simple, thorough and clear in its direction for usage?
- Is the scale aimed at the right thing? Is it put together in the right way?
- Have important variables been omitted from, or unsuitable variables been included in, the scale? Have suitable score ranges and weights been used for the component variables of the scale? How good is the quality of the basic data used in assigning scores?
- How much time and effort are required to obtain and organize the data needed for the scale?

Sensitivity: An index of the performance of a diagnostic test, calculated as the percentage of individuals with a disease who are classified correctly as having the disease, that is, the conditional probability of having a positive test result, given having the disease. A test is sensitive to the disease if it is positive for most individuals having the disease. Achievement of high sensitivity is important when case detection is of primary concern. For example, the ELISA test developed to diagnose HIV infections is said to have a sensitivity of 99.9%. *See also* **Bayes's theorem**, **negative predictive value**, **positive predictive value** and **specificity**. [Altman, D. G., Machin, D., Bryant, T. N. and Gardner, M. J., 2000, *Statistics with Confidence*, 2nd ed., BMJ Books, London.]

Sensitivity analysis: Essentially a series of analysis of a data set to assess whether altering any of the assumptions made leads to different final interpretations or conclusions. Particularly important when dealing with `clinical trials` in which there are `missing values` and various assumptions are posited about the missing data mechanism and how the different assumptions affect inferences about treatments effects. [*Statistics in Biopharmaceutical Research*, 2014, **6**, 338–48.]

Sequential allocation procedures: Procedures for allocating patients to treatments in a `clinical trial` where patients enter the trial sequentially over time. At the time of entry, values of prognostic factors that might influence the outcome of the trial are often known and procedures that utilize this information have received much attention. One of the most widely used of these procedures is permuted block allocation, in which strata are defined in terms of those patients that have the same values of all prognostic factors. In its simplest form, this method will randomly allocate a treatment to an incoming patient when balance exists among the treatments within the stratum to which the patient belongs. If such a balance does not exist then the treatment that will achieve balance will be allocated. A problem is that, at least in principle, an investigator with access to all previous allocations can calculate, for a known set of prognostic factors, the treatment allocation for the next patient and so possibly introduce selection `bias`. [*Statistics in Medicine*, 1986, **5**, 211–29.]

Sequential analysis: A procedure in which a statistical test of significance is conducted repeatedly over time as the data are collected. After each observation, the cumulative data are analyzed and one of the following three decisions is taken:

- Stop the data collection, reject the null hypothesis, and claim statistical significance.
- Stop the data collection, do not reject the null hypothesis, and state that the results are not statistically significant.
- Continue the data collection, since as yet the cumulated data are inadequate to draw a conclusion.

In some cases, namely *open sequential designs*, no provision is made to terminate the trial with the conclusion that there is no difference between the treatments. In others, namely *closed sequential designs*, such a conclusion can be reached. In *group sequential designs*, `interim analyses` are undertaken after each accumulation of a particular number of subjects into the two groups. Suitable values for the number of subjects can be found from the overall significance level, the expected treatment difference, and the required power. [Armitage, P., 1975, *Sequential Medical Trials*, 2nd ed., Blackwell, Oxford.]

Sequential sums of squares: A term encountered primarily in regression analysis for the contributions of variables as they are added to the model in a particular sequence. Essentially, the difference in the residual sum of squares before and after adding a variable. [Rawlings, J. O., Pantula, S. G. and Dickey, D. A., 2013, *Applied Regression Analysis: A Research Tool*, 2nd ed., Springer, New York.]

Serial correlation: The correlation often observed between pairs of measurements on the same subject in a longitudinal study. The magnitude of such correlation often depends on the time separation of the measurements. Typically, the correlation becomes less as the separation increases. The correlation needs to be modelled appropriately in the analysis of such data if correct inferences are to be made. *See also* **mixed-effects models** and **time series**. [Rawlings, J. O., Pantula, S. G. and Dickey, D. A., 2013, *Applied Regression Analysis: A Research Tool*, 2nd ed., Springer, New York.]

Serial dilution assay: A standard microbiological method for estimating the density (average number of organisms per unit volume) in a solution, under the assumptions that:

- The organisms are distributed randomly throughout the solution.
- Each sample from the solution, when incubated in the culture medium, is certain to exhibit fertility whenever the sample contains one or more organisms.

  Maximum likelihood estimation is used to provide an estimate of the solution average organisms per unit volume, which is usually known as the *most probable number*. [*Journal of Microbiological Methods*, 1988, **18**, 91–8.]

Serial interval: The period from the observation of symptoms in one case to the observation of symptoms in a second case infected directly from the first.

Serial measurements: Observations on the same subject collected over time. *See also* **longitudinal data**.

Serological data: Data produced in studies where the presence of antibodies in individuals is investigated using a serological test. For example, the proportion of individuals in different age groups who are seropositive may be recorded. [*Bulletin of the Society for Pathology*, 2000, **93**, 340–7.]

Sex-specific death rate: A death rate calculated separately for men and women. Men have a higher mortality rate than women because of the higher rates they suffer in the leading causes of death, namely cardiovascular and respiratory diseases, cancer and accidents. [*American Journal of Epidemiology*, 2002, **156**, 11–21.]

Sham procedures in medicine: Usually 'pretend' treatments given to a group of patients in a clinical trial against which the real or active therapy is tested. A drug trial, for example, often involves comparison of the active drug and a placebo, both manufactured to look identical. Such procedures become ethically more difficult to defend where surgery is involved; for example, transplanting foetal cells into the brain involves drilling small holes in the patient's head, and in any trial of the procedure such surgery would also be necessary for the control group, who do not actually receive the foetal cells. [*Critical Care Medicine*, 2003, **31**, 5126–30.]

Shelf life: The time interval that a drug product is expected to remain within the approved specifications after manufacture. For example, the shelf life of the drug azuffidine used to treat inflammatory bowel disease is three years.

Shrinkage: The phenomenon that generally occurs when an equation derived from, say, a `multiple linear regression` is applied to a new data set, in which the model predicts much less well than in the original sample. In particular, the value of the `multiple correlation coefficient` becomes less, that is, it 'shrinks'. [*Biometrics*, 1976, **32**, 1–49.]

Sickness absence: Absence from work attributed to medical incapacity.

Sigmoid: A description of a curve having an elongated *S*-shape.

Signed rank test: *See* **Wilcoxon's signed rank test**.

Significance level: The level of probability at which it is agreed that the null hypothesis will be rejected. Conventionally set at 0.05.

Significance test: A statistical procedure that, when applied to a set of observations, results in a `p-value` relative to some hypothesis. Examples include `Student's t-test`, `z-test` and `Wilcoxon's signed rank test`. [Altman, D. G., 2018, *Practical Statistics for Medical Research*, Chapman & Hall/CRC, Boca Raton, FL.]

Sign test: A test of the null hypothesis that positive and negative values among a series of observations are equally likely. The observations are often differences between a response variable observed under two conditions on a set of subjects. [Altman, D. G., 2018, *Practical Statistics for Medical Research*, Chapman & Hall/CRC, Boca Raton, FL.]

Simple random sampling: A form of `sampling design` in which the *n* sampling units are drawn for the population in such a way that every possible combination of the *n* units is equally likely. With this type of sampling design, the probability that the *i*th population unit is included in the sample (the *inclusion probability*) is the same for each unit. [Altman, D. G., 2018, *Practical Statistics for Medical Research*, Chapman & Hall/CRC, Boca Raton, FL.]

Simpson's paradox: The observation that a measure of association between two variables (e.g., type of treatment and outcome) may be identical within the levels of a third variable (e.g., sex) but can take on an entirely different value when the third variable is disregarded, and the association measure calculated from the pooled data. Such a situation can occur only if the third variable is associated with both of the other two variables. As an example, consider the following pair of `two-by-two contingency tables` giving information about amount of prenatal care and survival in two clinics: In both clinics, A and B, the `chi-squared test` for assessing the hypothesis of independence of survival and amount of care leads to

| Clinic A | Amount of care | Died | Infants' survival | |
			Survived	Total
	Less	3	176	179
	More	4	293	279
	Total	7	469	476

| Clinic B | Amount of care | Died | Infants' survival | |
			Survived	Total
	Less	17	197	214
	More	2	23	25
	Total	19	220	239

acceptance of the hypothesis. (In both cases, the statistic is almost zero.) If, however, the data are collapsed over clinics, then the resulting chi-squared statistic takes the value of 5.26, and the conclusion would now be that amount of care and survival are related. *See also* **collapsing categories** and **log-linear models**. [*Journal of the American Statistical Association*, 1993, **88**, 81–8.]

Simulation: The artificial generation of random processes to imitate the behaviour of particular statistical models. *See also* **Monte Carlo methods**. [Kleijnen, J. P. C. and Groenendaal, W., 1992, *Simulation, a Statistical Perspective*, John Wiley & Sons, New York.]

Simultaneous confidence interval: A confidence interval (perhaps more correctly a region) for several parameters being estimated simultaneously, that is, a multivariate parameter. *See also* **multiple comparison tests**. [Miller, R. G., 1981, *Simultaneous Statistical Inference*, 2nd ed., Springer, New York.]

Simultaneous inference: Inferences that involve hypothesis about more than a single parameter, that is, inferences on several parameters simultaneously. *See also* **Wald's test**. [Miller, R. G., 1981, *Simultaneous Statistical Inference*, 2nd ed., Springer, New York.].

Single-blinding: *See* **blinding**.

Single-case study: Synonym for **N of 1 clinical trial**.

Single linkage clustering: A method of cluster analysis in which the distance between two clusters is defined as the least distance between a pair of individuals, one member of the pair being in each group. [Everitt, B. S., Landau, S., Leese, M. and Stahl, D., 2011, *Cluster Analysis*, 5th ed., John Wiley & Sons, Chichester.]

Single-masked: Synonym for **single-blind**.

Single sample *t*-test: *See* **student's *t*-test**.

Distribution with positive skewness.

Distribution with negative skewness.

Figure 80 Examples of skewed distributions.

Singly censored data: Censored observations that occur in clinical trials where all the patients enter the study at the same time point, and where the study is terminated after a fixed time period. *See also* **progressively censored data**.

Sister dependence: The dependence of the times from the division of a mother cell to the division of each of the pair of sister cells created by the mother cell division. [*Cancer Research*, 1987, **47**, 206–9.]

Skewness: The lack of symmetry in a probability or frequency distribution. A distribution is said to have *positive skewness* when it has a long, thin tail at the right and to have *negative skewness* when it has a long thin tail to the left. Examples are shown in Figure 80. *See also* **kurtosis**. [Altman, D. G., 2018, *Practical Statistics for Medical Research*, Chapman & Hall/CRC, Boca Raton, FL.]

Ski-jump distribution: *See* **J-shaped distribution**.

Slope ratio assay: A general class of biological assay, where the dose–response relationship lines for the standard test stimuli are in the form not of two parallel regression lines but of two different lines with different slopes intersecting the ordinate at a point corresponding to zero doses of the stimuli. The relative potency of these stimuli is obtained by taking the ratio of the estimated slopes of the two lines. [Finney, D. J., 1978, *Statistical Methods in Biological Assay*, 3rd ed., Arnold, London.]

Slutzky–Yule effect: The oscillatory series often produced when a moving average is applied to a time series consisting of random observations. [Chatfield, C., 2019, *The Analysis of Time Series: An Introduction*, 7th ed., Chapman & Hall/CRC, Boca Raton, FL.]

Small area estimation: Procedures for using data from national surveys to derive estimates of characteristics of interest at the state or local level. [*Demography*, 1973, **10**, 137–59.]

Small expected frequencies: A term that is found in discussions of the analysis of contingency tables. It arises because the derivation of the chi-squared distribution, as an approximation for the distribution of the chi-squared test when the hypothesis of independence is true, is made under the assumption that the expected frequencies are not too small. Typically, this rather vague phrase has been interpreted as meaning that a satisfactory approximation is achieved only when expected frequencies are five or more. Despite the widespread acceptance of this 'rule', it is nowadays thought to be largely irrelevant, since there is a great deal of evidence that the usual chi-squared test can be used safely when expected frequencies are far smaller. *See also* **exact tests**. [Everitt, B. S., 1992, *The Analysis of Contingency tables*, 2nd ed., Chapman & Hall/CRC, Boca Raton, FL.]

> **Small expected frequencies:** Ignore the recommendation that expected frequencies need to be above five for the chi-squared test to be used, and never apply Yates's correction.

Smear-and-sweep: A method of adjusting death rates for the effects of confounding variables. The procedure is iterative, each iteration consisting of two steps. The first entails 'smearing' the data into a two-way classification based on two of the confounding variables, and the second consists of 'sweeping' the resulting cells into categories according to their ordering on the death rate of interest. [*Journal of Speech and Hearing Research*, 1980, **23**, 814–27.]

Smoothing: The removal of minor fluctuations from a series of observations, usually by applying some form of regression analysis, particularly locally weighted regression. *See also* **generalized additive model** and **moving average**. [Hardle, W., 1990, *Applied Nonparametric Regression*, Cambridge University Press, Cambridge.]

SMR: Acronym for **standardized mortality rate**.

Snedecor's F-distribution: Synonym for **F-distribution**.

Snowball sampling: A method of survey sample selection that is often used to locate rare or difficult-to-find populations. The procedure usually involves two stages:

• The identification of a sample of respondents with a particular characteristic
• Asking initial sample members to provide names of other potential sample members

For example, in sampling heroin addicts, an identified addict would be asked for the names of other addicts that he or she knows. Although the method is relatively low-cost and often effective for locating hard-to-find individuals, little is known about the statistical properties of the resulting samples. [*Sociological Methods and Research*, 1981, **10**, 141–63.]

Snowflakes: A graphical technique for displaying multivariate data. For q variables, a snowflake is constructed by plotting the magnitude of each variable along equiangular rays originating from the same point. Each observation corresponds to

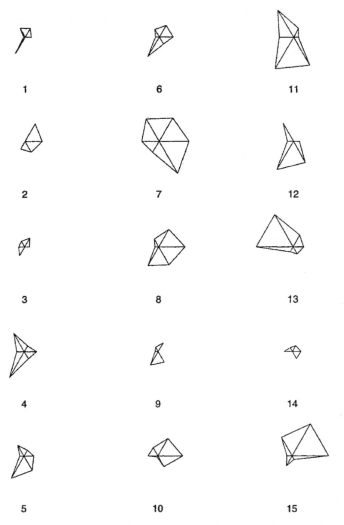

Figure 81 Set of snowflakes for 15 six-dimensional multivariate observations.

a particular-shaped snowflake and these are often displayed side by side for quick visual inspection. An example is shown in Figure 81.

Social classifications: Strata in society composed of individuals and families of equal economic and educational standing. Often needed in studies that aim to describe variations in health or healthcare use according to socioeconomic status. [*Epidemiologic Reviews*, 1988, **10**, 87–121.]

Sojourn time: The interval during which a particular condition is potentially detectable but remains undiagnosed. One example is the period during which a breast tumour is not palpable and has no symptoms but is detectable by mammography. The sojourn time is an important parameter of the potential effectiveness of a screening programme. [*American Journal of Epidemiology*, 1974, **100**, 357–66.]

Somer's d: A measure of association for a `contingency table` with ordered row and column categories that is suitable for the asymmetric case in which one variable is considered the response and one explanatory. *See also* **Kendall's tau statistic**. [Everitt, B. S., 1992, *The Analysis of Contingency Tables*, 2nd ed., Chapman & Hall/CRC, Boca Raton, FL.]

Sources of data: Usually refers to reports and government publications giving, for example, statistics on cancer registrations, number of abortions carried out in particular time periods, or number of deaths from AIDS. Examples of such reports are those provided by the World Health Organization, such as the *World Health Statistics Annual*, which details the seasonal distribution of new cases for about 40 different infectious diseases, and the *World Health Quarterly*, which includes statistics on **mortality** and **morbidity**.

Space–time clustering: An approach to the analysis of epidemics that takes account of three components:

- The time distribution of cases
- The space distribution
- A measure of the space–time interaction

The analysis uses the simultaneous measurement and classification of time and distance intervals between all possible pairs of cases. [*Statistics in Medicine*, 1995, **14**, 2382–92.]

Spatial data: A collection of measurements or observations on one or more variables taken at specified locations and for which the spatial organization of the data is of primary interest. For example, the number of deaths from respiratory cancer in different regions of a country. *See also* **disease cluster**, **disease mapping** and **scan statistic**. [Upton, G. and Fingleton, B., 1985, *Spatial Data Analysis by Example*, volume 1, John Wiley & Sons, Chichester.]

Spearman–Kärber estimator: An estimator of the `median effective dose` in bioassays having a binary variable as a response. [*Technology*, 1977, **11**, 714–19.]

Spearman's rank correlation: A measure of the relationship between two variables that uses only the ranks of the observations on each. In essence, `Pearson's product moment correlation` of the ranks on each of the two variables. [Altman, D. G., 2018, *Practical Statistics for Medical Research*, Chapman & Hall/CRC, Boca Raton, FL.]

Specificity: An index of the performance of a `diagnostic test`, calculated as the percentage of individuals without the disease who are classified as not having the disease, that is, the `conditional probability` of a negative test result given that the disease is absent. A test is specific if it is positive for only a small percentage of those without the disease. For example, the ELISA test developed to diagnose HIV infections is said to have a specificity of 99.9%. *See also* **negative predictive value** and **positive predictive value**. [Altman, D. G., Machin, D., Bryant, T. N. and Gardner, M. J., 2000, *Statistics with Confidence*, 2nd ed., BMJ Books, London.]

Specific variates: *See* **factor analysis**.

Spectral analysis: A procedure for the analysis of the frequencies and periodicities in `time series` data. The time series is effectively decomposed into an infinite number of periodic components, each of infinitesimal amplitude, so the purpose of the analysis is to estimate the contributions of components in certain ranges of frequency. Such an analysis may show that contributions to the fluctuations in the time series come from a continuous range of frequencies, and the pattern of spectral densities may suggest a particular model for the series. Alternatively, the analysis may suggest one or two dominant frequencies. [Chatfield, C., 2019, *The Analysis of Time Series: An Introduction*, 7th ed., Chapman & Hall/CRC, Boca Raton, FL.]

Sphericity: *See* **Mauchly test**.

Split-half method: A procedure used primarily in psychology to estimate the reliability of a test. Two scores are obtained from the same test, either from alternative items, the so-called *odd–even technique*, or from parallel sections of items. The correlation of these scores, or some transformation of them, gives the required reliability. *See also* **Cronbach's alpha**. [Dunn, G., 2004, *Statistical Evaluation of Measurement Errors*, Arnold, London.]

Split-mouth design: A design frequently used in dental `clinical trials` in which a mouth is divided into two or more experimental segments that are randomly assigned to different treatments. Has the advantage of removing a lot of inter-subject variability from the estimated treatment effect. [*Statistical Methods in Medical Research*, 2017, **26**, 2543–51.]

Split-plot design: A term originating in agricultural field experiments, where the division of a testing area or plot into a number of parts permitted the inclusion of an extra factor into the study. In medicine, similar designs occur when the same patient or subject is observed at each level of a factor, or at all combinations of levels of a number of factors. *See also* **longitudinal data**. [*American Statistician*, 1992, **46**, 155–62.]

Spread: Synonym for **dispersion**.

Spreadsheet: A rectangular array of cells, each of which may contain text or numbers or may be empty. The term is derived from the sheet of paper employed by an accountant to set out financial calculations. [*Journal of Medical Systems*, 1990, **14**, 107–17.]

Spurious correlation: A term introduced by Karl Pearson at the end of the nineteenth century to describe the situation in which a correlation is found to exist between two ratios or indices even though the original values are random observations on uncorrelated variables, for example computing rates using the same denominator. Specifically, if two variables X and Y are not related, then the two ratios X/Z and Y/Z will be related. [*Medical Care*, 1997, **35**, 77–92.]

Spurious precision: The tendency to report results to too many significant figures, due largely to copying figures directly from computer output without applying some sensible `rounding`. [*British Medical Journal*, 1998, **316**, 141–4.]

Square contingency table: A `contingency table` with the same number of rows as columns. Such tables arise in rater agreement studies and paired data studies. [Agresti, A., 2019, *An Introduction to Categorical Data Analysis*, John Wiley & Sons, New York.]

Square root transformation: A transformation involving taking the square roots of the original observations. Often used to make random variables suspected to have a `Poisson distribution` more suitable for analysis by techniques such as `analysis of variance`.

Stability analysis: A term usually applied to investigations carried out by pharmaceutical companies to determine the shelf life of their drug products. The procedure generally involves testing various batches of the product at several storage time points.

Staggered entry: A term often applied to studies of survival in which subjects are entered at times related to their own disease history but that are unpredictable from the point of view of the study. [*Annals of Mathematical Statistics*, 1997, **25**, 662–82.]

Staircase method: Synonym for **up-and-down method**.

Standard curve: The curve that relates the responses in an assay given by a range of standard solutions to their known concentrations. It permits the analytical concentration of an unknown solution to be inferred from its assay response by interpolation.

Standard design: Synonym for **Fibonacci dose-escalation scheme**.

Standard deviation (SD): The most commonly used measure of the spread of a set of observations. Equal to the square root of the `variance`. [Altman, D. G., 2018, *Practical Statistics for Medical Research*, Chapman & Hall/CRC, Boca Raton, FL.]

Standard error (SE): The standard deviation of an estimator or sample statistic. For example, the standard error of the sample mean of n observations is $\sigma/\sqrt{n}$, where σ^2 is the variance of the original observations. [Altman, D. G., 2018, *Practical Statistics for Medical Research*, Chapman & Hall/CRC, Boca Raton, FL.]

Standardization: A term used in a variety of ways in medical research. The most common usage is in the context of transforming a variable by dividing by its standard deviation to give a new variable with standard deviation unity. Also often used for the process of producing an index of mortality, which is adjusted for the age distribution in a particular group being examined. *See also* **standardized mortality rate**, **indirect standardization** and **direct standardization**.

Standardized mortality rate (SMR): The number of deaths, either total or cause-specific, in a given population, expressed as a percentage of the deaths that would have been expected if the age- and sex-specific rates in a 'standard' population had applied. In Canada in 2002, for example, the age-standardized mortality rate from all causes of death for men was 816.5 deaths per 100,000 population. The corresponding figure for women was 505.4 deaths. [Everitt, B. S. and Palmer, C. (eds.), 2011, *Encyclopedic Companion to Medical Statistics*, 2nd ed., John Wiley & Sons, Chichester.]

Standardized regression coefficient: *See* **beta coefficient**.

Standardized residual: *See* **residual**.

Standard normal distribution: A `normal distribution` with zero mean and unit variance.

Standard normal variable: A random variable having a `standard normal distribution`.

Standard scores: Variable values transformed to zero mean and unit variance.

Standards for Reporting of Diagnostic Accuracy (STARD): A checklist for reporting studies of diagnostic tests, arrived at by consensus of a large group of experts including statisticians and editors of medical journals. The checklist includes descriptions of populations and samples, the criteria for recruitment, expertise of the testers, etc. [*Clinical Chemistry*, 2003, **49**, 1–6.]

STARD: Abbreviation for **Standards for Reporting of Diagnostic Accuracy.**

Stationary series: A `time series` with mean and variance that are independent of time. The behaviour and appearances of such series, in stretches of sufficient length, are statistically identical. [Chatfield, C., 2019, *The Analysis of Time Series: An Introduction*, 7th ed., Chapman & Hall/CRC, Boca Raton, FL.]

Statistic: A numerical characteristic of a sample, for example the sample mean and sample variance. *See also* **parameter**.

Statistical software: A set of computer programs for performing a variety of statistical analyses and data manipulation operations. Widely used examples include:
- R
- SPSS: www.spss.com/
- SAS: www.sas.com/
- S-PLUS: www.insightful.com/
- STATA: www.stata.com/

Statistical surveillance: The continual observation of a `time series` with the goal of detecting an important change in the underlying process as soon as possible after it has occurred. An example of where such a procedure is of considerable importance is in monitoring foetal heart rate during labour. [*International Statistical Review*, 2003, **71**, 403–34.]

Statistician: A mathematician manqué who has abandoned the provable in favour of the probable. A being with the brain of an accountant and the soul of a philatelist. A charmless drudge. *Guernsey McPearson*.

A little harsh perhaps?

Steady state: A property of an `open population` where the number of people entering the population is balanced by the number exiting the population in any period of time within levels of age, sex and other determinants of risk.

Stem-and-leaf plot: A method of displaying data in which each observation is split into two parts, labelled the stem and the leaf, for example tens and units. The stems are arranged in a column, and the leaves are attached to the relevant stem. The resulting display gives the shape information usually provided by a histogram, whilst retaining the original observation values. Figure 82 shows an example. [Altman, D. G., 2018, *Practical Statistics for Medical Research*, Chapman & Hall/ CRC, Boca Raton, FL.]

Stepped wedge design: A design for a clinical trial in which patients start with the placebo, but at certain predefined time points one patient or a portion of the patients switches from placebo to the new treatment and remains on this treatment until the end of the study. The allocation of patients to treatment switches is random. This design is a special case of a crossover design but with treatment switches in one direction. [*Contemporary Clinical Trials*, 2007, **28**, 182–91.]

Stepwise regression: *See* selection methods in regression.

Stillbirth rate: The number of stillbirths divided by the number of live births and stillbirths in the same time period. Usually expressed per 1000 total births per year. The following table gives the rates for England, Wales, Scotland and Northern Ireland for both 1971 and 1992:[*Central African Journal of Medicine*, 1996, **42**, 89–92.]

	1971	1992
England	12.4	4.2
Wales	14.2	4.1
Scotland	13.1	5.4
Northern Ireland	14.3	4.7

Stochastic curtailment: A data monitoring technique for clinical trials in which power is recalculated as the trial progresses taking into consideration the data already observed (so-called *conditional power*). [Ellenberg, S. S., Fleming, T. R. and DeMets, D. L., 2002, *Data Monitoring Committees in Clinical Trials*, John Wiley & Sons, New York.]

Stochastic process: A series of random variables describing an empirical process whose development is governed by probability laws usually in time but sometimes in space and possibly even in both space and time. Examples in medicine include the development of epidemics and chronic diseases. [Chang, C. L., 1980, *An Introduction to Stochastic Processes and Their Applications*, Kneger, New York.]

Stopping rules: Procedures that allow interim analyses in clinical trials at predefined times, whilst preserving the type I error at some prespecified level.

```
14 : 2
14 : 555
14 : 67777
14 : 889
15 : 000000111111
15 : 222222222222333333333333333333
15 : 444444444444555555555555555555555
15 : 666666666666666666666677777777777777777777
15 : 88888888888888888888888888888889999999999999999
16 : 00000000000000000000011111111111111111111
16 : 22222222222222222233333333333333333333333333333
16 : 44444444444444444455555555555555555
16 : 666666666667777777
16 : 88888899999999
17 : 00000000000111
17 : 333
17 : 4
17 : 67
17 : 88
```

Figure 82 Stem-and-leaf diagram for the heights of 349 elderly women.

See also **sequential analysis**. [Armitage, P., 1975, *Sequential Medical Trials*, 2nd ed., Blackwell, Oxford.]

Stop screen design: *See* **screening studies**.

Strata: *See* **stratification**.

Stratification: The division of a population into parts known as strata, particularly for the purpose of drawing a sample, for example a population of patients stratified by GP practice attended. Stratification increases the efficiency of a `sampling design` with respect to count and estimator precision. [Thompson, S. K., 1992, *Sampling*, John Wiley & Sons, New York.]

Stratified analysis: A method for assessing the effect of a variable or risk factor on an outcome, while keeping another variable constant. For example, investigating the effect of smoking behaviour on death from lung cancer separately for men and women.

Stratified Cox's regression model: A model that can be used for the analysis of clustered time-to-event data, for example, when the data for each individual can be clustered into units such as clinics or families. [Gibbons, R. D. and Amatya, A. K., 2016, *Statistical Methods for Drug Safely*, CRC Press, Boca Raton, FL.]

Stratified medicine: Essentially a synonym for **precision medicine**.

Stratified log-rank test: A method for comparing the survival experience of two groups of subjects given different treatments, when the groups are stratified by age or some other prognostic variable. [Collett, D., 2015, *Modelling Survival Data in Medical Research*, 3rd ed., Chapman & Hall/CRC, Boca Raton, FL.]

Stratified randomization: A procedure designed to allocate patients to treatments in `clinical trials` to achieve approximate balance of important characteristics, without sacrificing the advantages of random allocation. *See also* **minimization**. [Gibbons, R. D. and Amatya, A. K., 2016, *Statistical Methods for Drug Safely*, CRC, Boca Raton, FL.]

Stratified random sampling: Random sampling from each strata of a population after stratification. [Foremann, E. K., 1991, *Survey Sampling Principles*, Marcel Dekker, New York.]

Stroke index: A global measure of disease activity in rheumatoid arthritis. The index is based on two objective laboratory measurements, one subjective clinical measurement and two semi-objective clinical measurements, chosen from 13 possibilities by using clinical judgement. [*Medicine and Science in Sports and Exercise*, 2002, **34**, 637–42.]

Structural equation modelling: A procedure that combines aspects of multiple linear regression and factor analysis to investigate relationships between latent variables and manifest variables. *See also* **path analysis**. [Bollen, K. A., 1989, *Structural Equations with Latent Variables*, John Wiley & Sons, New York.]

> **Structural equation modelling:** It is important to remember that even with such sophisticated models, correlation still does not necessarily imply causation.

Structural zeros: Zero frequencies occurring in the cells of contingency tables, which arise because it is theoretically impossible for an observation to fall in this cell. For example, if male and female students are asked about health problems that cause them concern, then the cell corresponding to, say, menstrual problems for men will have a zero entry. *See also* **incomplete contingency tables** and **sampling zeros**. [Agresti, A., 2019, *An Introduction to Categorical Data Analysis*, John Wiley & Sons, New York.]

Stuart–Maxwell test: A test of marginal homogeneity in a square contingency table. [Everitt, B. S., 1992, *The Analysis of Contingency Tables*, 2nd ed., Chapman & Hall/CRC, Boca Raton, FL.]

Studentization: The removal of a nuisance parameter by constructing a statistic whose sampling distribution does not depend on that parameter. [Cox, D. R., 2006, *Principles of Statistical Inference*, Cambridge University Press, Cambridge.]

Student's *t*-distribution: The probability distribution of the ratio of a standard normal variable to the square root of a variable with a chi-squared distribution. In particular, the distribution of the test statistics used in all forms of student's t-test. The distribution is bell-shaped and depends on the value of a single parameter. Some examples are shown in Figure 83. [Altman, D. G., 2018, *Practical Statistics for Medical Research*, Chapman & Hall/CRC, Boca Raton, FL.]

Student's *t*-test: Significance test for assessing a hypothesis about population means. One version is used in situations where it is required to test whether the mean of a population takes a particular value. This is generally known as a *single-sample t-test*.

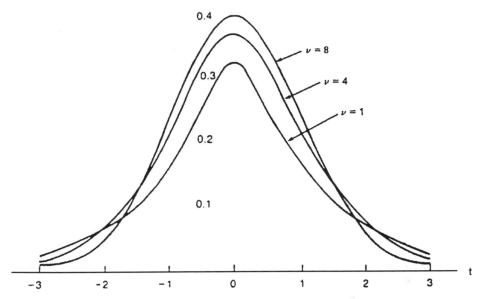

Figure 83 Examples of Student's *t*-distributions for various parameter values.

Another version is designed to test the equality of the means of two populations given independent samples from each, and is known as the *independent-samples t-test*. The latter assumes normality for each population and equality of population variances but is known to be relatively robust to moderate departures from either assumption. *See also* **matched-pairs *t*-test**. [Altman, D. G., 2018, *Practical Statistics for Medical Research*, Chapman & Hall/CRC, Boca Raton, FL.]

Sturdy statistics: Synonym for **robust statistics**.

Subgroup analysis: The analysis of particular subgroups of patients in a `clinical trial` to assess possible treatment–subgroup interactions. An investigator may, for example, want to understand whether a drug affects older patients differently from those who are younger. Essentially an investigation of possibly interesting *treatment × covariate interactions*. Analyzing many subgroupings for treatment effects can greatly increase overall `type I error` rates. *See also* **fishing expedition**. [*Controlled Clinical Trials*, 1989, **10**, 187S–94S.]

Subgroup analysis: According to Professor Stephen Senn, an aimless dredge.

Subjective endpoints: Endpoints in `clinical trials` that can be measured only by subjective clinical rating scales. [*Journal of Antimicrobiological Chemotherapy*, 1998, **41**, 467–86.]

Subjective probability: Synonym for **personal probability**.

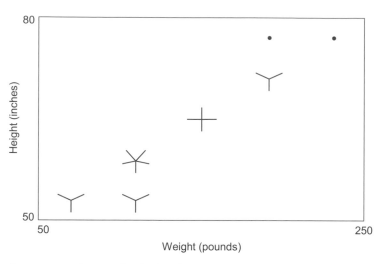

Figure 84 Sunflower plot for height and weight.

Sufficient statistic: A statistic that, in a certain sense, summarizes all the information contained in a sample of observations about a particular parameter. [Cox, D. R., 2006, *Principles of Statistical Inference*, Cambridge University Press, Cambridge.]

Summary measure analysis of longitudinal data: Synonym for **response feature analysis**.

Sunflower plot: A modification of the usual scatter diagram, designed to reduce the problem of overlap caused by multiple points at one position (particularly if the data have been rounded to integers). The scatterplot is first partitioned with a grid and the number of points in each cell of the grid is counted. If there is only a single point in a cell, then a dot is plotted at the centre of the cell. If there is more than one observation in a cell, then a sunflower icon is drawn on which the number of petals is equal to the number of points falling in that cell. An example is shown in Figure 84. [*Journal of the American Statistical Association*, 1984, **79**, 807–22.]

Supervised pattern recognition: *See* **pattern recognition**.

Suppressor variables: A variable in a regression analysis that is not correlated with the dependent variable but that is still useful for increasing the size of the multiple correlation coefficient by virtue of its correlations with other explanatory variables. The variable suppresses variance that is irrelevant to prediction of the dependent variable. [Lord, F. M. and Novick, M. R., 1968, *Statistical Theories of Mental Test Scores*, Addison-Wesley, Reading, MA.]

Surface models: A term used for those models for screening studies that consider only those events that can be observed directly, such as disease incidence rate, prevalence and mortality. *See also* **deep models**.

Surrogate endpoints: A term often encountered in discussions of clinical trials to refer to an outcome measure that an investigator considers is correlated highly with an endpoint of interest, but that can be measured at lower expense or at an earlier time. In some cases, ethical issues may suggest the use of a surrogate.

Examples include measurement of blood pressure as a surrogate for cardiovascular mortality, measurement of lipid levels as a surrogate for arteriosclerosis, and, in cancer studies, measurement of time to relapse as a surrogate for total survival time. Considerable controversy in interpretation can be generated when doubts arise about the correlation of the surrogate endpoint with the endpoint of interest, or over whether the surrogate endpoint should be considered as an endpoint of primary interest in its own right. The main danger of the use of surrogates is that they may not capture the combined risk–benefit of a treatment. [*Annals of Internal Medicine*, 1996, **125**, 605–13.]

Surrogate endpoints: Surrogate outcomes should only be used when it is certain that they are valid substitutes for the real outcome.

Surrogate observation: An observed variable that relates in some way to the variable of primary importance, which cannot itself be conveniently observed directly. *See also* **latent variable**.

Surveillance of disease: The continued watchfulness over the distributions and trends of disease incidence through the systematic collection, consolidation and evaluation of morbidity and mortality reports and other relevant data, with the aim of applying these data to prevention and control. In general, the observed number of cases of different types during a specified time interval is evaluated, and the question asked as to whether an increase (or decrease) has occurred which can signal that something has changed the risk situation in the population of interest. A statistical technique such as the cusum is used to compare the observed numbers during a surveillance process with the baseline data. [*Lancet*, 1995, **346**, 196.]

Survey: An investigation that collects planned information from individuals about their history, habits, knowledge, attitudes or behaviour. A health survey, for example, might include questions about smoking habits and exercise, as well as a variety of demographic and socioeconomic characteristics. [Hunt, S. M., McEwan, J. and McKenna, S. P., 1986, *Measuring Health Status*, Croom Helm, London.]

Survival curve: *See* **survival function**.

Survival function: The probability that the survival time of an individual is longer than some particular value. A plot of this probability against time is called a *survival curve* and is a useful component in the analysis of such data. *See also* **product limit estimator** and **hazard function**. [Collett, D., 2015, *Modelling Survival Data in Medical Research*, 3rd ed., Chapman & Hall/CRC, Boca Raton, FL.]

Survival time: Observations of the time until the occurrence of a particular event, for example recovery, improvement or death. Such data need special forms of analysis to deal with both possible skewness and censoring of the observations. *See also*

Cox's proportional hazards model. [Collett, D., 2015, *Modelling Survival Data in Medical Research*, 3rd ed., Chapman & Hall/CRC, Boca Raton, FL.]

Survivor function: Synonym for **survival function**.

Suspended rootogram: Synonym for **hanging rootogram**.

Switching effect: The effect on estimates of treatment differences of patient's changing treatments in a `clinical trial`. Such changes of treatment are often allowed in, for example, cancer trials, due to lack of efficacy and/or disease progression. [*Statistics in Medicine*, 2005, **24**, 1783–90.]

Symmetrical distribution: A `probability distribution` or frequency distribution that is symmetrical about some central value. The `normal distribution` is a well-known example, being symmetrical around its mean value.

Symmetrical matrix: A square matrix that is symmetrical about its leading diagonal, that is, a matrix with elements a_{ij} such that $a_{ij} = a_{ji}$. In statistics, `correlation matrices` and `variance-covariance matrices` are of this form.

Symmetry in square contingency tables: *See* **Bowker's test for symmetry**.

Symptom checklist: A brief multidimensional self-report inventory designed to screen for a broad range of psychological problems and symptoms of psychopathology. It can be useful in the initial evaluation of patients as an objective method of screening for psychological problems and to measure patient progress during treatment. *See also* **general health questionnaire**.

Syndromic Surveillance: The ongoing, systematic collection, analysis, interpretation and application of real-time indicators of diseases and outbreaks that allow for their detection. The surveillance is based on the ongoing, routine collection of 'health-related' data and aggregate laboratory test results, which is generally collected for some purpose other than surveillance. The data and associated surveillance are intended to provide leading indicators that precede diagnosis or case confirmation with the goal of providing early warning of an outbreak. [*Biosecurity and Bioterrorism: Biodefense Strategy, Practice and Science*, 2012, **1**, 247–53.]

Synergism: A term used when the joint effect of two treatments is greater than the sum of their effects when administered separately (*positive synergism*), or when the sum of their effects is less than when administered separately (*negative synergism* or *antagonism*). [*American Journal of Epidemiology*, 1978, **108**, 60–7.]

Systematic allocation: Procedures for allocating treatments to patients in a `clinical trial` that attempt to emulate random allocation by using some systematic scheme, such as giving treatment *A* to those people with even birth dates and giving treatment *B* to those with odd birth dates. Whilst unbiased in principle, problems arise because of the openness of the allocation system and the consequent possibility of abuse.

Systematic error: The `bias` that results when a data-collecting procedure or a method of analysis leads to results deviating from the true quantity to be estimated. Unlike random error, systematic error is not dealt with by increasing sample size; this serves only to obtain more precise biased estimates of the desired quantity.

Systematic review: A review of all studies conforming to a set of criteria and relating to a particular research question of interest. Particularly important in investigating the results from `clinical trials`. The most important aspects of such a review are how to choose the studies to be included and how to ensure that all relevant (and acceptable) studies are included. Once all selected studies are available, then the next stage generally involves a `meta-analysis` of the `effect sizes` extracted from each. *See also* **forest plot**. [Chalmers, I. and Altman, D., 1995, *Systematic Reviews*, British Medical Journal Publishing, London.]

Tango's index: An index for summarizing the occurrences of cases of disease in a stable geographical unit where the occurrences are grouped into discrete intervals. Can be used to detect `disease clusters` occurring over time. *See also* **ratchet scan statistic** and **scan statistic**. [*Statistics in Medicine*, 1993, **12**, 1813–28.]

Target population: The collection of individuals, items, measurements, etc. about which it is required to make inferences. Often, the population that is actually sampled differs from the target population, which may result in misleading conclusions being made. For example, if an investigator is interested in some aspect of characterizing the natural history of rheumatoid arthritis, then the target population will be all patients with the disease. If, however, the investigator examines only those cases arising from, say, the records office of a large university hospital, then it is likely that selective factors will cause the population that is actually sampled to differ from the target population for a number of reasons, including the fact that rheumatoid arthritis does not always require hospitalization. [Colton, T., 1974, *Statistics in Medicine*, Little, Brown & Company, Boston, MA.]

TD50: Abbreviation for **tumorigenic dose 50**.

Telephone sampling: The use of a telephone for sample survey data collection. Telephone surveys are commonly used in market research, primarily because good samples can be achieved at reasonable cost. Sampling can be via directories, which can lead to `bias` because many households are unlisted, or random digit dialling, in which random four digit numbers in known exchanges are generated to assure that both listed and unlisted households are included. [Laurakas, P. J., 1987, *Telephone Survey Methods: Sampling, Selection and Supervision*, Sage Publications, Thousand Oaks, CA.]

Test–retest reliability: An index of score consistency over a brief time period, typically several weeks, usually simply the `correlation coefficient` calculated between administration of the test twice with a certain amount of time between administrations. [*Medical Care Research and Review*, 2002, **59**, 184–96.]

Test statistic: A statistic used to assess a particular hypothesis in relation to some population. The essential requirement of such a statistic is a known `sampling distribution` when the null hypothesis is true. [Altman, D., 2018, Practical *Statistics for Medical Research*, Chapman & Hall/CRC, Boca Raton, FL.]

Tetrachoric correlation: An estimate of the correlation between two random variables having a `bivariate normal distribution`, obtained from the information from a double dichotomy of their bivariate distribution, that is, four counts giving the number of observations above and below a particular value for each variable. For example, height and weight of a sample of individuals might only be recorded in terms of the numbers of people above and below some particular value on each variable. The tetrachoric correlation can be estimated by `maximum likelihood estimation`. [Everitt, B. S. and Palmer, C. (eds.), 2011, *Encyclopedic Companion to Medical Statistics*, 2nd ed., John Wiley & Sons, Chichester.]

The popularity paradox: The greater the harm through overdiagnosis and overtreatment from `screening studies`, the more people there are who believe they owe their health, or even their life, to the programme. [Raffle, A. and Gray, M., 2007, *Screening: Evidence and Practice*, Oxford University Press, Oxford.]

Therapeutic ratio: The ratio of efficacy response over toxicity response. High values indicate that a treatment is beneficial with only a small chance of toxicity. A quantitative measure of the relative safety of a drug. [*Nature Reviews, Drug Discovery*, 2012, **11**, 751–61.]

Therapeutic trial: Synonym for **clinical trial**.

Therapeutic window: The prescribable dose range in which a treatment's benefits may outweigh its side effects. [*Neurology*, 1998, **50**, 599–603.]

Three-group resistant line: A method of `linear regression` that is resistant to `outliers` and observations with large `influence`. Basically, the method involves dividing the data into three groups and then finding the median of each group. A straight line is then fitted through these medians. [*Crop Science*, 2001, **41**, 1931–9.]

Three-period crossover design: A design in which two treatments, *A* and *B* are given to subjects in the order *A*, *B*, *B* or *B*, *A*, *A*. Two sequence groups are formed by random allocation. The additional third observation period alleviates many of the problems associated with the analysis of the usual form of the `crossover design` having only two observations on each participant. In particular, an appropriate three-period crossover design allows for use of all the data to estimate and test direct treatment effects, even when `carry-over effects` are present. [*Statistics in Medicine*, 1996, **15**, 127–44.]

Threshold-crossing data: Measurements of the time when some variable of interest crosses a threshold value. Because patient examinations occur only periodically, the exact time of crossing the threshold is often unknown. In such cases, it is known only that the time falls within a specified interval, so the observation is an `interval-censored` observation. [*Statistics in Medicine*, 1993, **12**, 1589–603.]

Threshold limit value: The maximum permissible concentration of a chemical compound present in the air within a working area (as a gas, vapour or particulate matter), which, according to current knowledge, generally does not impair the health of employees or cause undue annoyance. For example, the currently applied value for organophosphorous pesticides is 10 mg/m^3.

Threshold model: A model that postulates that an effect occurs only above some threshold value, for example a model that assumes that the effect of a drug is zero below some critical dose level. Also used as a synonym for `genetic liability` model.

Tietze–Potter method: A procedure for estimating the net `discontinuation rates` in studies of the effectiveness of contraceptives. [*Statistics in Medicine*, 1986, **5**, 475–89.]

Time-by-time analysis of longitudinal data: The separate analysis of the available data at each time point in a longitudinal study, for example a series of `Student's t-tests` to assess the differences between two treatments means at each time point in a `clinical trial`. A flawed method since at no stage does this analysis use the information that indicates which observations are from the same individual.

Consequently, the standard errors used will be based, incorrectly, on between-subject variation. [Everitt, B. S. and Pickles, A., 2004, *Statistical Aspects of the Design and Analysis of Clinical Trials*, Imperial College Press, London.]

> **Time-by-time analysis of longitudinal data:** Should be used only rarely as far better methods for analyzing longitudinal data are now readily available.

Time-dependent covariates: Covariates whose values change over time, as opposed to covariates whose values remain constant over time (*time-independent covariates*). A pretreatment measurement of some characteristic is an example of the latter; age and weight are examples of the former.

Time-independent covariates: *See* **time-dependent covariates**.

Time series: Values of a variable recorded, usually at a regular interval, over a long period of time. The observed movement and fluctuations of many such series are composed of four different components: `secular trend`, `seasonal variation`, `cyclical variation` and irregular variation. An example from medicine is the `incidence` of a disease recorded yearly over a period of time (see Figure 85). Such data usually require special methods for their analysis because of the presence of `serial correlation` between the separate observations. *See also* **autocorrelation** and **spectral analysis**. [Chatfield, C., 2019, *The Analysis of Times Series: An Introduction*, 7th ed., Chapman & Hall/CRC, Boca Raton, FL.]

Time-to-event variable: Quintessentially a synonym for **survival time**.

Time trade-off technique: *See* **Von Neumann–Morgenstern standard gamble**.

Time-varying covariates: Synonym for **time-dependent covariates**.

Titration study: An investigation in which a patient receives a higher dose of a compound according to a set of predetermined rules if he or she fails to achieve a satisfactory

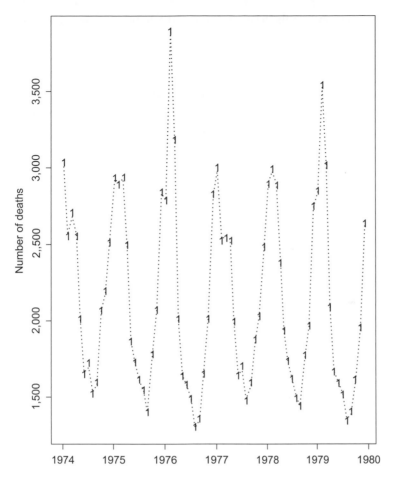

Figure 85 Time series of monthly deaths from lung cancer in the United Kingdom in the period 1974–9.

response at the current dose level and has not had any unacceptable reaction to the drug. Definition of a response is usually in terms of some objective physiological measurement, for example the reduction of blood pressure below a certain level. Such a study might be used, for example, to investigate whether a dose of some drug of interest can be found to treat cancer pain adequately. [*Journal of Human Hypertension*, 2001, **15**, 475–80.]

T_{max}: A measure traditionally used to compare treatments in `bioequivalence trials`. The measure is simply the time at which a patient's highest recorded value occurs. *See also* C_{max}, **area under curve** and **response feature analysis**.

Tobit model: A type of censored regression model. [*Econometrica*, 1958, **26**, 24–36.]

Tobit regression model: Measures of substance concentration in urine, serum, etc. often have an assay limit of detection. When concentration levels fall below this limit, the exact measures cannot be obtained; instead the measures are censored as only

partial information that the levels are under the limit is known. Tobit regression models are often used to analyze such data. [*American Journal of Epidemiology*, 2014, **179**, 1018–24.]

Tolerance: A term used in `stepwise regression` for the proportion of the sum of squares about the mean of an explanatory variable not accounted for by other variables already included in the regression equation. Small values indicate possible `multicollinearity` problems. *See also* **variance inflation factor**. [Rawlings, J. O., Pantula, S. G. and Dickey, D. A., 2013, *Applied Regression Analysis: A Research Tool*, 2nd ed., Springer, New York.]

Tolerance interval: Statistical intervals that contain at least a specified proportion of a population either on average or with a stated confidence value. Used to summarize uncertainty about values of a random variable, usually a future value. *See also* **reference interval**. [Guttman, I., 1970, *Statistical Tolerance Regions*, Hafner, Darien, CT.]

Total fertility rate: The average number of children that would be born per woman if all women lived to the end of their childbearing years and bore children according to a given set of age-specific fertility rates. An important fertility measure that provides an accurate answer to the question of how many children a woman has, on average. For example, in 2001, in Afghanistan the figure was 5.79 children per woman and in Belgium it was 1.61 children per woman. Although still high in many parts of the world, total fertility rates have been declining rapidly over the last decade. [*World Population Review*, 2020.]

Total sum of squares: The sum of the squared deviations of all the observations from their mean.

Townsend index: An index designed to measure material deprivation of an area. The index is calculated as an unweighted sum of four standardized census variables corresponding to area-level proportions of unemployment, car ownership, crowding and home ownership. [*International Journal of Health Services*, 1985, **15**, 637–63.]

Tracking: A term sometimes used in discussions of `longitudinal data` to describe the ability to predict subsequent observations from earlier values. Informally, this implies that subjects that have, for example, the largest values of the response variable at the start of the study tend to continue to have the larger values. More formally, a population is said to track with respect to a particular observable characteristic if, for each individual, the expected value of the relevant deviation from the population mean remains unchanged over time. [Everitt, B. S. and Pickles, A., 2004, *Statistical Aspects of the Design and Analysis of Clinical Trials*, revised ed., Imperial College Press, London.]

Training set: *See* **discriminant analysis**.

Transformation: A change in the scale of measurement of some variable(s). Examples are the `square root transformation` and `logarithmic transformation`. Generally applied to allow the observations to satisfy more clearly the assumptions

1.0
0.95

0.8

0.6

Power

0.4

0.2

0

50%   60%   70%   80%   90%   100%

Percentage of patients on the new treatment

Figure 86 Treatment allocation ratio influences the power of a study. The diagram shows a reduction in power as the proportion of participants on the new treatment is increased. (Taken from *Clinical Trials* by S. J. Pocock with the permission of the publisher Wiley.)

needed by some statistical technique to be applied to the data. [Altman, D., 2018, Practical *Statistics for Medical Research*, Chapman & Hall/CRC, Boca Raton, FL.]

Transition models: *See* conditional regression models.

Translational medicine: A term that describes research wherein a basic laboratory discovery becomes applicable to the diagnosis, treatment or prevention of a specific disease, that is, the translation of basic research discoveries into clinical applications. [Chow, S.-C., 2011, *Controversial Statistical Issues in Clinical Trials*, CRC, Boca Raton, FL.]

Transmission probability: A term used primarily in investigations of the spread of AIDS for the probability of contracting infection from an HIV-infected partner in one intercourse. [*American Journal of Epidemiology*, 2002, **155**, 159–68.]

Transmission rate: The rate at which an infectious disease agent is spread through the environment or to another person.

Treatment allocation ratio: The ratio of the number of subjects allocated to the two treatments in a `clinical trial`. Equal allocation is most common in practice, but it may be advisable to allocate patients randomly in other ratios when comparing a new treatment with an old treatment, or when one treatment is much more difficult or expensive to administer. The change of detecting a real difference between the two treatments is not reduced much as long as the ratio is not more extreme than 2:1, as can be seen in Figure 86. [Pocock, S. J., 1983, *Clinical Trials*, John Wiley & Sons, Chichester.]

Treatment × covariate interaction: *See* **subgroup analysis**.

Treatment cross-contamination: Any instance in which a patient assigned to receive a particular treatment in a `clinical trial` is exposed to one of the other treatments during the course of the trial. [*Journal of Prosthetic Dentistry*, 1983, **49**, 576.]

Treatment period interaction: Synonym for **carry-over effect**.

Treatment received analysis: Analyzing the results of a `clinical trial` by the treatment received by a patient rather than by the treatment allocated at randomization as in `intention-to-treat analysis`. Not to be recommended because patient `compliance` is very likely to be related to outcome. [*Statistics in Medicine*, 1991, **10**, 1595–605.]

Treatment switching: Describes a situation in a randomized `clinical trial` where patients switch from their randomly assigned treatment onto an alternative, generally from the control group on to the experimental treatment. Such switching is most common in clinical trials of cancer treatments primarily for ethical reasons. The analysis of trials in which switching has occurred is always not straightforward because a standard `intention-to-treat analysis` does not measure the comparative effectiveness of the treatment due to the control group being contaminated by the experimental treatment. [*Medical Decision Making*, 2014, **34**, 387–402.]

Treatment trial: Synonym for **clinical trial**.

Trend: Movement in one direction of the values of a variable over a period of time.

Triangular test: A term used for a particular type of closed sequential design in which the boundaries that control the procedure have the shape of a triangle. [*Statistics in Medicine*, 1994, **13**, 1357–68.]

Trim and fill method: An attempt to achieve a more objective approach to the interpretation of a `funnel plot`, that imputes estimates of `effect sizes` for studies thought to have been included from a `meta-analysis`. [*Journal of the American Statistical Association*, 2000, **95**, 89–98.]

Trimmed mean: *See* **alpha-trimmed mean**.

Triple scatterplot: Synonym for **bubble plot**.

Trohoc study: A term used occasionally for retrospective study, derived from spelling cohort backwards. To be avoided at all costs!

Trough-to-peak ratio: A measure used most often in `clinical trials` of antihypertensive drugs and their effect on blood pressure. The latter usually achieves a maximum (the peak effect) and then decreases to a minimum (the trough effect). The `Food and Drug Administration` recommends that the ratio of peak to trough should be at least 0.5. Statistical properties of the ratio are complicated by the known correlation of trough and peak values. [*Journal of Hypertension*, 2001, **19**, 703–11.]

Truncated data: Data for which sample values larger (truncated on the right) or smaller (truncated on the left) than a fixed value either are not recorded or are not observed.

***t*-test:** *See* **student's *t*-test.**

Two-phase studies: In public health and medical research, it is often the case that certain necessary data elements are too expensive or time-consuming to collect on all participants. In such cases a two-phase approach may be used; at phase one it is assumed that certain covariates are available for all participants. Some of these covariates are then used to stratify the phase one sample. Then within each phase one strata, a subsample of participants is identified, and the expensive measures collected, forming the phase two data. Estimation and inference given data from a two-phase study is well established and described in the reference. [*Statistics in Medicine*, 1991, **10**, 739–47.]

Tumorigenic dose 50 (TD50): The daily dose of a compound required to halve the probability of remaining tumourless at the end of a standardized lifetime. [*Annals of Neurology*, 2001, **50**, 458–62.]

Tumour lethality function: A term used in animal tumorigenicity experiments for the ratio of the death rates for tumour-bearing and tumour-free animals. [*Journal of the Royal Statistical Society, C*, 2000, **49**, 157.]

Turnbull estimator: A method for estimating the survival function for a set of survival times when the data contain `interval-censored` observations. *See also* **product limit estimator**. [*Journal of the Royal Statistical Society, Series B*, 1976, **38**, 290–5.]

Twin analysis: The analysis of data on identical and fraternal twins to make inferences about the extent and overlaps of genetic involvement in the determinants of one or more traits. Such analysis usually makes the assumption that the shared environment experiences relevant to the traits in question are equally important for both types of twin. [Sham, P., 1998, *Statistics in Human Genetics*, Arnold, London.]

Twin concordance: Synonymous with **concordance**.

TWiST: A quality-of-life-oriented endpoint for comparing therapies given by the time without symptoms of disease and toxicity of treatment. Calculated for each patient by subtracting from the overall time to symptomatic disease relapse any previous time that the patient experiences treatment toxicity. [*Quality of Life Research*, 2002, **11**, 37–45.]

Two-armed bandit allocation: A procedure for forming treatment groups in a `clinical trial`, in which the probability of assigning a patient to a particular treatment is a function of the observed difference in outcomes of patients already enrolled in the trial. The motivation behind the procedure is to ensure more ethical allocation of patients while retaining a given probability of selecting correctly the better treatment at the end of the trial. *See also* **minimization** and **play-the-winner rule**. [*Journal of the Royal Statistical Society, Series D*, 1978, **27**, 97–102.]

	Variable 1	
	0	1
Variable 2 0	A	b
1	C	d

For example, smoking and age

	Age	
Amount of smoking	Under 40	Over 40
Less than 20 cigarettes per day	50	15
More than 20 cigarettes per day	10	25

Two-by-two (2 × 2) contingency table: A `contingency table` with two rows and two columns formed from cross-classifying two `binary variables`. The general form of such a table is: [Everitt, B. S., 1992, *The Analysis of Contingency Tables*, 2nd ed., Chapman & Hall/CRC, Boca Raton, FL.]

Two-by-two crossover design: *See* **crossover design**.

Two-phase sampling: A sampling scheme involving two distinct phases. In the first phase, information about particular variables of interest is collected on all members of the sample. In the second phase, information about other variables is collected on a subsample of the individuals in the original sample. An example of where this type of sampling procedure might be useful is when estimating `prevalence` on the basis of results provided by a fallible, but inexpensive and easy-to-use, indicator of the true disease state of the sampled individuals. The diagnosis of a subsample of the individuals might then be validated through the use of an accurate diagnostic test. This type of sampling procedure is often referred to wrongly as `two-stage sampling`, which in fact involves a completely different design. [*Survey Methodology*, 1990, **16**, 105–16.]

Two-sided test: A test in which the alternative hypothesis is not directional, for example that one population mean is not equal to another. *See also* **one-sided test**.

Two-stage sampling: A procedure used most often in the assessment of quality assurance before, during and after the manufacture of, for example, a drug product. Typically, this would involve sampling randomly a number of packages of some drug, and then sampling a number of tablets from each of these packages.

Two-stage stopping rule: A procedure sometimes used in `clinical trials` in which results are first examined after only a fraction of the planned number of subjects in each group have completed the trial. The relevant `test statistic` is calculated and the trial is stopped if the difference between the treatments is significant at stage 1 level a_1. Otherwise, additional subjects in each treatment group are recruited, the test statistic is calculated again, and the groups are compared at stage 2, level a_2, where a_1 and a_2 are chosen to given an overall significance level of a. *See also* **interim analyses**. [*Biometrics*, 1984, **40**, 791–5.]

Two-way classification: The classification of a set of observations according to two criteria, as, for example, in a `contingency table` constructed from two variables.

Type I error: The error that results when the null hypothesis is rejected falsely.

Type II error: The error that results when the null hypothesis is accepted falsely.

Type III error: It has been suggested by a number of authors that this term be used for identifying the poorer of two treatments as the better.

Ultrasound growth measurements: Such measurements are monitored to evaluate if a foetus is growing normally compared with a defined standard chart at a specified gestational age. For example, during pregnancy foetal anthropometric measures consisting of head circumference, biparietal diameter, occipito-frontal diameter. Abdominal circumference and femur length are measured using ultrasound to monitor attained foetal size at a given gestational age. [*Statistical Methods in Medical Research*, 2020, **29**, 2795–813.]

Umbrella ordering: A commonly observed response pattern in a one-factor design with ordered treatment levels in which the response variable increases with an increase in treatment level up to a certain point, then decreases with further increase in the treatment level. [*Journal of the American Statistical Association*, 1981, **76**, 175–81.]

Unanimity rule: A requirement that all of a number of diagnostic tests yield positive results before declaring that a patient has a particular complaint. *See also* **majority rule**. [*Statistics in Medicine*, 1988, **7**, 549–58.]

Unbalanced designs: Synonym for **non-orthogonal designs**.

Unbiased: *See* **bias**.

Uncertainty analysis: Synonym for **sensitivity analysis**.

Uncle test: A question that might be posed to doctors about to take part in a clinical trial to assess whether it is ethical for them to participate, for example, 'Would you be willing to randomize a close relative of yours, or even yourself, into any arm of the study?' [*Statistical Methods in Medical Research*, 2002, **11**, 1–22.]

Unequal allocation: A procedure often used in clinical trials to improve the acceptability of the trial by increased allocation to the experimental group, increasing the patient's exposure to the treatment, mitigating the higher dropout in one of the groups and reducing the cost of the treatment by placing fewer patients on the more expensive treatment. *See also* **adaptive randomization designs**, **covariate-adaptive randomization** and **Bayesian adaptive randomization**. [*Contemporary Clinical Trials*, 2006, **27**, 1–12.]

Unidentified model: *See* **identification**.

Uniform distribution: The `probability distribution` of a random variable having constant probability over an interval. The most commonly encountered uniform distribution is one over the interval zero to one.

Uniformly most powerful test: A test of a given hypothesis that is at least as powerful as another for all values of the parameter under consideration, and more powerful for at least one value of the parameter. [Casella, G., 2008, *Statistical Inference*, 2nd ed., Cengage Learning, Boston, MA.]

Unimodal distribution: A `probability distribution` or frequency distribution having only a single mode. The `normal distribution` and `Student's t-distribution` are two examples. [Altman, D., 2018, *Practical Statistics for Medical Research*, Chapman & Hall/CRC, Boca Raton, FL.]

Unit normal variable: Synonym for **standard normal variable**.

Univariate data: Data involving a single measurement on each subject or patient.

Universe: A little-used alternative term for **population**.

Unsupervised pattern recognition: *See* **pattern recognition**.

Up-and-down method: A method most associated with estimating the `lethal dose 50` in toxicity studies, but that has also been used in a variety of different medical areas, including visual and auditory investigations and taste-testing in diabetics.

The method consists of the following steps: after a series of equally spaced dosage levels has been chosen, the first trial is performed at some dosage level and then trials take place sequentially. Each subsequent trial is performed at the next lower or

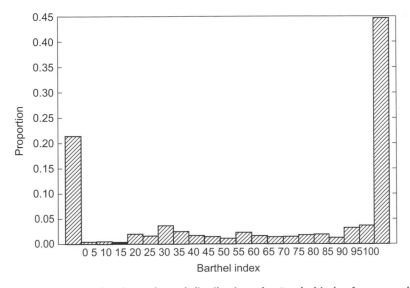

Figure 87 Example of a U-shaped distribution: the Barthel index for a sample of individuals.

the next higher dosage level according to whether the immediately preceding trial did or did not evoke a positive response. [*Pain*, 1988, **32**, 55–63.]

U-shaped distribution: A `probability distribution` or frequency distribution shaped more or less like a letter U, although not necessarily symmetrical. Such a distribution has its greatest frequencies at the two extremes of the range of the variable. An example of such a distribution is shown in Figure 87.

Utility analysis: A method for decision-making under uncertainty based on a set of axioms of rational behaviour. Often used in interventions or programmes designed to improve health. [*Medical Care*, 1994, **32**, 183–8.]

Vague prior: A term used for the `prior distribution` in `Bayesian methods` in the situation when there is complete ignorance about the value of a parameter. [*American Journal of Epidemiology*, 2005, **162**, 694–703.]

Validity: The extent to which a measuring instrument is measuring what was intended, or the degree to which the inference drawn from a study is warranted.

Validity checks: A part of data editing in which a check is made that only allowable values or codes are given for the answers to questions asked of subjects. A negative height, for example, would clearly not be an allowable value.

Variable: Some characteristic that differs from subject to subject or from time to time.

Variable selection: *See* **selection methods in regression**.

Variance: A measure of the spread or dispersion of a random variable around its mean. Generally assessed by the sum of squared deviations of a set of sample observations from their arithmetic mean divided by $n - 1$, where n is the sample size. This provides an unbiased estimator of the population value. [Altman, D. G., 2018, *Practical Statistics for Medical Research*, Chapman & Hall/CRC, Boca Raton, FL.]

Variance components: A term generally used for the variances of random effects in statistical models, for example `mixed-effects models`. Particularly important in quantitative genetics where phenotypic variation is often partitioned into genetic variation, environmental variation, and the interaction of genetic and environmental variation. [Searle, S. R., Casella, G. and McCulloch, C. E., 1992, *Variance Components*, John Wiley & Sons, New York.]

Variance–covariance matrix: A `symmetrical matrix` in which the off-diagonal elements are the `covariances` (sample or population) of pairs of variables, and the elements on the main diagonal are the variances (sample or population) of the variables. [Everitt, B. S. and Dunn, G., 2010, *Applied Multivariate Data Analysis*, 2nd ed., Wiley, Chichester.]

Variance function: *See* **generalized linear model**.

Variance inflation factor: An indicator of the effect that the other explanatory variables have on the variance of a regression coefficient of a particular variable, given by the reciprocal of one minus the square of the `multiple correlation coefficient` of the variable with the remaining explanatory variables. Large values indicate possible `multicollinearity` problems. A rough rule of

Figure 88 Venn diagram.

thumb is that values greater than 10 are a cause of concern. *See also* **tolerance**. [Lewis-Beck, M. S., 1993, *Regression Analysis*, Sage Publications, London.]

Variance ratio distribution: Synonym for *F*-**distribution**.

Variance ratio test: Synonym for *F*-**test**.

Variance-stabilizing transformations: Transformations designed to give approximate independence between mean and variance as a preliminary to, for example, analysis of variance. The arc-sine transformation is an example. [*Bioinformatics*, 2002, **18**, 596–604.]

Varimax rotation: A method for factor rotation that, by maximizing a particular function of the initial factor loadings, attempts to find a set of factors that are easy to interpret. [Everitt, B. S. and Dunn, G., 2010, *Applied Multivariate Data Analysis*, 2nd ed., Wiley, Chichester.]

Variogram: A graphical device used in the analysis of time series, or longitudinal studies and, in particular, of spatial data. Consists of a plot of the variance of the difference in the observed variable values at separate times or at sites against their distance apart. The plot is often helpful in describing the association among repeated values. [*Biometrics*, 2001, **57**, 211–18.]

Vector: A matrix having only one row or column.

Venn diagram: A graphical representation of the extent to which two or more quantities or concepts are mutually inclusive and mutually exclusive. An example is shown in Figure 88.

Virtually safe dose (VSD): The exposure level to some toxic agent corresponding to an acceptably small risk of suffering an ill effect. From a regulatory perspective, this typically means an increased risk of no more than 10^{-6} or 10^{-4} above background. Often used to judge the safety of foodstuffs. In the USA, for example, one study found that the amount of dioxin in one serving of a particular brand of ice-cream was 190 times higher than the accepted virtually safe dose. [*Biometrics*, 1998, **54**, 558–69.]

Visual analogue scales: Scales used to measure quantities such as pain or satisfaction. The patient is shown a straight line, the ends of which are labelled with extreme states. The patient is then asked to mark the point on the line that represents their perception of their current state. For example, such a scale for pain might be:

No pain _____ Unbearable pain

See also **adjectival scales** and **semantic differential scale**. [*Archives of Disease in Childhood*, 2002, **86**, 416–18.]

Vital index: Synonym for **birth–death ratio**.

Vital statistics: A select group of statistical data concerned with events related to the life and death of human beings, for example death rates and divorce rates.

Volunteer bias: A possible source of bias in clinical trials (and other studies) that involve participants who volunteer because of the known propensity of volunteers to respond better than other patients to treatment. A classic nonclinical trial example is the people who formed the sample for the Kinsey Report.

[Bland, M., 2001, *An Introduction to Medical Statistics*, 3rd ed., Oxford University Press, Oxford.]

Volunteer bias: Never trust a volunteer!

Von Neumann–Morgenstern standard gamble: A suggested procedure for assessing the risk that seriously ill patients will take when offered treatment that offers potential benefit in quality of life, but with the trade-off that there is a finite possibility that the patient may not survive the treatment. The patient is asked to consider the following situation:

You have been suffering from angina for several years. As a result of your illness, you experience severe chest pain after even minor physical exertion, such as climbing the stairs or walking one block in cold weather. You have been forced to quit your job and spend most days at home watching TV. Imagine that you are offered the possibility of an operation that will result in complete recovery from your illness. However, the operation carries some risk. Specifically, there is a probability *P* that you will die during the course of the operation. How large must *P* be before you will decline the operation and choose to remain in your present state?

Because few patients are accustomed to dealing with probabilities, an alternative procedure called the *time trade-off technique* is often suggested, which begins by estimating the likely remaining years of life for a healthy subject, using actuarial tables. The previous question is rephrased as follows:

Imagine living the remainder of your natural span [an estimated number of years would be given] in your present state. Contrast this with the alternative that you remain in perfect health for fewer years. How many years would you sacrifice if you could have perfect health? [*Health Services Research*, 1994, **29**, 207–24.]

Vote counting: The practice of taking a simple tally of the number of positive studies, decided by significance dichotomized at the 5% level of each study, in a `meta-analysis` and the result taken as evidence for efficacy, safety, of the lack of either or both for the treatment under investigation. Such a practice is associated with many problems, for example, it ignores sample size, and the results of a series of small studies may provide a high or low vote count, which is discordant with the greatest mass of the data which might be restricted to a few large and well-controlled studies. [Gibbons, R. D. and Amatya, A. K., 2016, *Statistical Methods for Drug Safety*, CRC, Boca Raton, FL.]

VSD: Abbreviation for **virtually safe dose**.

Vulnerable-population trials: `Clinical trials` in which the study participants are considered vulnerable, with limited capacity for protecting themselves, for example, by refusing further treatment. An example might be a study of antidepressant therapy in children. Such trials require an increased level of control and monitoring. [Ellenberg, S. S., Fleming, T. R. and DeMets, D. L., 2002, *Data Monitoring Committees in Clinical Trials*, Wiley, New York.]

W

Wait-list controls: Subjects in a clinical trial that receive the intervention, but only after its affect has been assessed in subjects assigned to the experimental group. [*Psychosomatic Medicine*, 2000, **62**, 614–22.]

Wald's test: A test for the hypothesis that a set of related parameters all take the value zero.

Wald–Wolfowitz test: A distribution-free method for testing the null hypothesis that two samples come from identical populations. The test is based on a count of the number of runs. [Hollander, M. and Wolfe, D. A., 1999, *Nonparametric Statistical Methods*, John Wiley & Sons, New York.]

Ward's method: An agglomerative hierarchical clustering method in which a sum-of-squares criterion is used to decide on which individuals or clusters should be fused at each stage in the procedure. *See also* **single linkage clustering**, **average linkage clustering**, **complete linkage cluster analysis** and **K-means cluster analysis**. [Everitt, B. S., Landau, S., Lees, M. and Stahl, D., 2011, *Cluster Analysis*, 5th ed., John Wiley & Sons, New York.]

Warning lines: Lines on a control chart indicating a mild degree of departure from a desired level of control.

Washout period: An interval introduced between the treatment periods in a crossover design in an effort to eliminate possible carry-over effects. [Senn, S., 2008, *Statistical Issues in Drug Development*, 2nd ed., John Wiley & Sons, Chichester.]

Weibull distribution: A probability distribution that occurs in the analysis of survival data and has the important property that the corresponding hazard function can be made to increase with time, decrease with time, or remain constant, depending on the values of a particular parameter that characterizes the distribution. [*British Journal of Cancer*, 1954, **8**, 1–12.]

Weighted average: An average of quantities to which have been attached a series of weights in order to make proper allowance for their relative importance. For example, a set of mean values may be combined using a weighted average in which the weights are the sample sizes on which each mean is based.

Weighted kappa: A version of the kappa coefficient that permits disagreements between raters to be weighted differentially, to allow for differences in how serious such disagreements are judged to be. [*Canadian Journal of Statistics*, 1999, **27**, 3–23.]

Weighted least squares: A method of estimation in which estimates arise from minimizing a weighted sum of squares of the differences between the response variable and its predicted value in terms of the model of interest. Often used when the variance of the response variable is thought to change over the range of values of the explanatory variable(s), in which case the weights are generally taken as the reciprocals of the variance. *See also* **least squares estimation** and **iteratively reweighted least squares**. [Rawlings, J. O., Pantula, S. G. and Dickey, D. A., 2013, *Applied Regression Analysis: A Research Tool*, Springer, New York.]

Weight variation tests: Tests designed to ensure that manufacturers control the variation in the weight of the tablet form of drugs that they produce. The *British Pharmacopoeia* tests, for example, use a sample of 20 tablets from any batch.

Each table is weighed singly and the average for 20 tablets is found from the data. No tablet should deviate from the average by more than double the percentage given in the table, and no more than two tablets should deviate from the average by the tabulated percentage: [*Chemical and Pharmaceutical Bulletin*, 2001, **49**, 1412–19.]

Average weight of tablet	Percentage
≤80 mg	10
80–250 mg	7.5
>250 mg	5

White noise sequence: A sequence of independent random variables that all have a normal distribution with zero mean and the same variance.

Wilcoxon's rank sum test: An alternative name for the **Mann–Whitney test**.

Wilcoxon's signed rank test: A distribution-free method for testing the difference between two populations using matched samples. The test is based on the absolute differences of the pairs of observations in the two samples, ranked according to size, with each rank being given the sign of the original difference. The test statistic is the sum of the positive ranks. [Hollander, M. and Wolfe, D. A., 1999, *Nonparametric Statistical Methods*, John Wiley & Sons, New York.]

Wilk's lambda: *See* **multivariate analysis of variance**.

William's agreement measure: An index of agreement that is useful for measuring the reliability of individual raters compared with a group. The index is the ratio of the proportion of agreement (across subjects) between the individual rater and the rest of the group to the average proportion of agreement between all pairs of raters in the rest of the group. *See also* **kappa coefficient**. [*British Journal of Psychology*, 1976, **2**, 89–108.]

Within-groups mean square: *See* mean squares.

Within-group sum of squares: *See* analysis of variance.

World Health Quarterly: *See* sources of data.

World Health Statistics Annual: *See* sources of data.

Worm count: A method of surveillance of helminth infection of the gut that depends on counts of worms, or their cysts or ova, in quantitatively titrated samples of faeces. [*International Journal for Parasitology*, 2001, **31**, 720–7.]

Wright's inbreeding coefficient: The probability that two allelic genes united in a zygote are both descended from a gene found in an ancestor common to both parents. [*Molecular Ecology*, 1995, **4**, 239–47.]

Yates's contingency correction: When testing for independence in a contingency table, a continuous probability distribution, namely the chi-squared distribution, is used as an approximation to the discrete probability of observed frequencies, namely the multinomial distribution. To improve this approximation, Yates suggested a correction that involves subtracting 0.5 from the positive discrepancies (observed − expected) and adding 0.5 to the negative discrepancies before these values are squared in the calculation of the usual chi-squared test. If the sample size is larger, then the correction will have little effect on the value of the test statistic. Now no longer really needed since exact tests can be used. [Everitt, B. S., 1992, *The Analysis of Contingency Tables*, 2nd ed., Chapman & Hall/CRC, Boca Raton, FL.]

Years of potential life lost: A measure of the total number of life years lost due to premature death in a population from a certain cause. Premature death is usually defined as death earlier than some given value, for example, 65 or 75 years, or less than the appropriate average life expectancy. An indicator of premature mortality that gives more importance to the causes of death that occurred at younger ages than those that occurred at older ages. [*British Medical Journal*, 1990, **301**, 429–32.]

Yea-saying: Synonym for **acquiescence bias**.

Youden's index: An index that captures the performance of a diagnostic test into a single measure namely (sensitivity + specificity − 1). The index has a value between zero and one. In a perfect test, the index takes the value one and it has value zero when the test gives the same proportion of positive results for groups with and without the disease of interest. [*Cancer*, 1950, **3**, 32–5.]

Z

Zelen's single-consent design: An alternative to simple random allocation for forming treatment groups in a clinical trial. Begins with the set of N eligible patients. All N of these patients are then subdivided randomly into two groups, say groups G_1 and G_2 of sizes n_1 and n_2. The standard therapy is applied to all patients assigned to G_1. The new therapy is assigned only to those patients in G_2 who consent to its use. The remaining patients who refuse the new treatment are treated with the standard therapy. The main advantages of the design are that almost all eligible individuals are included in the trial and that it allows the evaluation of the true effect of offering experimental interventions to patients. The main disadvantages are that such trials have to be open-label trials and that the statistical power of the study may be affected as a high proportion of participants choose to have the standard treatment. [*New England Journal of Medicine*, 1979, **300**, 1242–5.]

Zero-inflated data: Such data are characterized by the presence of a large portion of zero-values, in addition to continuous non-zero, that is, positive values. Examples include monthly medical costs and daily alcohol drinks. Such data are commonly analyzed by a pair of regression models, the first a logistic regression model for the probability of having a nonzero response and the second a linear regression model for the actual values of the response when it is non-zero. [*Statistics in Medicine*, 2016, **35**, 5070–93.]

Zero-inflated Poisson regression: A model for count data with excess zeroes, for example, the frequency of using medical services shows many zeroes in healthcare systems because a large number of people do not access medical services. [*Technometrics*, 1992, **34**, 1–14.]

Zero-sum game: A game played by a number of people in which the winner takes all the stakes provided by the losers so that the algebraic sum of gains at any stage is zero. Many decision problems can be modelled as such games involving two people. [*New Scientist*, 1990, **4**, 1.]

Z-scores: Synonym for **standard scores**.

z-test: A test for assessing the hypothesis that the mean of a normal distribution takes a particular value, or for assessing whether the means of two normal distributions with the same known variance are equal.

z-transformation: *See* Fisher's z-transformation.

Zygosity determination: The determination of whether a pair of twins are identical or fraternal. It can be achieved to a high (over 95%) level of certainty by questionnaire, but any desired level of accuracy can be achieved by typing a number of genetic markers to see whether the genetic sharing is 100% or only 50%. Important in `twin analysis`. [Sham, P., 1998, *Statistics in Human Genetics*, Arnold, London.]